Biological Aspects of Alcoholism

Acknowledgments

The editors wish to express their appreciation to the authors for their timely contributions. They are also indebted to Melissa Hickey and Kathy Fassler for skillful assistance in the preparation of the manuscripts.

WHO Expert Series on Neuroscience[1]

The WHO's Mental Health Programme has three major objectives which it hopes to achieve in cooperation with its Member States. These are, first, to prevent or control mental and neurological disorders and psychosocial problems; second, to ensure a broad utilization of mental health knowledge in general health care; and third, to help countries in dealing with psychosocial aspects of overall development.

The WHO Expert Series on Neuroscience[1] is intended to help mainly in the achievement of the first two of these objectives. It is one of the many efforts the Organization has undertaken to promote the exchange of information and collaborative research on mental and neurological disorders.

The themes for inclusion in the Series are selected by the Heads of the WHO Collaborating Centres for Research and Training in Mental Health and Neuroscience located in some 34 countries, and the texts are produced by experts participating in the WHO programme.

Series Editors: Norman Sartorius and Leonid L. Prilipko

Current Volumes

Vol. 1   Haag, H., Rüther, E., Hippius, H. *Tardive Dyskinesia*

Vol. 2   Grof, P., Akther, M.I., Campbell, M., Gottfries, C.G., Khan, I., Lapierre, Y., Lemberger, L., Müller-Örlinghausen, B., and Woggon, B.
Clinical Evaluation of Psychotropic Drugs for Psychiatric Disorders

Vol. 3   Moussaoui, D., Racagni, G.
Anxiety: Clinical, Biological and Pharmacotherapeutic Aspects

Vol. 4   Tabakoff, B., Hoffman, P. (Eds)
Biological Aspects of Alcoholism

Vol. 5   Maj, M., Starace, F., Sartorius, N.
Mental Disorders in HIV-1 Infection and AIDS

---

[1] Taking into consideration that advances in neuroscience have a great potential for the prevention, control and treatment of mental and neurological disorders, as well as for the promotion of mental health, it was decided to continue the WHO Expert Series on Biological Psychiatry under the new title: "WHO Expert Series on Neuroscience", for all volumes published in 1995 and thereafter.

Biological Aspects of Alcoholism

WHO Expert Series on Biological Psychiatry
Volume 4

Edited by
Boris Tabakoff and Paula L. Hoffman
University of Colorado Health Science Center, Denver, CO

Coordinating Editors
Norman Sartorius and L. Prilipko

Hogrefe & Huber Publishers
Seattle • Toronto • Bern • Göttingen

Library of Congress Cataloging-in-Publication Data
Tabakoff, B. (Boris)
Biological Aspects of Alcoholism / Boris Tabakoff, Paula L. Hoffman
p. cm.— (WHO expert series on biological psychiatry; v. 4)
Includes bibliographical references and index.
ISBN 0-88937-130-X
1. Alcoholism—Pathophysiology.   2. Alcoholism—Genetic aspects.
3. Alcohol—Physiological effect.   I. Hoffman, P. L. (Paula L.)   II. Title.
III. Series.
[DNLM: 1. Alcoholism—metabolism.   2. Alcoholism—genetics
3. Alcohol, Ethyl—metabolism.   4. Sex Factors.   5. Ethnic Groups.
W1 WH48 v. 4 1995 / WM 274 T112b   1995]
RC565.T23   1995
616.86'107— dc20
DNLM/DLC
for Library of Congress

94-19261
CIP

Canadian Cataloguing in Publication Data
Tabakoff, Boris, 1942-
Biological aspects of alcoholism
(WHO expert series on biological psychiatry ; v.4)
Includes bibliographical references and index.
ISBN 0-88937-130-X
1. Alcohol - Physiological effect.   I. Hoffman, Paula L.
II. Title.   III. Series.
QP801.A3T3 1995   616.86'1   C94-931337-8

ISBN 0-88937-130-X
Hogrefe & Huber Publishers, Seattle •Toronto • Bern • Göttingen
ISBN 3-456-82540-4
Hogrefe & Huber Publishers, Göttingen • Bern • Seattle •Toronto

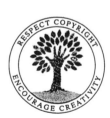

© Copyright 1995 by Hogrefe & Huber Publishers
USA: P.O. Box 2487, Kirkland, WA 98083-2487,
Phone (206) 820-1500, Fax (206) 823-8324
CANADA: 12 Bruce Park Avenue, Toronto, Ontario M4P 2S3,
Phone (416) 482-6339
SWITZERLAND: Länggass-Straße 76, CH-3000 Bern 9,
Phone (031) 300-4500, Fax (031) 300-4590
GERMANY: Rohnsweg 25, D-37085 Göttingen,
Phone (0551) 49609-0, Fax (0551) 49609-88

Printed in USA

Preface

The manufacture, sale and consumption of alcoholic beverages are legally and culturally ingrained activities in much of the world. Alcohol (ethanol) consumption is on the ascent in developing countries and is also increasing in countries such as Japan, which traditionally have had low levels of alcohol consumption. Although the consumption of alcohol is an innocuous part of the lives of many people, a significant portion of the world population suffers the results of excessive alcohol consumption, including behavioral and physical consequences of acute alcohol intoxication (violent acts, accidents, etc.), damage to organs, dependence on alcohol and the societal and family disruptions produced by alcohol abuse and alcoholism. Alcohol abuse is a contributing factor in a number of health problems and various studies have demonstrated that 25 to 30 per cent of general hospital admissions in the U.S.A. screen positively for alcoholism.

The initial determinants of alcohol consumption by an individual are many-fold, but the etiology of alcohol abuse and alcoholism involves the interactions of environmental and biological factors. Research over the past two decades has provided important insight into the cellular and molecular sites of ethanol's actions and into the individual differences in biology which sensitize certain segments of the population to the acute and chronic effects of ethanol. More recent data has focussed attention on biological systems which may be markers or determinants of a genetic predisposition to alcoholism. This progress in the understanding of the *biology of alcoholism* provides an imperative to all health professionals to incorporate the new knowledge into their strategies for the prevention, treatment and further research on alcohol abuse and alcoholism.

The contents of this book are meant to provide, in a single text, a review of the current status of a large segment of biological research on alcoholism. Such a review will be relevant to trainees in the psychological and medical disciplines, practicing alcoholism treatment professionals and addiction researchers. It is hoped that the focus of this text on the biology of alcoholism can add to the knowledge of the environmental contributors to development of addiction and provide for the interested reader an integrated view of the addiction process and the organismic consequences of ethanol's action. The initial chapters of this text have been organized to provide an overview of the evolution of biological concepts of alcohol dependence, the evolution of theories on genetic contributions to development of alcoholism and the evolution of concepts of biological contributions to heterogenous typologies of alcoholism. A detailed account of the metabolic fate of ingested alcohol and the metabolic anomalies produced by alcohol is presented as a backdrop to information on how individual differences in alcohol metabolism can impact on drinking practices and alcohol-induced pathologies. The metabolic anomalies produced by ethanol ingestion are also considered as possible biological markers of alcohol consumption which can be used clinically to identify problem drinkers and to monitor abstinence in alcoholism treatment settings. Subsequent chapters focus on the issue of genetic (biological) factors which predispose individuals to alcoholism and on the importance of typology of alcoholism in considerations of genetic influences in the etiology of alcoholism. Recent data on genetic polymorphisms of neural receptors for transmitters such as dopamine in alcoholics are discussed to provide perspective on the determinants of alcoholism and on the use of such genetic polymorphisms as "markers" of predisposition to alcoholism. Discussion is also included on genetic polymorphisms in the enzymes that metabolize ethanol, which can, in certain instances, provide protection from development of alcoholism.

Since the process of addiction is centered in the brain, the neurobiology of ethanol's actions is discussed in detail. Current information on neural systems which are particularly sensitive to ethanol's acute and chronic effects provides insights into the generation of intoxication by ethanol and the development of physical dependence on ethanol. Neurotransmitter systems which play a major role in the actions of other drugs which have properties similar to those of ethanol, e.g.: benzodiazepines, are major targets of ethanol's actions. Yet, ethanol acts through rather distinct molecular mechanisms and has an overall spectrum of action dissimilar from the other dependence producing sedative/hypnotic drugs. The development of tolerance to and physical dependence on alcohol is generated by adaptation of neurons to the chronic presence of ethanol in brain, but this chronic exposure of neurons to ethanol also produces neural damage and cell death. The pathological consequences of alcohol abuse on brain function are some of the most devastating features of alcoholism. The neurologic pathologies many times produce incapacitation requiring long-term hospitalization and, in more minor manifestations, produce cognitive problems which interfere with normal function and with attempts at treatment and rehabilitation.

The earlier chapters on the genetics and typology of alcoholism consider important gender differences in the predisposition to alcohol-related problems, and the topic of gender-specific issues in alcoholism receives greater attention in a chapter devoted to women's drinking practices, including the social and psychological determinants and the biological consequences of these drinking patterns. One of the possible consequences of alcohol consumption by women who are pregnant is damage to the fetus, and research on the fetal alcohol syndrome is discussed in the context of the complexities of gender, timing of drinking during pregnancy and quantitative issues of alcohol consumption. The information on gender-specific effects of alcohol reinforces the importance of individual differences in the biological effects of ethanol and the consequences of alcohol abuse.

The strategies for treatment of alcoholism are relying increasingly on medications which are not only targeted to alleviate withdrawal signs and symptoms but also are targeted at reducing relapse and/or reducing alcohol consumption. The chapter on pharmacological treatment of alcoholism reviews the therapeutic approaches ranging from use of agents that produce an aversion to ethanol to those purported to reduce craving, and also makes the point that proper matching of patient characteristics to therapy is an important element in success of treatment.

Although the emphasis of this text is on the biological aspects of alcohol abuse and alcoholism, the final chapter well emphasizes the importance of interactions of biology and environment. The relationship of situational variables to alcohol craving, and the role that learning or conditioning play in the motivation to take a drink or in the inability to terminate a drinking bout is discussed at some length. This chapter enunciates how contemporary learning theory is applicable to predicting the association of specific events with craving or relapse, and also provides insights into why only some individuals abuse alcohol and cannot maintain sobriety.

The theme of individual differences in biology and in situational variables as predisposing elements for alcoholism emerges strongly from this text. Rather than generating anxiety over the possible confusion such variability may produce in treatment, prevention, and further research on alcoholism, the text attempts to provide information and guidance on the way that knowledge of individual and group differences can generate optimal success in the clinic and in the laboratory. For both students and specialists, this text holds revealing insights into biological determinants, and the interaction of biology with environment, that produce the multifaceted entity we refer to as alcoholism.

Boris Tabakoff, Ph.D.
Paula L. Hoffman, Ph.D.

Table of Contents

Neurobiology of Alcohol's Actions and the Addictive Process 189
J. E. Dildy-Mayfield and R. A. Harris

The Psychobiology of Conditioning, Reinforcement and Craving 225
M. Vogel-Sprott

Neurologic Pathology of Alcohol Abuse 245
Peter L. Carlen and Enrique Menzano

Emerging Approaches to Pharmacotherapy of Alcohol Abuse and Dependence

Historical Perspective on the Biology of Alcohol Abuse and Dependence

John B. Saunders
Centre for Drug and Alcohol Studies, Royal Prince Alfred Hospital
and Departments of Medicine and Psychiatry, University of Sydney,
Sydney, New South Wales, Australia

Alcohol abuse and dependence have posed an unusual challenge to researchers over the 200 years they have been subjected to scientific enquiry. Are they discrete clinical syndromes which run true in different populations? Are they indeed diseases, in the conventional medical sense of that term? Or are these terms merely convenient labels for an array of drinking problems which are as varied as human beings themselves? If alcohol abuse and dependence are discrete clinical entities, are they primarily of biological origin? Or are they manifestations of an underlying psychological disorder? Perhaps drinking problems are simply maladaptive behaviors which are determined by social factors with no significant biological contribution.

Each of these viewpoints has its adherents and its tradition of research. Indeed, many of these schools of thought barely admit of each others' existence. In describing the contribution of biological research, the present review will adopt the standpoint that alcohol abuse and dependence develop as a result of a complex interaction between the pharmacological properties of alcohol[1], the characteristics and needs of the individual, and various environmental influences. Biological mechanisms of alcohol abuse and dependence

---

[1] The unqualified term "alcohol" refers to ethyl alcohol (ethanol)

1

must therefore be placed in this wider context. Before examining some of the major themes in biological research, I shall briefly review how our conceptual understanding of these conditions has developed over the years.

Nature of Alcohol Abuse and Dependence

The term "alcoholism" was introduced by Magnus Huss in 1823 to describe a condition of recurrent drunkenness which ran a progressive course over many years, and resulted in a variety of harmful consequences. For much of the time since then alcoholism was regarded as a discrete disease entity of biological causation and predictable natural history. In the 1930s and 1940s several investigators (including Silkworth (1937), Lemere et al. (1943) and Brocklehurst (1949), proposed that it was an allergic disease akin to food allergy or an idiosyncratic drug reaction. In some formulations, a site of action in the brain was proposed, for example in the medulla immediately surrounding the fourth ventricle (Brocklehurst, 1949). The disease concept of alcoholism was embraced by the self-help movements of the 1930s, and was promoted widely by the most successful of these movements, Alcoholics Anonymous.

The disease concept reached its apotheosis with the publication by Jellinek in 1960 of "The Disease Concept of Alcoholism". Jellinek described five sub-types of alcoholism. Alpha alcoholism was defined as a "purely psychological reliance upon the effect of alcohol to relieve bodily or emotional pain". Beta alcoholism was identified as a continuous type of heavy drinking which led to medical complications such as cirrhosis and peripheral neuropathy, but where psychological or physical dependence were minimal or absent. Gamma alcoholism was thought to typify abnormal drinking behavior in Anglo-Saxon countries. It was characterized by increased tolerance to alcohol, withdrawal symptoms, craving and loss of control over drinking. "There is a definite progression from psychological to physical dependence." Delta alcoholism was similar to gamma alcoholism, but "instead of loss of control there is inability to abstain". This was considered to be the predominant species of alcoholism in wine producing countries. Epsilon alcoholism or "dipsomania" was the term applied to intermittent binge drinking, which is interspersed with periods of abstinence or, more rarely, low level drinking.

Sociological and epidemiological research from the 1960s onwards challenged the disease concept. Community surveys of alcohol consumption and related problems showed that consumption was distributed as a continuum, not bimodally as would be expected if there were separate populations of "alcoholics" and "normal drinkers" (Cahalan, Cisin & Crossley, 1969; Wilson, 1980). Alcohol-related problems too showed a continuous distribution. Indeed, it was calculated that only a minority of alcohol-related problems in the community as a whole occurred in those classified as alcoholic. From these studies a model of alcohol problems was developed which, rather than being syndromal in nature, was conceptualized as an array of diverse effects of alcohol, disaggregated not clustered, and highly influenced by cultural and other societal factors (Room, 1991). The disease concept was dismissed as a "myth" (Fingarette, 1988; Peele, 1989) and some rejected the view that alcohol had addictive properties.

A major conceptual advance occurred in 1976, with the publication by Edwards and Gross (1976) of their description of the "alcohol dependence syndrome". This comprises a discrete cluster of behaviors and symptoms which includes a subjective compulsion to consume alcohol, preoccupation with drinking, tolerance, and withdrawal symptoms when alcohol intake is stopped or reduced. Not all these features need be present; rather, dependence is conceptualized as existing in various degrees of severity. The dependence syndrome does not include any medical or other disorders caused by drinking. There was a further elaboration of this model into a bi-axial concept of a dependence syndrome and "alcohol-related disabilities", which were defined as the physical, psychological and social consequences of alcohol use (Edwards, Gross, Keller, Moser & Room, 1977). Thus the dependence syndrome is a "purer" concept than alcoholism, definitions of which typically encompass the consequences as well as the action of heavy drinking (Saunders, 1986).

The dependence syndrome has formed the basis of the classification of alcohol use disorders in the 10th revision of the International Classification of Diseases (ICD-10), published by the World Health Organization (1992), and the latest revision of the Diagnostic and Statistical Manual (DSM-IIIR) (American Psychiatric Association, 1987). The current operational criteria require three (of 8 or 9) elements to have occurred in the previous 12 months.

W.H.O. has now introduced the concept of a hierarchy of diagnoses, which recognizes the variety and dimensionality of drinking problems. They include hazardous alcohol use (which confers the *risk* of harmful consequences), dysfunctional use (alcohol consumption which is causing social problems), and harmful use (which is

causing actual physical or psychological damage), as well as dependence. This reflects the shift away from alcohol dependence (or alcoholism) as the exclusive concern towards a focus on early
intervention for hazardous and harmful alcohol use. Alcohol abuse
is the DSM-IIIR term which covers a maladaptive pattern of drinking
of lesser severity than dependence.

Biological research has in general not paid much attention to
clinical typologies until recent years. For example, although the
Jellinek classification was very influential in other spheres, it did not
become a focus for much biological research. This concentrated on
identifying biological concomitants of "alcoholism" which was often
loosely defined, or investigating discrete phenomena such as tolerance and physiological dependence (both manifestations of
neuroadaptation) or specific physical or neuropsychiatric sequelae.
Only in the past decade has biological research related its findings to
well-defined clinical (DSM or ICD) diagnoses, or typologies (such as
that developed by Cloninger). There has also been relatively little
research into cognitive processes underlying drinking behavior. This
is not surprising: it will require a degree of technical sophistication
which is quantally greater than we presently possess.

This review will now explore some of the main themes in biological research and indicate how they have developed over the last half
century. Necessarily, the review is selective. It will concentrate on
mechanisms of the core syndromes of alcohol abuse and dependence, and will make only relatively brief reference to physical and
neuropsychiatric sequelae. "Alcohol abuse" will be used as a convenient shorthand term to encompass problem drinking (including
hazardous and harmful drinking) which does not meet the criteria
for dependence, while alcoholism, which was the term used in much
of the work cited, will indicate a relatively severe drinking problem,
typically with evidence of physiological dependence.

Genetic Factors

Alcohol abuse and dependence are well-known to cluster in families.
Early theories of familial transmission were bound up with Victorian
concepts of moral degeneracy, of "the sins of the father visiting upon
the sons". These theories became assimilated with Social Darwinism
and the growing eugenics movement. With the decline in alcohol
problems following the First World War and, in the U.S.A. the enact-
ment of prohibition, interest in the genetics of alcoholism declined.
The growing popularity of the disease concept in the 1930s rekindled

interest in the mode of transmission, but it was not until the 1970s that the genetics of alcoholism was the focus of much enquiry.

It is relatively easy to document that alcohol abuse and dependence cluster in families. It is more difficult to disentangle whether this is related to genetic factors or reflects environmental influences such as modelling of drinking behavior on that of family members. Proponents of the disease model generally assumed that it was a largely inherited condition. Others were dismissive of genetic theories. The statement of Kessel and Walton (1965) that "alcoholism is passed on in the same way that money is inherited, not in the same way that, say, eye colour is", is fairly typical of this viewpoint.

There are several techniques for separating a genetic component from environmental influences. They include studies of children adopted away from an alcoholic biological parent, comparisons of monozygotic and dizygotic twins, and identification of biochemical and physiological markers in persons at high risk for developing alcohol abuse and dependence. The results of such studies are outlined below; for a more comprehensive review, see the chapter by Parsian and Cloninger (this volume).

Several investigators have taken advantage of the excellent adoption registries in Scandinavia to examine the influence of parental alcoholism on the development of drinking problems in adopted-away children. Goodwin and colleagues (1973) reported that sons of alcoholic biological fathers who were adopted out of the parental home were four times more likely to become alcohol dependent in adult life than adopted-away sons of non-alcoholic fathers. These findings were subsequently confirmed in Swedish and U.S.A. adoption studies and a genetic predisposition, albeit a weaker one, was subsequently identified in female adoptees (Cloninger, Bohman & Sigvardsson, 1981; Cadoret, O'Gorman, Troughton and Heywood, 1985).

Cloninger and colleagues (1981) extended this work with a sophisticated cross-fostering analysis. Subjects were subdivided according to whether there was evidence of a biological predisposition to drinking problems (alcohol abuse in the biological father or mother, parental history of alcoholism treatment, occupational status and criminal behavior) or an environmental one (alcohol abuse in an adoptive parent, socio-economic status of the adoptive home, residential stability). Two subtypes of alcoholism were identified. Type 1 alcohol abuse occurred in both sexes; it was moderately heritable and its expression was strongly influenced by environmental factors. It was characterized by relatively late onset of drinking problems, low risk taking, marked psychological dependence, and remorse about drinking. Type 2 alcohol abuse occurred only in men, was much more highly heritable and was not dependent on environmental factors for its expression, other than the mere availability of alcohol. This subtype was associated with early onset of drinking problems, impulsive behavior, criminal activities and a relatively low psychological dependence. This typology has been developed further, with the description of putative neurochemical mechanisms involved in the expression of each of these subtypes (Cloninger, 1989).

Twin studies provide another paradigm for investigating genetic influences on drinking behavior and susceptibility to alcohol abuse. In essence, if monozygotic twin pairs show greater concordance for alcohol abuse than dizygotic pairs, that is strong presumptive evidence for a genetic influence. Several such studies have been reported since the 1960s and in the main have shown such findings (Saunders, 1982). Over the past 10 years, more sophisticated biometric genetic models have been developed to address significant drawbacks of twin studies, including the fact that monozygotic twins are more likely to share their environment than dizygotic pairs, and therefore be subjected more to the influence of the drinking behavior of family members.

Recently, twin studies have expanded from ascertainment of monozygotic and dizygotic pair concordance for alcohol abuse and dependence to include measurement of multiple psychological, social and biological characteristics related to alcohol (Martin, 1991; Heath, Meyer, Jardine& Martin, 1991). The intention is to determine which specific characteristics or events lead to specific outcomes, and to relate each to genetic or familial modes of transmission or to purely individual experiences. Such studies require large numbers of twins from the general population and sophisticated data analysis, but will allow tests of detailed hypotheses about each of the dimensions of alcohol-related behavior and alcohol-related disease rather than only measuring the "heritability" of a clinical endpoint.

Trait Markers of Alcohol Abuse

At about the time the first studies of the heritability of alcohol abuse were reported, interest was developing in genetic markers of susceptibility. Several putative markers of susceptibility were reported in the 1960s and 1970s: they included ABO and other blood groups, colour blindness, taste sensitivity, and hair colour and other anthropometric characteristics (Cruz-Coke& Varela, 1966). Many of these associations were not confirmed in replicate studies. Others proved to be spurious. They illustrate the problem in trying to identify biological markers in persons who have already developed alcohol abuse, that the so-called markers could be secondary to the effects of alcohol. For example, the association with colour blindness was subsequently found to be due to alcohol's effects on colour vision.

A more rigorous approach would be to investigate a series of candidate markers in a cohort of subjects who are followed up into adult life to distinguish those who develop alcohol abuse from those who do not. Cohort studies such as these are expensive and time-consuming, and have not been employed extensively. They are also highly dependent on reliable follow-up, which is difficult to ensure over the 25 or more years that would be necessary.

A technique which has been employed more extensively is to search for biological markers in persons who are considered to be at high risk of alcohol abuse, for example the offspring of alcoholic parents. Begleiter and colleagues identified differences in event-related potentials between the preadolescent sons of alcoholics (before the sons had begun to drink alcohol) and matched sons of non-alcoholics (Begleiter, Porjesz, Bihari & Kissin, 1984). Among the sons of alcoholics, the P300 wave (a positive wave which occurs approximately 300 milliseconds after an anticipated stimulus) was reduced in amplitude. This has been interpreted as indicating reduced ability on the part of sons of alcoholics to selectively attend to anticipated stimuli, and may indicate a more generalized deficit in information processing.

There has also been considerable investment in identification of peripheral blood markers of susceptibility to alcohol abuse and dependence. Subnormal levels of platelet monoamine oxidase (MAO) activity in alcohol dependent persons have been reported by several groups (Whitfield, 1991), the lowest levels being found in alcoholics of the Type 2 subgroup. Levels remain low even after prolonged abstinence from alcohol (Sullivan, Stanfield, Maltbie, Hammett & Cavener, 1978). There are indications that relatives of alcoholics have subnormal values too, which would strongly support a genetic basis for this finding. However, it remains to be established whether MAO is a real marker of susceptibility to alcohol abuse or rather to a particular personality type characterized by impulsive behavior and risk taking. A recent discovery is a subnormal level of platelet adenylate cyclase activity (following stimulation with caesium fluoride) in alcohol dependent persons which persists for at least a year following detoxification from alcohol (Tabakoff et al., 1988). Again, this would suggest a primary genetic defect.

The most recent proposed marker of alcoholism is the A1 allele of the dopamine D_2 receptor. This allele was found in 70% of chronic alcoholics and only 20% of non-alcoholic control subjects (Blum et al., 1990). Although this finding was greeted by some as support for the single gene theory of alcoholism, a simple calculation reveals that at any reasonable estimate of the prevalence of alcoholism, the majority of the subjects with the A1 allele would be non-alcoholic. More detailed discussions of this and related studies can be found in the chapters by Parsian and Cloninger and by Sherman et al. (this volume).

These studies can be regarded as providing promising evidence of the existence of markers of susceptibility to alcohol abuse. The findings cannot be accepted as definitive yet. However, it is worthwhile considering the implications of having such markers and their potential utility. Screening for high risk youth and counselling of them and their families would represent a practical outcome of this research. If an allelic variant of a single gene, or a small number of genes, were identified as predisposing to alcohol abuse, somatic gene therapy would offer at least a hypothetical treatment. For the moment this represents a pipedream rather than a practical proposition.

Responses to Alcohol

Many popular theories of alcoholism have been based on the belief that alcohol abusers respond to alcohol in a way that is qualitatively or quantitatively different from that of non-alcoholic individuals. Again the difficulty in examining this proposition is that differences in response to alcohol might just be secondary to the effects of long-term drinking. Giving alcohol in controlled experiments to children of alcoholics before they had been exposed to alcohol poses insurmountable ethical, as well as legal, problems.

Schuckit and colleagues have overcome this difficulty by examining the response to alcohol in young men who had recently started drinking but had not developed any problems. Those who had a positive family history for alcoholism showed a lesser response to alcohol than their counterparts with a negative family history (Schuckit, Gold & Risch, 1987). For example, the serum cortisol and prolactin responses to an alcohol challenge were blunted in subjects with a family history of alcoholism, subjective feelings of intoxication were less and there was greater tolerance to the effects of alcohol on psychomotor performance.

Alcohol Metabolism

Susceptibility to the effects of alcohol could be related to individual variation in its metabolism. In 1965 von Wartburg, Papenberg and Aebi described an "atypical" form of alcohol dehydrogenase, which was considerably more active at physiological pH. They proposed that this aberrant form might predispose to the toxic effects of alcohol, in that it would result in more rapid metabolism of alcohol to acetaldehyde, a toxic and highly reactive compound. This finding stimulated a line of investigation into the pathways of alcohol metabolism and into variation in the principal enzymes concerned with alcohol metabolism.

The composition and genomic origin of the enzymes which are principally concerned with the oxidation of alcohol, alcohol dehydrogenase (ADH), the "microsomal ethanol oxidizing system" (MEOS), and aldehyde dehydrogenase (ALDH) have been elucidated over the past 30 years. In 1971 Smith, Hopkinson & Harris identified the genetic basis of the principal (class 1) isoenzymes of ADH. These comprised dimeric forms which were coded by three gene loci, which they labelled ADH1, ADH2, and ADH3 respectively. The "atypical" enzyme of von Wartburg was identified as being due to a single base pair substitution at the ADH2 locus. However, it did not appear to be related clearly to alcohol sensitivity, such as the alcohol-flush reaction, or to tissue toxicity such as liver damage (Ricciardi, Saunders, Williams & Hopkinson, 1983). For more detailed discussion of ADH isozymes, see the chapter by Ehrig and Li (this volume).

Attention then turned to alternative pathways such as MEOS, which is one of the cytochrome-p450 based oxidases. The role of this enzyme in human alcohol metabolism has been the subject of considerable controversy. It is probably responsible for only a small proportion of alcohol metabolism in non-alcoholic subjects and at moderate blood alcohol concentrations. There is growing evidence that in alcohol abusers it plays a greater role and in them may result in the generation of acetaldehyde in amounts that overcome aldehyde oxidative capacity. According to this hypothesis, the resulting accumulation of acetaldehyde would result in formation of free radicals and consequent tissue injury (Lieber, 1991). However, at the present time one must conclude that "the jury is still out".

The second enzyme in the alcohol oxidative pathway, ALDH, also exists in multiple molecular forms. Research into their genetic basis and physiological effects has been particularly productive. ALDH consists of at least five isoenzymes, of which one is located within mitochondria, whereas the others are found largely, if not exclusively, in the cytosol. An inactive variant of the mitochondrial isoenzyme has been identified in up to 50% of subjects from Chinese, Japanese and other South-east Asian populations (Harada, Agarwal & Goedde, 1981). This isoenzyme, having a low Km for acetaldehyde, is responsible for the bulk of acetaldehyde oxidation in humans. In persons who have an inactive mitochondrial isoenzyme, acetaldehyde accumulates whenever alcohol is ingested and an unpleasant facial flushing reaction results. This is analogous to the reaction experienced by persons being treated with the alcohol-sensitizing drug disulfiram (Antabuse), which is itself an ALDH inhibitor.

There is now compelling evidence that the presence of this inactive isoenzyme is a significant factor explaining the comparatively low prevalence of alcohol abuse and dependence in oriental populations. Harada and colleagues reported that only 2% of alcoholic patients in a treatment centre in Japan had the inactive mitochondrial isoenzyme compared with 50% of the general population (Harada, Agarwal, Goedde & Ishikawa, 1983). This finding was the first convincing evidence of a single gene defect which influences the drinking behavior of whole populations.

Isoenzyme variants of ADH and ALDH have now been reported in European subjects and there is provisional evidence that some may be associated with the alcohol-flush reaction in these populations (Yoshida, Dave, Ward & Peters, 1989).

Neurobiological Mechanisms

The neurobiological basis for the effects of alcohol and the development of tolerance and dependence has been extensively investigated since the 1950s. For many years little headway seemed to be made. Studies of neurotransmitter levels and turnover during alcohol intoxication and withdrawal produced conflicting results. Indeed, one might apply Keller's dictum to much of this early work: "Whenever a biological variable is measured in an alcoholic, it is present in either a higher concentration, a lower concentration, or about the same concentration compared with non-alcoholics".

One of the main difficulties was that no specific receptor for alcohol in the central nervous system could be identified. A fruitful line of investigation was established in the early 1970s by Goldstein, who examined alcohol's effects not on specific receptor systems but on biological membranes in general. Alcohol was known to intercalate into lipid bilayers, and the degree of perturbation produced by various aliphatic alcohols was correlated with their lipid solubility. An analogy was drawn with general anesthetics whose potency paralleled their lipophilicity. Goldstein and her colleagues demonstrated that alcohol increased the degree of fluidization of biomembranes. Furthermore, membranes extracted from animals who had been chronically exposed to alcohol (and rendered tolerant and dependent) showed a decreased fluidization and resistance to the perturbating effects of alcohol (Chin & Goldstein, 1977; Goldstein, 1987). Subsequently alterations in the composition of neuronal membranes were identified, there being a reduction in the normal ratio of polyunsaturated to saturated fatty acids.

Thus, the leading theory by the early 1980s was that the primary site of action of alcohol was within the lipid matrix of neuronal membranes. Chronic exposure would lead to changes in membrane lipid composition and a decrease in fluidization, and thus induce a state of neuroadaptation. This would restore the membrane to a more functional state in the presence of alcohol. As a result of this change, the structure and function of macromolecules within the membrane would be altered, with attendant effects on receptors, membrane-bound enzymes, and ion channels *inter alia*.

This immensely attractive hypothesis provided a great stimulus to neurobiological research on alcohol. However, its status remains that of a hypothesis and there are now several pieces of evidence that indicate the need for its reevaluation. There is doubt whether the biophysical properties and chemical composition of membrane lipids are indeed altered at concentrations of alcohol which cause intoxication in humans. Secondly, there is wide variation in the responsiveness of neurones to alcohol, indicating a considerable degree of specificity in alcohol's effects. Thirdly, the changes in lipid composition may be specific to the phosphatidyl fraction. On the other hand, it has not yet been possible to identify any membrane receptor responsible for alcohol's actions on the release or response to any specific neurotransmitter. No receptor or ion channel has yet been identified that possesses a high affinity binding site for alcohol.

Over the past decade, research has switched back to examining alcohol's effects on specific neurotransmitters (Shanley, 1991), though there is now a greater focus on the microenvironment of receptor-ion channel complexes. These studies are outlined below. For a more detailed discussion, see the chapter by Dildy-Mayfield and Harris (this volume). Alcohol acutely has been found to stimulate GABA-mediated neurotransmission, GABA being the principal inhibitory neurotransmitter in the central nervous system. This is effected by opening of chloride channels. Chronic exposure results in a conformational change in the GABA-benzodiazepine-chloride channel complex and induces what has been described as a functional uncoupling of this complex resulting in decreased responsiveness to alcohol (Allan and Harris, 1987).

Alcohol also affects calcium channels at physiologically relevant concentrations. Acutely it inhibits calcium flux across nerve terminals consequent upon depolarization. Chronically alcohol induces synthesis of calcium channels and there is increased calcium flux upon depolarization (Littleton & Little, 1987). This hypothesis proposes that when alcohol is removed, the increased calcium flux continues unabated and induces an alcohol withdrawal syndrome. Calcium channel blockers of the dihydropyridine type prevent the withdrawal syndrome in experimental animals in which physical dependence on alcohol has been induced (Little, Dolin & Halsey, 1986).

Other receptors are linked not to ion channels but to second messenger systems, such as adenylate cyclase, through guanine nucleotide binding proteins. Levels of (caesium flouride-stimulated) adenylate cyclase activity are subnormal both in cerebral tissue from experimental animals rendered alcohol dependent and in platelets from human alcoholics compared with non-alcoholics (Tabakoff et al., 1988).

Chronic alcohol consumption has also been found to influence receptor density. Following chronic exposure to alcohol, there is induction of NDMA-type glutamate receptors (Grant, Valverius, Hudspith & Tabakoff, 1990). Given that glutamate is the principal excitatory neurotransmitter in the brain, it is argued that this will result in a central nervous system hyperactivity syndrome when alcohol is no longer present. Glutamate neurotransmission is also implicated in neuronal plasticity (and therefore learning processes) and toxicity (which might result in cell death and impairment of cognitive and other functions).

Neurobiological research has leant heavily on the availability of animal models of tolerance and dependence. Inevitably, these have been somewhat limited in their genesis. Defining the neurobiological basis of clinical syndromes in humans is difficult because of limitations in the experimental techniques available.

Laboratory Markers of Alcohol Consumption

In the earlier section on genetics and alcohol, several biological "markers" of susceptibility to alcohol abuse and dependence were described. Another group of markers are those which reflect recent alcohol intake or the effects of alcohol on tissues. These are the "state markers."

The availability of valid laboratory measures of recent alcohol consumption would be extremely useful for screening, diagnosis and monitoring response to therapy. An important function would be to corroborate self-reported alcohol consumption, which although more accurate than many would suppose, can still be very misleading in a significant minority of drinkers. The first markers of alcohol consumption were described somewhat over 20 years ago, and two of the first to be reported, serum gamma glutamyl-transferase (GGT) activity and erythrocyte mean cell volume (MCV), are among the best established (Rosalki & Rau, 1972; Wu, Chanarin & Levi, 1974; Whitfield, 1981).

The clinical usefulness of these markers depends very much on the target condition. In the early studies their sensitivity and specificity were judged with reference to the diagnosis of alcoholism. Sensitivities for both GGT and MCV of around 80% were reported. With the broadening of the concept of problem drinking to encompass hazardous consumption and alcohol abuse as well as dependence, and the increasing emphasis on early intervention, there has been considerable interest in employing them as screening tools for these conditions. Unfortunately, their sensitivity in detecting hazardous consumption and alcohol abuse is much less, figures of 15-30% being typical (Chick, Kreitman & Plant, 1982; Bernadt, Mumford, Taylor, Smith and Murray, 1982; Saunders and Aasland, 1987). Thus they compare poorly with questionnaires such as the "CAGE" and the "AUDIT", which was developed specifically to screen for hazardous consumption and alcohol abuse (Saunders & Aasland, 1987). Other longstanding markers such as the serum aminotransferases and uric acid are equally unimpressive in this population.

The search for more sensitive (and specific) markers has proceeded apace. One of the most promising is desialated transferrin, also known as carbohydrate deficient transferrin (CDT). This is an isoform of transferrin found in increased concentration in alcohol abusers. It is formed probably as a result of interference by alcohol or acetaldehyde in hepatic glycosylation of transferrin. CDT has been reported to be more sensitive and specific than any of the conventional markers (Stibler, Borg & Joustra, 1986). Plasma levels of acetaldehyde-protein adducts and antibodies to these adducts have been proposed as screening tests (Israel, Hurwitz, Niemela & Arnon, 1986), but there remain problems in establishing a valid quantitative assay.

Alcohol as a Cause of Human Disease

Although the adverse effects of alcohol on behavior and social functioning are unarguable, it is only in the past 25 years that its role as a cause of human disease has been widely accepted. Cirrhosis is a good illustration of this point. Until the 1960s cirrhosis occurring in alcohol abusers was generally termed "fatty nutritional cirrhosis" (Lieber, 1977). It was considered to be due to nutritional deficiency, which of course is very common in this population. Animal models of dietary deficiency demonstrate a range of liver damage (from fatty liver to cirrhosis) which has similarities with human alcoholic liver disease. This of course was comforting for those who wished to believe that they could continue drinking alcohol and as long as they maintained a nutritious diet would be spared its physical complications.

Much of the evidence for alcohol's central role as a cause of human disease has originated in Lieber's laboratory in New York. He and his co-workers developed an alcohol containing liquid diet, which they demonstrated would cause fatty liver and fatty-fibrotic change in several animal species. This group later developed a baboon model, and showed that cirrhosis of the liver could be induced after approximately two years of continuous administration of the liquid diet (Lieber, de Carli & Rubin, 1975). Importantly, histological abnormalities were not seen in pair-fed animals who had the same calorie intake but no alcohol.

The mechanisms by which alcohol induces tissue injury have been subject to extensive investigation. Several forms of damage, including fatty liver and hyperlipidemia, have been linked to the change in redox potential (specifically an alteration in the ratio of oxidized nicotine adenine dinucleotide (NAD^+) to the reduced form (NADH)), which fuels several secondary reactions involving the synthesis of fatty acids, glycerophosphate, and ultimately triglyceride (Lieber, 1977; Lieber, 1991; Salaspuro, Shaw, Jayatilleke, Ross & Lieber, 1981).

Acetaldehyde has long been implicated as a cause of tissue injury. It is a highly reactive compound, which causes peroxidation of lipids and forms Schiff's bases with protein amino groups, resulting in protein denaturation and enzyme inactivity. The problem which has beset researchers for decades is that acetaldehyde is an extremely difficult compound to assay reliably. Most theories of tissue injury have implicated it by association rather than on the basis of sound empirical evidence. A role for free radicals in alcohol-induced tissue injury has also been theoretically attractive but it is only in the last five years that it has received much empirical support (Nordmann, Ribiere& Rouach, 1988).

Adducts which acetaldehyde forms with plasma proteins, tissue proteins and haemoglobin have been proposed as a mechanism of injury. These adducts which are detectable in peripheral blood and organs such as the liver have been postulated to act as an acetaldehyde-transport mechanism, allowing acetaldehyde to dissociate in tissues and react with tissue macromolecules and thereby exert its toxic effects.

Dose Response Relationships in Alcoholic Tissue Injury

When alcohol was implicated as a cause of tissue damage, it became important for public health reasons to define the levels of alcohol intake and the patterns of drinking that were injurious. This area of research had its origins in Europe, particularly France (at the Institute National de la Sante et Recherche Medicale) and Germany. A series of influential studies conducted by Pequignot, Tuyns and Sarles in particular have examined the risk of morbidity from various diseases at various levels of alcohol intake. In the first study of this type, reported by Pequignot in 1958, the alcohol intake of patients with cirrhosis (who had presented with ascites) was compared with that of controls hospitalized for non-alcohol related disease. The "cirrhosis morbidity quotient" was calculated for several levels of intake, and it was calculated that the risk of cirrhosis increased (in relation to the baseline rate of occurrence due presumably to non-alcohol related disease) when daily alcohol intake exceeded 80 g. (Pequignot, 1960).

In subsequent studies, the alcohol intake and dietary history of patients with various disease states known or suspected to be due to alcohol (such as cirrhosis, pancreatitis, and oesophageal cancer) were compared with those of controls drawn from the general population. For cirrhosis the hazardous level of alcohol consumption was revised downwards to 40 g. per day for men and 20 g. per day for women (Pequignot, Chabert, Eydoux & Courcoul, 1974). For oesophageal cancer the threshold levels were similar; furthermore, an interactive effect of alcohol and tobacco smoking on cancer risk was identified (Pequignot and Tuyns, 1984). For pancreatitis and in one study for cirrhosis, the risk increased once any regular daily alcohol intake was recorded (Pequignot, Tuyns & Berta, 1978). How these very low levels of alcohol intake could lead to disease, given what we know about the mechanisms of tissue injury, is not apparent. It raises the possibility that alcohol may interact with other environmental factors (such as dietary constituents, including carcinogens, hepatitis and other viruses).

A similar design has been adopted by many centres to examine for the risk of other types of malignant disease, hypertension, coronary heart disease, and cerebrovascular disease. Over the past decade, evidence has accumulated for a *protective* effect of alcohol in low dose on the development of coronary heart disease. Specifically, the cumulative prevalence of fatal and non-fatal coronary events is lower in subjects consuming 10-20 g. alcohol per day than in total abstainers. At first it was assumed that this was a spurious effect, explained on the basis that many abstainers would have significant pre-existing disease. It is now apparent that this explanation is not tenable, and that coronary heart disease is less common in moderate drinkers than in lifelong abstainers (Beaglehole & Jackson, in press). The exact mechanism for the protective effect has not been clearly defined, although it may reflect increased synthesis of high density lipoprotein-cholesterol (HDL-C), at least one component of which retards the development of atherosclerosis.

Pharmacological Treatments

The ultimate goal of research into biological mechanisms of alcohol abuse and dependence is to identify treatments which would assist a problem drinker to cease (or in some cases reduce) alcohol consumption, ensure safe and effective relief of withdrawal symptoms, cure associated physical and psychological disorders, prevent relapse (unfortunately a common event in those with established dependence), and prevent the onset of hazardous drinking and dependence in high risk individuals.

It would be agreeable to think that the pharmacological treatments currently available represent the logical outcome of a brilliantly conceived and well-executed program of research into the biology of abuse and dependence. Although there are some examples of this, for the most part current treatments are the result of serendipity or adoption of existing drugs on the basis of reasoning by analogy.

The most satisfactory area of treatment is detoxification: there are now well-established protocols for the effective relief and prevention of withdrawal symptoms (Sellers& Kalant, 1976). Most involve the use of a benzodiazepine, with which alcohol shows cross tolerance and cross dependence, presumably through their effects on GABA-mediated neurotransmission. Calcium channel blockers relieve withdrawal symptoms, as described earlier. However, they are not as effective in the prevention of fits or in treating delirium tremens as the benzodiazepines.

Of the drugs prescribed to promote long-term abstinence, the supreme example of serendipity is disulfiram (Antabuse). In the 1940s, rubber workers who were exposed to disulfiram-like compounds experienced unpleasant facial flushing when they drank alcohol. Disulfiram was subsequently introduced as an alcohol-sensitizing drug for the treatment of alcohol dependence. It was found to be an aldehyde dehydrogenase inhibitor and causes accumulation of acetaldehyde after alcohol is consumed. It has remained in use to this day and there is some evidence from randomized controlled trials of modest efficacy in the first three months of treatment, though this seems to be because of fear of an aversive reaction rather than any pharmacological effect (Fuller et al., 1986).

In the 1980s, interest turned to drugs which would have application for the person with hazardous consumption and alcohol abuse, reflecting the switch to intervention at an earlier stage. Presently, the most promising would seem to be the serotonin reuptake inhibitors. These were introduced for clinical trials when evidence of subnormal serotonergic neurotransmission in animal models of alcohol abuse was found. Controlled trials among subjects with alcohol abuse have shown that cumulative alcohol intake is significantly reduced compared with periods when a placebo preparation is taken (Naranjo et al., 1987; Sellers & Romach, 1991). The current status of other drugs used in the treatment of alcohol abuse and dependence is the subject of a recent review by the author (Saunders, 1989).

It is fair to say that to date the payoff in terms of useful pharmacological agents has not been as great as one might have hoped for.

However, with our greater understanding of the role of individual neurotransmitters in alcohol abuse and dependence, the availability of molecular biology techniques, and a focus on key clinical issues such as compliance, craving and the reinstatement phenomenon (an important determinant of relapse in alcohol dependent persons), there are good prospects of significant therapeutic advances.

Acknowledgements

Dr. J.B. Whitfield and Dr. K. Conigrave provided many helpful comments on an earlier version of this manuscript. The Centre for Drug and Alcohol Studies is supported by a research unit grant from the Drug and Alcohol Directorate, NSW Health Department, which is gratefully acknowledged.

References

Allan, A.M. & Harris RA. (1987). Acute and chronic ethanol treatments alter GABA receptor operated chloride channels. *Pharmacology, Biochemistry and Behavior*, 27:665-670.

American Psychiatric Association. (1987). *Diagnostic and Statistical Manual of Mental Disorders*,Third Edition, Revised. Washington, DC: American Psychiatric Association.

Beaglehole, R. & Jackson, R. Alcohol consumption, cardiovascular disease and total mortality. *Drug and Alcohol Review*, in press.

Begleiter, H., Porjesz, B., Bihari, B., Kissin, B. (1984). Event-related brain potentials in boys at risk for alcoholism. *Science*, 225:1493-1496.

Bernadt, M.W., Mumford, J., Taylor, C., Smith, B. and Murray, R.M. (1982). Comparison of questionnaires and laboratory tests in the detection of excessive drinking and alcoholism. *Lancet*, i:325-328.

Blum, K., Noble, E.P., Sheridan, P.J., Montgomery, A., Richie, T., Jagadeeswaran, P., Nogami, H., Briggs, A.H. and Cohn, J.B. (1990). Allelic association of human dopamine D_2 receptor gene in alcoholism. *Journal of the American Medical Association*, 263:2055-2060.

Brocklehurst, T. (1949). Alcoholic addiction: its classification and cure. *South African Medical Journal*, 23:771-774.

Cadoret, R.J., O'Gorman, T.W., Toughton E & Heywood E. (1985). Alcoholism and antisocial personality. Interrelationships, genetic and environmental factors. *Archives of General Psychiatry*, 42:161-167.

Cahalan, D., Cisin, I.H. & Crossley, H.M. (1969). *American Drinking Practices. A National Survey of Drinking Behavior and Attitudes. Monograph # 6.* New Brunswick: Rutgers Center of Alcohol Studies.

Chick, J., Kreitman, N. & Plant, M. (1981). Mean cell volume and gamma glutamyl transpeptidase as measures of drinking in working men. *Lancet*, i:1249-1251.

Chin, J.H. & Goldstein, D.B. (1977). Drug tolerance in biomembranes: a spin label study of the effects of ethanol. *Science*, 196:684-685.

Cloninger, C.R., Bohman, M. & Sigvardsson, S. (1981). Inheritance of alcohol abuse. *Archives of General Psychiatry*, 38:861-868.

Cruz-coke, R. and Varela, A. (1966). Inheritance of alcoholism. *Lancet*, ii:1281-1284.

Edwards, G. & Gross, M.M. (1976). Alcohol dependence: provisional description of a clinical syndrome. *British Medical Journal*, i:1058-1061.

Edwards, G., Gross, M.M., Keller, M., Moser, J and Room, R. (1977), *Alcohol Related Disabilities (WHO Offset Publication No. 32).* Geneva: World Health Organization.

Fingarette, H. (1988). *Heavy Drinking: The Myth of Alcoholism as a Disease.* London: University of California Press.

Fuller, R.K., Branchey, L., Brightwell, D.R. et al. (1986). Disulfiram treatment of alcoholism. A Veterans Association Cooperative Study. *Journal of the American Medical Association*, 256:1499-1455.

Goldstein, D.B. (1987). Ethanol-induced adaptation in biological membranes. *Annals of the New York Academy of Sciences*, 492:103-111.

Goodwin, D.W., Schulsinger, F., Hermansen, L., Guze, S.B. and Winokur, G. (1973). Alcohol problems in adoptees raised apart from alcoholic biological parents. *Archives of General Psychiatry*, 28:238-243.

Grant, K.A., Valverius, P., Hudspith, M. and Tabakoff, B. (1990). Ethanol withdrawal seizures and the NMDA receptor complex. *European Journal of Pharmacology*, 176:289-296.

Harada, S., Agarwal, D.P. & Goedde, H.W. (1981). Aldehyde dehydrogenase deficiency as a cause of facial flushing reaction to alcohol in Japanese. *Lancet*, ii:982.

Harada, S., Agarwal, D.P., Goedde, H.W. & Ishikawa, B. (1983). Aldehyde dehydrogenase isoenzyme variations and alcoholism in Japan. *Pharmacology, Biochemistry and Behavior*, 18 (Suppl. 1):151-153.

Heath, A.C., Meyer, J., Jardine, R. & Martin, N.G. (1991). The inheritance of alcohol consumption patterns in a general population twin sample. II. Determinants of consumption frequency and quantity consumed. *Journal of Studies on Alcohol*, 52:425-433.

Israel, Y., Hurwitz, E., Nielema, O. & Arnon, R. (1976). Monoclonal and polyclonal antibodies against acetaldehyde containing epitopes in acetaldehyde-protein adducts. *Proceedings of the National Academy of Sciences, USA*, 83:7923-7927.

Jellinek, E.M. (1960). *The Disease Concept of Alcoholism*. New Brunswick: Hillhouse Press.

Kessel, N. and Walton, H. (1965). *Alcoholism*. Harmondsworth, Middlesex: Penguin Books:71.

Lemere, F., Voegtlin, W.L., Broz, W.R., O'Hollaren, P. & Tupper, W.E. (1943). Heredity as an etiologic factor in chronic alcoholism. *Northwestern Medicine*, 42:110-111.

Lieber, C.S. (1977). Pathogenesis of alcoholic liver disease: an overview. In: M.M. Fisher and J.G. Rankin (Eds.) *Alcohol and the Liver*. New York: Plenum Press.

Lieber, C.S. (1991). Metabolism of ethanol and associated hepatotoxicity. *Drug and Alcohol Review*, 10:175-202.

Lieber, C.S., de Carli, L.M. & Rubin, E. (1975). Sequential production of fatty liver, hepatitis and cirrhosis in subhuman primates fed ethanol with adequate diets. *Proceedings of the National Academy of Sciences, USA*, 72:437-441.

Little, H.J., Dolin, S. & Halsey, M.J. (1986). Calcium channel antagonists decrease ethanol withdrawal syndrome. *Life Sciences*, 39: 2059-2065.

Littleton, J.M. & Little, H.J. (1987). Dihydropyridine-sensitive Ca^{++} channels in brain are involved in the central nervous system hyperexcitability associated with alcohol withdrawal states. *Annals of the New York Academy of Sciences*, 522:199-202.

Martin, N.G. (1991). Twin studies of alcohol consumption, metabolism and sensitivity. In: H Begleiter and CR Cloninger (Eds.), *Genetics and Biology of Alcoholism Banbury Report No. 33*, (pp. 15-29).

Naranjo, C.A., Sellers, E.M., Sullivan, J.T., Woodley, D.V., Kadlec, K. & Sykora, K. (1987). The serotonin uptake inhibitor citalopram attenuates ethanol intake. *Clinical Pharmacology and Therapeutics*, 41: 266-274.

Nordmann, R., Ribiere, C. & Rouach, H. (1988). Free radical and oxidative stress: their implication in the metabolism and toxicity of ethanol. In: Kuriyama K, Takada A and Ishii H. (Eds.) *Biomedical and Social Aspects of Alcohol and Alcoholism* (pp. 17-27). Amsterdam: Excerpta Medica.

Peele, S. (1989). The diseasing of America: addiction treatment out of control. Lexington: Lexington Books.

Pequignot, G. (1960). Enquete par interrogatoire sur les circonstances dietetiques de la cirrhose alcoolique en France. *Annales Medico Chirurgicales du Centre*, 17:1-21.

Pequignot, G., Chabert, C., Eydoux, H. & Courcoul, M.A. (1974). Augmentation du risque de cirrhose en fonction de la ration d'alcool. *Revue de l'Alcoolisme*, 20:191-202.

Pequignot, G. & Tuyns, A.J. (1984). Thresholds for damage. In: *Pharmacological Treatments for Alcoholism*, Edwards G, Littleton J, eds. London: Croom Helm: 219-228.

Pequignot, G., Tuyns, A.J. & Berta, J.L. (1978). Ascitic cirrhosis in relation to alcohol consumption. *International Journal of Epidemiology*, 7:113-120.

Ricciardi, B.R., Saunders, J.B., Williams, R. and Hopkinson, D.A. (1983). Hepatic ADH and ALDH isoenzymes in different racial groups and chronic alcoholism. *Pharmacology, Biochemistry and Behavior*, 18 (Suppl. 1):61-65.

Room, R. (1991). Drug policy reform in historical perspective: movements and mechanisms. *Drug and Alcohol Review*, 10:37-43.

Rosalki, S.B. & Rau, D. (1972). Serum gamma glutamyl transpeptidase activity in alcoholism. *Clinica Chimica Acta*, 39:41-47.

Salaspuro, M.P., Shaw, S., Jayatilleke, E., Rose, N.A. & Lieber, C.S. (1981). Attenuation of the ethanol-induced hepatic redox change after chronic alcohol consumption in baboons: metabolic consequences in vivo and in vitro. *Hepatology*, 1:33-38.

Saunders, J.B. (1982). Alcoholism: new evidence for a genetic contribution. *British Medical Journal*, 284:1137-1138.

Saunders, J.B. (1986). Changing perspectives on alcohol and drug problems. *Australian Drug and Alcohol Review*, 5:51-56.

Saunders, J.B. (1989). The efficacy of treatment for drinking problems. *International Review of Psychiatry*, 1:121-138.

Saunders, J.B & Aasland, O.G. (1987). *World Health Organization Collaborative Project on Identification and Treatment of Persons with Harmful Alcohol Consumption. Report on Phase 1. Development of a Screening Instrument*. Geneva: World Health Organization.

Schuckit, M.A, Gold, M.A. & Risch, S.C. (1987). Plasma cortisol levels following ethanol in sons of alcoholics and controls. *Archives of General Psychiatry*, 44:942-945.

Sellers, E.M. & Kalant, H. (1976). Alcohol intoxication and withdrawal. *New England Journal of Medicine*, 294:757-762.

Sellers, E.M. & Romach, M.K. (1991). Pharmacotheraphy of alcohol and drug problems. *Drug and Alcohol Review*, 10:215-224.

Shanley, B.C. (1991). Alcohol and the brain: recent advances in biomedical research. *Drug and Alcohol Review*, 10:75-78.

Silkworth, W.D. (1937). Alcoholism as a manifestation of allergy. *Medical Recorder*, 145:249-251.

Smith, M., Hopkinson, D.A. & Harris, H. (1971). Developmental changes and polymorphism in human alcohol dehydrogenase. *Annals of Human Genetics*, 24:251-271.

Stibler, H., Borg, S. & Joustra, M. (1986). Micro anion exchange chromatography of carbohydrate deficient transferrin in serum in relation to alcohol consumption. *Alcoholism: Clinical and Experimental Research*, 10:535-544.

Sullivan, J.L., Stanfield, C.N., Maltbie, A.A., Hammett, E. and Cavener, J.O. (1978). Stability of low blood platelet MAO activity in human alcoholics. *Biological Psychiatry*, 13:391-397.

Tabakoff, B., Hoffman, P.L., Lee, T.M., Saito, T., Willard, B. & de Leon-Jones, F. (1988). Differences in platelet enzyme activity between alcoholics and non-alcoholics. *New England Journal of Medicine*, 318:134-139.

von Wartburg, J.P., Papenberg, J. & Aebi, H. (1965). An atypical human alcohol dehydrogenase. *Canadian Journal of Biochemistry*, 43:889-898.

Whitfield, J.B. (1981). Alcohol related biochemical changes in heavy drinking. *Australian and New Zealand Journal of Medicine*, 11:132-139.

Whitfield, J.B. (1991). Biological markers of alcoholism. *Drug and Alcohol Review*, 10:127-135.

Wilson, P. (1980). *Drinking in England and Wales*. London: HMSO.

World Health Organization. (1992). *International Classification of Diseases. 10th Revision*. Geneva: World Health Organization.

Wu, A., Chanarin & Levi, A.J. (1974). Macrocytosis of chronic alcoholism. *Lancet*, i:829-830.

Yoshida, A., Dave, V., Ward, R.J. & Peters, T.J. (1989). Cytosolic aldehyde dehydrogenase (ALDH$_1$) variants found in alcohol flushers. *Annals of Human Genetics*, 53:1-7.

Metabolism of Alcohol and Metabolic Consequences

Torsten Ehrig and Ting-Kai Li
Department of Biochemistry and Molecular Biology and Department
of Medicine, Indiana University School of Medicine,
Indianapolis, Indiana, USA

The principal site of ethanol oxidation is the liver due to the abundance of alcohol metabolizing enzymes in this organ. Metabolic consequences of alcohol ingestion are therefore found mainly in the liver. Ethanol is oxidized in the hepatocyte to acetate by three enzyme systems: alcohol dehydrogenase (ADH) and, to a lesser extent, the microsomal ethanol oxidizing system (MEOS), convert ethanol to acetaldehyde, which is then metabolized to acetate by aldehyde dehydrogenase (ALDH). Each of these systems has a distinct subcellular localization. ADH is found in the cytosol, MEOS in the microsomal fraction, and the ALDH isoenzyme relevant for alcohol metabolism in mitochondria. During ethanol oxidation, NADH is produced in the cytosol, and the reducing equivalents are transported into the mitochondrion for regeneration by the mitochondrial respiratory chain. The transport occurs via various shuttle systems. The steady-state concentrations of intermediary metabolites depend on the relative activities of these metabolic systems. There is now growing evidence that directly relates the formation of acetaldehyde in the liver to alcoholic liver disease. An increase in the hepatic NADH/NAD$^+$ ratio leading to triglyceride accumulation may also play an etiologic role, although the significance of fatty liver in the onset of alcoholic liver disease is not clear. This review describes the kinetic properties of alcohol metabolizing enzymes in humans with a specific emphasis towards the consequences of producing potentially pathogenic metabolites. The possible significance of genetic variants of both the ADH and ALDH systems for interindividual differences in pathologic response to chronic alcohol ingestion will be addressed. Since the rat is a well-studied model system of alcohol metabolism, alcohol metabolizing enzyme systems in the rat will be compared with those in humans.

Hepatic Systems of Ethanol Metabolism

Alcohol dehydrogenase (ADH)

Genetic model. Mammalian alcohol dehydrogenases are dimeric molecules with subunits of 40,000 daltons. Based on comparisons of the primary sequences (Jornvall et al., 1987a,b; Kaiser et al., 1988) and of differences in the steady-state kinetic behavior of the different isoenzyme forms, mammalian ADH has been subdivided into three classes, designated class I, II and III (Wagner et al., 1984). There is about 60-70% sequence identity among the isoenzymes of different classes. In humans, one class II isoenzyme (Jornvall et al., 1987b), one class III isoenzyme (Kaiser et al., 1988), and a multitude of isoenzymes in class I (Bosron et al., 1983a; Yin et al., 1984a; Burnell et al., 1989) have been isolated. Three different gene loci, ADH_1, ADH_2 and ADH_3, code for the three major subunit types of class I ADH, α, β and γ, respectively (Smith, 1986), as shown in Table 1. The class I chains combine randomly to form all possible combinations of dimers. Polymorphisms in the ADH_2 and ADH_3 genes have been identified, and the known alleles code for β_1, β_2 and β_3 chains (Bosron et al., 1983b; Yin et al., 1984b) and γ_1 and γ_2 chains (Smith, 1986). The translated amino acid sequences of the alleles differ by exchanges of one or two amino acids. Genotyping techniques using the polymerase chain reaction (PCR) allow the determination of the ADH haplotypes from an ordinary blood sample (Gennari et al., 1988; Xu et al., 1988). Sequence and X-ray crystallographic data indicate that the mutations, except for a probably kinetically unimportant exchange at position 349 between γ_1 and γ_2, involve the coenzyme binding site (Jörnvall et al., 1987a; Burnell et al., 1987; Ehrig et al., 1988; Hurley et al., 1990). These mutations affect in a major way not only the kinetic constants for coenzyme binding, but also for substrate binding and maximal velocity (V_{max}).

Table 1
Genetic model of human ADH liver isoenzymes

Class	I			II	III
Locus	ADH_1	ADH_2	ADH_3	ADH4	ADH5
Peptide	α	b_1	g_1	p	c
		b_2	g_2		
		β_3			

Class II and class III isoenzymes exist only as homodimers—the π and χ peptides are sufficiently different from each other and from the α, β and γ peptides that heterodimers across the classes are not found (Jörnvall et al., 1987a). The postulated structural gene loci coding for the class II and III π and χ peptides have been named ADH_4 and ADH_5 (Smith, 1986). Recently, an ADH gene which is quite different from those shown in Table I based on the sequence alignments has been cloned and named ADH 6 (Yasunami et al., 1991). Molecular and catalytic properties of this enzyme are unknown. There is also a unique form of ADH in stomach, σ-ADH, which has tentatively been assigned to class II ADH (Moreno & Pares, 1991). The class III isoenzyme has recently been identified as the glutathione-dependent formaldehyde dehydrogenase (Koivusalo & Uotila, 1990).

Human liver homogenates that have isoenzymes with the β_2 subunit exhibit high activity *in vitro* (vonWartburg et al., 1965). Such livers have an approximately 5-fold higher ADH activity per g liver tissue than those that have only the β_1 subunit (vonWartburg & Schurch, 1968). These livers, because of their high *in vitro* activity, were initially called "atypical" livers. Subsequently, it was found that livers containing isoenzymes with β_3 subunits were even more "atypical". Since the differences among the β ADH subunits have now been characterized at the protein and DNA level, current usage no longer employs the kinetic properties as the primary identifier of the different genetic variants.

In the rat, the multitude of liver ADH isoenzymes has been less extensively studied than in humans. Sequence data (Crabb & Edenberg, 1986) and kinetic data (Julia et al., 1987) allow tentative assignment of the different isoenzymes to the three classes. Starch gel electropohoresis shows one class II enzyme and several class I and III forms in the liver (Crabb et al., 1983; Julia et al., 1987). The

multiplicity of class I forms probably arises from sulfhydryl oxidation rather than from genetic polymorphism (Crabb et al., 1983).
Ethnic distribution of ADH2 and ADH3 alleles. As shown in Table
2, there are marked differences in allele frequency among different
ethnic populations both at the ADH_2 and ADH_3 locus. The ADH_22 allele is most prominent in Oriental populations, and the ADH_23 allele
has thus far been found only in the Black American population. North
American Indians, although considered members of the Mongoloid
major mating population, do not exhibit the ADH_22 allele. ADH genotyping in various ethnic groups is discussed in greater detail in the
chapter by Sherman et al. (this volume).

*Table 2: Ethnic distribution of ADH allele frequencies and occurrence of
deficient $ALDH_2$*

Allele	$ADH_2{}^1$	$ADH_2{}^2$	$ADH_2{}^3$	$ADH_3{}^1$	$ADH_3{}^2$	deficient $ALDH_2$
Peptide	β_1	β_2	β_3	g_1	γ_2	(%)
Caucasians	0.90-0.96	0.04-0.10	<0.05	0.53-0.60	0.40-0.47	0
Orientals	0.32-.38	0.62-0.68	<0.05	0.91-0.95	0.05-0.09	44
Black Amerians	0.85	<0.05	0.15	0.85	0.15	0
North American Indians[a]	1.00	0.00	0.00	0.07-0.57	0.43-0.93	0-16
South American Indians[b]						0c / 41[d]

Data taken from Rex, et al, 1985, Bosron, et al, 1988, and references cited therein; v
onWartburg & Schürch (1968); O'Dowd, et al. (1990).
[a]Sioux, Navajo, Pueblo and Oklahoma
[b]Mapuche
[c]as determined by genotyping for the Glu-Lys 487 exchange
[d]as determined by activity stain of electrophoresis

Catalytic properties. The catalytic properties of ADH isoenzymes
have been well-studied in humans. There are significant steady-state
kinetic differences among the isoenzymes. Kinetic constants of homodimeric isoenzymes are given in Table 3. Only homodimers are
listed, since heterodimers behave like a mixture of parental homodimers (Bosron et al., 1983a). Most of the human ADH isoenzymes are
saturated with ethanol at commonly found intoxicating ethanol con-

Table 3
Steady-state kinetic constants of homodimeric isoenzymes of human liver ADH

Species	Human							Rat
Class	I						II	I
Isozyme	$\alpha\alpha$	$\beta_1\beta_1$	$\beta_2\beta_2$	$\beta_3\beta_3$	$\gamma_1\gamma_1$	$\gamma_2\gamma_2$	$\pi\pi$	c
K_m EtOH (mM)	4.2	0.049	0.94	36	1.0a	0.49a	34	0.48
K_m Acetald (mM)	4.3	0.085	0.24	3.4	0.33	0.24	30	0.037
K_m NAD (μM)	13	7	180	710	8	9	14	33
K_m NADH (μM)	11	6	105	260	7		16	4
K_i NAD (μM)	32	90	340	2300			86	58
K_i Acetald (μM)	150[b]	2.9[b]	44[b]		20[b,d]		9000	12
K_i NADH (μM)	0.4	0.19	9.7	56	0.98	1.6	1.9	0.9
V_{max} forwd (U/mg)	0.6	0.23	8.6	7.9	2.2	0.87	0.5	3.9

Values taken from Bosron et al. (1979, 1983a), Yin et al. (1984a), Burnell et al. (1989) & Crabb et al. (1983).

All values for human enzymes at pH 7.5, for rat enzyme at pH 7.3.

[a]values are $S_{0.5}$-values.

[b]Bosron, Magnes and Li, unpublished results.

[c]reported as a mixture of different molecular forms.

[d]for ethanol range 0.2-2 mM

centrations, giving rise to the well-known pseudo zero-order (i.e. independent of ethanol concentration) elimination pharmacokinetics. The class II ADH and the β_3-containing isoenzymes, both of which have a high K_m of 36 mM for ethanol, will not be saturated at these concentrations and can be expected to introduce some ethanol-concentration-dependence to the elimination kinetics. As another consequence of the high K_m of the class II isoenzyme, it has been estimated that it would contribute up to about 40% to the total ADH activity at the highly intoxicating ethanol concentration of 60 mM, but only about 26% at a moderately intoxicating concentration of 10 mM (Li et al., 1977). The class III isoenzyme has a K_m value for ethanol of above 1 M (Wagner et al., 1984) and, therefore, would not contribute significantly to alcohol metabolism.

The steady-state kinetics of most ADH isoenzymes are compatible with a compulsory mechanism with coenzyme binding first (Bosron et al., 1979, 1983a; Yin et al., 1984a; Burnell et al., 1989; Crabb et al., 1983; Brändén et al., 1975). The activity of α and β homodimers conforms to Michaelis-Menten kinetics. The $\gamma\gamma$ isoenzymes show a nonlinear kinetic behavior, possibly indicating subunit interactions (Bosron et al., 1983a; Mardh et al., 1986a). The kinetic constants for the different isoenzymes vary widely (Table 3). Of most interest from the genetic viewpoint are the kinetic differences among the allelic isoenzymes. Table 3 shows that differences are particularly large for the allelic forms of the β subunit. Using an extension of the Michaelis-Menten equation which takes into account the presence of two substrates (ethanol and NAD^+) and of two products (Crabb et al., 1983; Segel, 1975), the kinetic constants given in Table 3 in combination with the equilibrium constant of the reaction (Baecklin, 1958) allow an estimation of the metabolic activity of the isoenzymes under substrate and product concentrations likely to prevail *in vivo*. The intrahepatic concentrations of ethanol and NAD^+ during alcohol metabolism can be estimated to a reasonable accuracy, whereas the concentrations of acetaldehyde and NADH are much less certain. (See sections "Experimental data in the rat" and "Experimental data in humans.") Nevertheless, assuming intrahepatic ethanol and NAD^+ concentrations of 20 and 0.5 mM, respectively, and acetaldehyde and NADH concentrations of 14 and 3 µM, respectively, the *in vitro* data would predict the following behavior *in vivo*. The β_1 subunit will metabolize at a rate close to its V_{max}, and the β_2 subunit at about 65% of V_{max}, mainly as a consequence of incomplete substrate saturation. The inhibition constant for acetaldehyde of the β_3 subunit has not been determined (Table 3), but, based on substrate saturation alone, it is clear that this subunit at most can operate at about 10% of its V_{max} under *in vivo* substrate concentrations. A particularly high ethanol elimination capacity can therefore be expected for "atypical" livers, since the β_2 subunit has both a high V_{max} (Table 3), and operates not too far below V_{max}. At conditions measuring V_{max}, "atypical" livers have a 5-fold higher ADH activity than livers containing only β_1 subunits (vonWartburg and Schurch, 1968). Assuming from the kinetic constants in Table 3 that the isoenzymes in a "typical" liver operate close to V_{max}, and the β_2 subunits in "atypical" livers at about 65% of V_{max}, one can estimate that the *in vivo* ethanol elimination capacity of an "atypical" liver should be about 3 times higher than that of a "typical" liver. In the section

"Conclusions about the metabolic state of alcohol dehydrogenase," these extrapolations from *in vitro* data to expected *in vivo* behavior of the isoenzymes will be compared to actual alcohol elimination rates measured *in vivo*.

For the allelic pair γ_1 - γ_2, similar differences in the ethanol elimination capacity, although probably less pronounced, can be expected. Available *in vitro* kinetic data (Table 3), although incomplete, suggest that both forms will operate close to V_{max} under substrate and product concentrations *in vivo*, so that the presence of the subunit with the higher V_{max} (γ_1, Table 3) should lead to a higher ethanol elimination capacity.

As with humans, ethanol is mainly oxidized by hepatic class I ADH in the rat (Julia et al., 1987). The steady-state kinetic properties of rat ADH are, in general, similar to those for the human isoenzymes. Kinetic constants of rat class I ADH are usually reported for a mixture of unresolved molecular forms (as in Table 3), since they exhibit very similar kinetic constants (Crabb et al., 1983). The kinetic values in Table 3 show that rat class I ADH will be fully saturated by NAD^+ and ethanol during alcohol metabolism. The K_m/K_i ratios for ethanol/acetaldehyde and $NAD^+/NADH$ are somewhat lower, but still comparable to the corresponding values in human enzymes, indicating a similar susceptibility to inhibition by products.

Microsomal ethanol oxidizing system (MEOS)

Among several microsomal cytochrome P450 isoenzymes with alcohol degrading activity, the major active component seems to be a microsomal cytochrome P450 isoenzyme with high V_{max} towards ethanol (Lasker et al., 1987). According to current nomenclature, this ethanol-inducible form is designated P450IIE1 (Lieber, 1988). As an undifferentiated group, the alcohol metabolizing P450 isoenzymes are known as the Microsomal Ethanol Oxidizing System (Lieber and DeCarli, 1970, 1972; Teschke et al., 1975; Tsutsumi et al., 1989). The K_m value for P450IIE1 towards ethanol is about 10 mM; accordingly, it will not be saturated during ethanol metabolism. In contrast to the alcohol dehydrogenase reaction which generates the high-energy-compound NADH from NAD^+, the microsomal ethanol metabolism converts the high-energy compound NADPH to $NADP^+$. This has been implicated to explain the observation that isocaloric substitution of ethanol for carbohydrates in alcoholics resulted in weight loss (Lieber, 1988). The ethanol metabolizing capacity of MEOS in rats is about 20 - 25% of that of the ADH isoenzymes, but chronic ingestion of ethanol or drugs can lead to a proliferation of the endoplasmic reticulum and about a 2-fold increase in MEOS activity (Lieber and DeCarli, 1972; Lieber, 1988). Exact estimates of the contribution of MEOS to the ethanol metabolizing capacity in humans are not available.

Aldehyde dehydrogenase (ALDH)

Several ALDH isoenzymes with different subcellular locations and widely varying kinetic properties have been described. With the structural information currently available, mammalian ALDH enzymes can be assigned to one of three classes (Weiner & Flynn, 1988). Human ALDH1 (E1) and ALDH2 (E2) are assigned to classes I and II, respectively. In the rat, the mitochondrion is the exclusive site of an aldehyde dehydrogenase with low K_m (Tottmar et al., 1973), which is generally believed to be responsible for acetaldehyde oxidation at the low acetaldehyde concentrations prevailing during ethanol metabolism *in vivo*. This conclusion derives from studies in the rat showing that acetaldehyde metabolism affected the β-hydroxybutyrate/acetoacetate ratio (indicative of the mitochondrial $NADH/NAD^+$ ratio) but not the lactate/pyruvate ratio (indicative of the cytosolic $NADH/NAD^+$ ratio) (Eriksson, 1973). Further evidence is that cycloserine, an inhibitor of a mitochondrial shuttle system to transport reducing equivalents between cytosol and mitochondrial matrix, did not affect the oxidation of acetaldehyde (Parrilla et al., 1974). In humans, the only isoenzyme with a low K_m value, ALDH2 (Table 4), is probably also located in the mitochondrion. Its importance for acetaldehyde oxidation in alcohol metabolism is underscored by the accumulation of acetaldehyde in individuals with the "Oriental" variant of ALDH2 (Mizoi et al., 1983). This "Oriental" enzyme is coded for by an allele of ALDH2 and has a lysine for glutamine substitution at position 487. This mutation reduces the enzymatic activity to near zero (Yoshida et al., 1983; Impraim et al., 1982; Ikawa et al., 1983; Jörnvall et al., 1987a).

Table 2 shows that the ALDH2-deficiency occurs with high frequency in Oriental populations. Among the several North American Indian tribes studied, only the Oklahoma Indians showed a substantial occurrence of deficient ALDH (16%), whereas in other tribes the frequency was low (Bosron et al., 1988; Zeiner et al., 1984; Goedde et al., 1986). Among South American Indians (Mapuche) a high percentage was phenotypically deficient (Goedde et al., 1986), but genotyping did not show the above-mentioned amino acid exchange at

Table 4
Steady-state kinetic constants of ALDH isozymes.

Isozyme	E1 (ALDH1)	E2 (ALDH2)	E3	E4
K_m Acetaldehyde (μM)	30	3	40-50	5000
K_m NAD (μM)	40	70	14	41

pH ranges from 7.0 to 7.4.
Values taken from Greenfield and Pietruszko (1977), Forte-McRobbie et al.(1986) and Kurys et al. (1989).

position 487 typical of the "Oriental" variant, suggesting that, in these cases, a different mutation may have led to a functionally deficient enzyme (O'Dowd et al., 1990). The genetic characteristics of ADH and ALDH are further detailed in the chapter by Sherman et al. (this volume).

Localization of ADH, ALDH and MEOS in the hepatic lobule

The distribution of ADH and ALDH within the hepatic lobule is controversial. Periportal, perivenous and balanced distributions of ADH, and balanced and perivenous distributions of ALDH in the rat have been reported (Chen et al., 1992; Vaananen et al., 1984; Morrison and Brock, 1967; Kato et al., 1990; Bengtsson et al., 1981). Results in humans indicate a predominantly centrilobular localization of ADH and a balanced distribution of ALDH (Morrison & Brock, 1967; Buehler et al., 1982). All authors agree that MEOS has a centrilobular localization both in rats and humans (Ingelman-Sundberg et al., 1988; Chen et al., 1988; Tsutsumi et al., 1989).

Reoxidation of NADH

NADH generated by the ADH and ALDH reactions is reoxidized by the electron transport chain in the mitochondria. Reducing equivalents generated in the cytosol by ADH have to be transported into the mitochondria by shuttle systems. The kinetic behavior of these steps is the least well characterized in ethanol metabolism. Data on the human system are totally absent, and the following is a description of the NADH reoxidation pathway in the rat. The rate-limiting step of NADH reoxidation seems to be the transport of reducing equivalents from the cytosol into the mitochondria by shuttle-systems rather than the oxidation of NADH via the electron transport chain itself. Among the multitude of shuttle-systems described, the malate-aspartate-shuttle transports about 50% of the reducing equivalents, and the glycerophosphate- and fatty acid-shuttle another 50% (Dawson, 1979). Higgins (1979) has suggested that the response of the shuttle transport velocity as a function of the cytosolic NADH concentration is characterized by a high K_m and not saturable at NADH concentrations found in the cytosol. This view is in agreement with the proposal that the kinetics of the malate-aspartate shuttle are determined by the steady-state kinetics of cytosolic and mitochondrial malate dehydrogenases. These enzymes will not be saturated by substrates *in vivo* and can, therefore, respond to an elevated cytoplasmic NADH concentration by a higher rate leading to an increased shuttle activity (Crow et al., 1982; Wiseman et al., 1991).

Metabolite Steady-State Concentrations in the Liver

Experimental data in the rat

Most data concerning hepatic metabolite steady-state concentrations during ethanol metabolism have been obtained in the rat. In rat liver, the cytosolic concentration of NAD^+ is about 500 µM (Sies, 1982). From the equilibrium constant of the lactate dehydrogenase reaction (Williamson et al. 1967), the concentration of free NADH in the cytosol can be estimated from the lactate/pyruvate ratio. The lactate/pyruvate ratio in the absence of ethanol ranges from about 5 to 12 (Williamson et al., 1969; Forsander et al., 1964, 1965; Lindros et al., 1971; Lumeng et al., 1980), corresponding to a free NADH concentration of around 0.5 µM. This value refers to the fraction of free NADH. The total NADH concentration is considerably higher, since a large fraction of NADH is bound to enzymes (Sies, 1982). In the presence of ethanol, the lactate/pyruvate ratio rises to 12-100 (Williamson et al., 1969; Forsander et al., 1965a, 1965b; Lindros et al., 1972; Lumeng et al., 1980) corresponding to a concentration of free NADH of up to 5 µM. There is also a rise in the mitochondrial $NADH/NAD^+$ ratio during ethanol metabolism, since the hepatic β-hydroxy-butyrate/acetoacetate ratio rises from about 1 to 5 - 7 (Forsander et al., 1965a). Acetaldehyde concentrations during ethanol metabolism are more difficult to estimate due to possible artefactual formation of acetaldehyde from ethanol during the sampling and assay procedure (Erikson 1983). Reported hepatic values range from 9 up to over 200 μM (Erikson, 1973; Lindros et al., 1972; Erikson et al. 1975; Lumeng et al., 1980). Concentrations below 100 μM are in best agreement with the metabolic simulations described in conclusions below.

Experimental data in humans

In contrast to the situation in the rat, data for metabolite concentrations in human livers are scarce. Nevertheless, values of the lactate/pyruvate ratio and of the acetaldehyde concentration in the hepatic vein during ethanol metabolism have been obtained in a few individuals. In healthy, nonalcoholic individuals, lactate/pyruvate ratios of about 10 - 30 in the absence of ethanol, and of about 80 - 100 during ethanol consumption have been observed (Tygstrup et al., 1965; Nuutinen et al., 1984; Seligson et al., 1959). These values are thus comparable to those in the rat liver. The mean hepatic vein acetaldehyde concentration was 14 μM, with, however, large interindividual variations (Nuutinen et al., 1984). The ADH phenotype of the individuals (i.e. the ADH isoenzyme composition in their livers) was, of course, unknown. Since the test subjects were most likely Caucasians, most of them were probably bearing the "typical" (containing β_1 subunits), and a smaller number, if any, the "atypical" phenotype (homozygous for β_2). Intrahepatic acetaldehyde concentrations around 14 μM would be consistent with a mitochondrially located acetaldehyde oxidation, since the kinetic constants of ALDH given in Table 4 show that, at this concentration, only the mitochondrially located ALDH2 will be saturated.

Conclusions about the metabolic state of alcohol dehydrogenase

Using substrate and product concentration values as described, the ethanol oxidation rate has been calculated from the *in vitro* steady-state kinetic data for rat ADH (Crabb et al., 1983; Crow et al., 1982). The activity thus obtained agrees with the experimental *in vivo* ethanol elimination rate in the rat and corroborates the general validity of metabolic simulations based on *in vitro* properties of enzymes, as far as average metabolite concentrations are concerned. These calculations show that, during ethanol metabolism, ADH in the rat operates at about 80% of its theoretically maximal velocity. This means that ADH is the major rate-limiting step in the catalytic sequence. The enzyme is practically completely saturated by the substrates ethanol and NAD^+. Product inhibition is largely responsible for the depression of activity to about 80%.

An obviously very similar situation is found in humans with the "typical" phenotype. A comparison of the theoretically maximal *in vitro* activity of "typical" livers with the ethanol elimination rates in drinking experiments shows that ADH operates close to the maximal activity and is, therefore, the major rate-limiting step of ethanol metabolism as in the rat (vonWartburg et al., 1965). That human ADH in "typical" livers is only minimally inhibited by products *in vivo* is also consistent with the kinetic constants given in Table 3 assuming the NADH and acetaldehyde concentrations as described above. A caveat to the described simulations of ethanol metabolism is that they have assumed an even distribution of the metabolic processes within the liver lobule and, therefore, allow only the estimation of average metabolite concentrations. It is possible that these simulations underestimate the concentration of, for example, acetaldehyde in certain locations of the hepatic lobule.

There is only little experimental evidence as to the degree this situation will change in individuals with isoenzymes comprising β_2 or β_3 subunits. Current research aims at evaluating the alcohol elimination rate as a function of the ADH and ALDH isoenzyme pattern, and only preliminary conclusions can be drawn from the data available today. In the previous section, "Catalytic properties," it was stated that the ethanol elimination capacity of a human liver as expected from the *in vitro* ADH activity is about 3-fold higher for livers containing the β_2 subunit compared to livers containing the β_1 subunits, if intrahepatic concentrations of acetaldehyde and NADH of 14 and 3 µM are assumed. However, preliminary results of drinking experiments indicate that the ethanol elimination rate of Asians homozygous for the β_2 allele, 0.34 mg/dl/min (Thomasson et al., 1990), is about twice that found for Caucasians (assumed to represent the elimination rate of individuals with the β_1 allele). This suggests that in individuals with the β_2 subunit the intrahepatic concentrations of acetaldehyde and/or NADH during alcohol metabolism may be actually higher than the values assumed above, and would slow down the ADH reaction by exerting product inhibition on ADH. In this metabolic situation, the ALDH activity and/or mitochondrial NADH reoxidation capacity would assume a larger share of the control over the metabolic flux through the ethanol elimination pathway. In view of the possible pathogenic roles of acetaldehyde and an increased $NADH/NAD^+$ ratio ("Metabolic conse-quences), it seems possible that individuals with the "atypical" phe-notype may have a higher risk to develop alcoholic liver disease. However, more research is necessary so that the *in vivo* elimination rates can be compared in groups of the same ethnic origin to elimi-nate the influence of other genetic background factors.

Similarly, a comparison of the allelic pairs β_1 - β_3 and γ_1 - γ_2 reveals differences in V_{max} (Table 3) that may lead to differences in the $NADH/NAD^+$ ratio and acetaldehyde concentration during alcohol metabolism. It seems likely that, in analogy to the situation with the β_1 - β_2 pair, the allele coding for the higher-V_{max} subunits (β_3 and γ_1) will be associated with higher *in vivo* product concentrations. How-ever, the magnitude of the effect will probably be smaller than in the case of the β_1 - β_2 pair. It remains to be determined whether or not the extreme variability of hepatic vein acetaldehyde concentrations after ethanol ingestion in the above cited study by Nuutinen et al. (1984), can be correlated with individual differences in the ADH isoenzyme pattern. Variations in the ADH phenotype clearly should not affect acetaldehyde concentrations as drastically as in the case of the "Ori-ental" variant of ALDH (Mizoi et al., 1983), although the ADH phe-notype appears to modulate the severity of the flushing reaction caused by the "Oriental" ALDH (Thomasson et al., 1990).

Metabolic states with high acetaldehyde concentrations

Although average acetaldehyde concentrations in the hepatic vein are around 14 µM, and in peripheral blood below the detection limit of about 2 µM during ethanol metabolism in Caucasians (Erik-son, 1983), these values may vary considerably. Striking is the large interindividual variability of acetaldehyde concentrations in hepatic veins of nonalcoholic individuals. In the test group cited above, the mean acetaldehyde concentration in the hepatic vein was 14 µM, but the individual values varied from close to zero to 170 µM (Nuutinen et al., 1984). Under certain circumstances, extremely high acetalde-hyde concentrations are found even in the peripheral blood, using methods that avoid artefactual acetaldehyde formation. In chronic alcoholics acetaldehyde in peripheral blood may reach values as high as 100 µM (Lindros et al., 1980). It has been suggested that a reduction of $ALDH_2$ activity in alcoholics is responsible for this phenomenon (Nuutinen et al., 1983, 1984). High acetaldehyde con-centrations are also characteristic of individuals with the "Oriental"

variant of ALDH, where mean peripheral blood acetaldehyde concentrations of over 30 µM, with maximal values of over 100 µM, are observed as a consequence of the reduced activity of ALDH2 (Mizoi et al., 1983). The metabolic states of the alcohol degrading enzymes and resulting metabolite steady-state concentrations under such high acetaldehyde concentrations are not well understood.

Genotype and Alcoholism

As described above, a deficiency in the mitochondrial ALDH in Asian populations leads to elevated peripheral acetaldehyde concentrations. The deficient ALDH is found in Japanese and Chinese alcoholics only in low frequency as compared with nonalcoholic controls (Shibuya & Yoshida, 1988). This suggests that elevated acetaldehyde concentrations constitute a protective factor against alcoholism, because excessive peripheral acetaldehyde concentration produces an aversive reaction called the alcohol-flush reaction. Individuals suffering from this reaction experience facial and anterior chest wall flushing and palpitations as the predominant symptoms. When severe, headaches, nausea, vomiting, brawny edema and hypotension can ensue. Recently, an association between ADH genotype and prevalence of alcoholism has also been demonstrated showing that, when compared with a control population, the ADH_22 and ADH_31 alleles are less frequently found than the ADH_21 and ADH_32 alleles, respectively (Thomasson et al., 1991; Table 5). The ADH_22 and ADH_31 alleles code for those subunits (β_2, γ_1) which can be expected to lead to higher hepatic NADH and/or acetaldehyde concentrations (see above section, "Conclusions about the metabolic state of alcohol dehydrogenase"). A possible interpretation is therefore that individuals with the ADH_22 and ADH_31 alleles produce acetaldehyde at a higher rate, thereby exerting a protective effect as does decreased metabolism of acetaldehyde in ALDH2 deficiency (Thomasson et al., 1991). This hypothesis needs further clarification by measuring acetaldehyde concentrations in genotyped individuals.

Metabolic Consequences

Ethanol ingestion alters a wide variety of hepatic and extrahepatic metabolic systems, as has been reviewed recently (Lieber, 1991a, b). Here, we will focus mainly on those metabolic changes in the liver that are an immediate consequence of the metabolic activity of alco-

Table 5
Human ADH and ALDH genotype and phenotype frequencies among alcoholics and nonalcoholics.

	Genotype (phenotype); frequency		
ADH2 gene allele	1-1 ($\beta_1\beta_1$)	1-2 ($\beta_1\beta_2$)	2-2 ($\beta_2\beta_2$)
Nonalcoholics	0.06	0.40	0.53
Alcoholics	0.37	0.31	0.33
ADH3 gene allele	1-1 ($\gamma_1\gamma_1$)	1-2 ($\gamma_1\gamma_2$)	2-2 ($\gamma_2\gamma_2$)
Nonalcoholics	0.89	0.11	0.00
Alcoholics	0.61	0.33	0.06
ALDH2 gene allele	1-1 (normal)	1-2 (deficient)	2-2 (deficient)
Nonalcoholics	0.52	0.36	0.12
Alcoholics	0.88	0.12	0.00

Data taken from Thomasson et al. (1991).

Phenotypes are deduced from the genotypes assuming codominant expression of ADH alleles (Gennari et al., 1988) and dominant expression of the ALDH2 2 allele (Crabb et al., 1989).

hol and aldehyde dehydrogenase and, therefore, are most likely to correlate with genetically determined isoenzyme patterns.

Increased NADH/NAD⁺ ratio

Alcohol metabolism leads to a reversible accumulation of triglycerides in the hepatocyte even after a single drinking episode (Wiebe et al., 1971) and, after prolonged alcohol intake, a fatty liver may result. This accumulation is the effect of decreased utilization of fatty acids rather than of increased synthesis since alcohol intake in the rat does not affect fatty acid synthesis (Guynn et al., 1973). Ethanol metabolism inhibits β-oxidation (Grunnet & Kondrup, 1986; Latipää et al., 1986; Fellenius and Kiessling, 1973; Ontko, 1973) and the citric acid cycle (Ontko, 1973; Fellenius and Kiessling, 1973) in the liver cell. Inhibition of the citric acid cycle has been explained by inhibition of α-ketoglutarate dehydrogenase by the elevated NADH/NAD⁺ ratio (Ontko, 1973). Inhibition of β-oxidation is also the consequence of an elevated NADH/NAD⁺ ratio, but the site of control has not been established (Latipää et al., 1986). The role of fatty liver in the etiology of alcoholic hepatitis and alcoholic cirrhosis is not clear. In recent years, attention has shifted from fatty liver towards acetaldehyde as the causative agent due to growing evidence that implicates this compound.

Increase in acetaldehyde concentration

Acetaldehyde is a reactive compound and forms adducts with a variety of proteins and other substances *in vitro*. More important are observations *in vivo* that acetaldehyde modifies proteins after chronic ingestion of ethanol. The *in vivo* modification process may be different from *in vitro* modification due to cell compartmentation, and perhaps also to the fact that acetaldehyde released from the generating enzyme may be present as a more reactive precursor (Behrens et al., 1988). Structures modified *in vivo* in the rat include an ethanol-inducible P450 isoenzyme (Behrens et al., 1988), hemoglobin (Niemelä et al., 1990), liver cytosolic proteins (Lin et al., 1988, 1989; Worrall et al., 1990), and liver plasma membranes (Barry et al., 1987). The number of identified proteins seems to depend strongly on the antibody preparation used for their detection (Behrens et al., 1988: Lin et al. 1989; Worrall et al., 1990), so that it is at present not possible to specify the number of proteins involved. A single modified cytosolic protein was identified in one study (Lin et al., 1988, 1989), and at least nine different cytosolic liver proteins have been detected in another study (Worrall et al.,1990). The pathological significance of these findings has been addressed by several recent investigations. Hepatocytes from alcoholic patients exhibit epitopes that are recognized by antibodies raised in animals against acetaldehyde-protein adducts (Niemela et al., 1991). The structures modified by acetaldehyde act as neoantigens *in vivo* and elicit an immune response (Hoerner et al., 1988; Niemelä et al., 1987). Thus, there is growing evidence that acetaldehyde may be a causative agent of alcoholic liver disease by modifying proteins on the cell surface of hepatocytes and initiating a cytotoxic response.

The acetaldehyde-modified epitopes occur predominantly with centrilobular localization, which correlates well with the observed centrilobular localization of alcoholic hepatitis (Niemelä et al., 1991). This suggests that, during ethanol metabolism, acetaldehyde concentrations are highest in the centrilobular region. This may be due to buildup of a sinusoidal acetaldehyde gradient along the blood flow within the sinuses. It still has to be clarified what the lobular distribution of ADH and ALDH are and whether or not this would lead to an increased localized production of acetaldehyde. Only in the case of MEOS has a clear pericentral localization been established, which may contribute to a higher centrilobular production of acetaldehyde (Tsutsumi et al., 1989).

To what extent functional impairment of modified proteins contributes to liver cell necrosis remains to be seen. In addition to its protein modifying activity, acetaldehyde has recently also been implicated in the etiology of alcoholic liver fibrosis by stimulating collagen synthesis in hepatic fat-storing cells (Moshage et al., 1990).

Competition of ethanol with other substrates

Alcohol metabolizing enzymes have a broad substrate specificity and may participate in metabolic pathways other than ethanol elimination. Human ADH isoenzymes catalyze the interconversion of alcohols and aldehydes in the metabolism of serotonin, dopamine and norepinephrine, which may explain the interference of ethanol with the metabolism of these substances (Consalvi et al., 1986; Mardh and Vallee, 1986; Mardh et al., 1986b; Mardh et al., 1985). Furthermore, human class I isoenzymes containing the γ chain metabolize androgenic steroids (McEvily et al., 1988) and are allosterically inhibited by testosterone (Mardh et al., 1986a). The physiological significance of these findings is, however, not clear, since physiological concentrations of androgens are far below the K_m of ADH.

Interference with the metabolism of biogenic amines may also take place at the level of ALDH since human aldehyde dehydrogenase catalyzes oxidation of aldehydes in the metabolism of biogenic amines (Ambroziak & Pietruszko, 1987; MacKerell et al., 1986).

References

Ambroziak, W. & Pietruszko, R. (1987). Human aldehyde dehydrogenase: metabolism of putrescine and histamine. *Alcohol. Clin. Exp. Res.,* 11:528-532.

Backlin, C.-I. (1958). The equilibriuim constant of the system ethanol, aldehyde, DPN+, DPNH and H+. *Acta Chem. Scand.*12:1279-1285.

Barry, R.E., Williams, A.J. & McGivan, J.D. (1987) The detection of acetaldehyde/liver plasma membrane protein adduct formed *in vivo* by alcohol feeding. *Liver* 7:364-368.

Bengtson, G., Kiessling, K.-H., Smith-Kielland, A. & Morland, J. (1981) Partial separation and biochemical characteristics of periportal and perivenous hepatocytes from rat liver. *Eur. J. Biochem.* 118:591-597.

Behrens, U.J., Hoerner, M., Lasker, J.M. & Lieber, C.S. (1988). Formation of acetaldehyde adducts with ethanol-inducible P450IIE1 *in vivo. Biochem. Biophys. Res. Commun.*, 154:584-590.

Bosron, W.F., Li, T.-K., Dafeldecker, W.P. & Vallee, B.L. (1979). Human liver π-alcohol dehydrogenase: kinetic and molecular properties. *Biochemistry*, 18:1101-1105.

Bosron, W.F., Magnes, L.J. & Li, T.-K. (1983a). Kinetic and electrophoretic properties of native and recombined isoenzymes of human liver alcohol dehydrogenase. *Biochemistry*, 22:1852-1857.

Bosron, W.F., Magnes, L.J. & Li, T.-K. (1983b). Human liver alcohol dehydrogenase: ADHIndianapolis Results from genetic polymorphism at the ADH2 gene locus. *Biochem. Genet.*, 21:735-744.

Bosron, W.F. & Li, T.-K. (1987). Catalytic properties of human liver alcohol dehydrogenase isoenzymes. *Enzyme*, 37:19-28.

Bosron, W.F., Rex, D.K., Harden, C.A., Li, T.-K. and Akerson, R.D. (1988) Alcohol and aldehyde dehydrogenase isoenzymes in Sioux North American Indians. *Alcohol. Clin. Exp. Res.*, 12:454-455.

Brändén, C.-I., Jörnvall, H., Eklund, H. & Furugren, B. (1975). Alcohol Dehydrogenase. P.D. Boyer, Ed., The Enzymes, Vol. XI. (pp. 103-190). New York: Academic Press.

Buehler, R. Hess, M. & vonWartburg, J.-P. (1982). Immunohistochemical localization of human liver alcohol dehydrogenase in liver tissue, cultured fibroblasts, and hela cells. *Am. J. Pathol.*, 108:89-99.

Burnell, J.C., Carr, L.J., Dwulett, F.J.. Edenberrg, H.J., Li, T.-K. & Bosron, W.F. (1987) The human C5b3 subunit differs from β_1 by a Cys for Arg 369 substitution which decreases NAD(H) binding. *Biochem. Biophys. Res. Commun.*, 146:1227-1233.

Burnell, J.C., Li, T.-K. & Bosron, W.F. (1989). Purification and steady-state characterization of human liver $\beta_3\beta_3$ Alcohol Dehydrogenase. *Biochemistry*, 28:6810-6815.

Chen, L., Sidner, R.A. & Lumeng, L. (1992). Distribution of alcohol dehydrogenase and the low Km form of aldehyde dehydrogenase in isolated perivenous and periportal hepatocytes in rats. *Alcohol. Clin. Exp. Res.*, 16:23-29.

Chen, L., Lumeng, L. & Wannamaker, S.A. (1988). Microsomal ethanol oxidizing system in perivenous and periportal hepatocytes. *Clin. Res.*, 36:394.

Consalvi, V., Mardh, G.& Vallee, B.L. (1986). Human alcohol dehydrogenases and serotonin metabolism. *Biochem. Biophys. Res. Commun.*, 139:1009-1016.

Crabb, D.W., Bosron, W.F. & Li,T.-K. (1983). Steady-state kinetic properties of purified rat liver alcohol dehydrogenase: application to predicting alcohol elimination rates *in vivo. Arch. Biochem. Biophys.*, 224:299-309.

Crabb, D.W. & Edenberg, H.J. (1986) Complete amino acid sequence of rat liver alcohol dehydrogenase deduced from the cDNA Sequence. *Gene,* 48:287-291.

Crabb, D.W., Edenberg, H.J., Bosron, W.F. & Li, T.-K. (1989) Genotypes for aldehyde dehydrogenase deficiency and alcohol sensitivity. *J. Clin. Invest.,* 83:314-316.

Crow, K.E., Cornell, N.W. & Veech, R.L. (1977). The rate of ethanol metabolism in isolated rat hepatocytes. *Alcohol. Clin. Exp. Res.,* 1:43-47.

Crow, K. E., Braggins, T.E., Batt, R.D. & Hardman, M.J. (1982). Rat liver cytosolic malate dehydrogenase: purification, kinetic properties, role in control of free cytosolic NADH concentration. *J.Biol. Chem.,* 257:14217-14255.

Dawson, A.G. (1979). Oxidation of cytosolic NADH formed during aerobic metabolism in mammalian cells. *Trends in Bioch. Sci.,* 4:171-176.

Ehrig, T., vonWartburg, J.-P. & Wermuth, B. (1988) cDNA sequence of the β2-subunit of human liver alcohol dehydrogenase. *FEBS Lett.,* 234:53-55.

Erikson, C.J.P. (1973). Ethanol and acetaldehyde metabolism in rat strains genetically selected for their ethanol preference. *Biochem. Pharmacol.,* 22:2283-2292.

Eriksson, C.J., Marselos, M. & Koivula, T. (1975) Role of cytosolic rat liver aldehyde dehydrogenase in the oxidation of acetaldehyde during ethanol metabolism In Vivo. *Biochem. J.,* 152:709 712.

Erikson, C.J.P. (1983). Human blood acetaldehyde concentration during ethanol oxidation (Update 1982). *Pharmacol. Biochem. Behav.,* 18:141-150.

Fellenius, E. & Kiessling, K.-H. (1973). Effect of ethanol on fatty acid oxidation in the perfused livers of starved, fed, and fat-fed rats. *Acta Chem. Scand.* 27:2781-2790.

Forsander, O.A., Mäenpää, P.H. & Salaspuro, M.P. (1965a). Influence of ethanol on the lactate/pyruvate and β-hydroxybutyrate/acetoacetate ratios in rat liver experiments. *Acta Chem. Scand.* 19:1770-1771.

Forsander, O.A., Raiha, N., Salaspuro, P. & Mäenpää, P. (1965b). Influence of ethanol on the liver metabolism of fed and starved rats. *Biochem J.* 94:259-265.

Forte-McRobbie, C. & Pietruszko, R. (1986). Purification and characterization of human liver "High K_m" aldehyde dehydrogenase and its identification as glutamic -semialdehyde dehydrogenase. *J. Biol. Chem.*, 261:2154-2163.

Gennari, K., Wermuth, B., Muellener, D., Ehrig, T. & vonWartburg, J.-P. (1988). Genotyping of human class I alcohol dehydrogenase. analysis of enzymatically amplified DNA with allele-specific oligonucleotides. *FEBS Lett*, 228:305-309.

Goedde, H.W., Agarwal, D.P., Harada, S., Rothhammer, F., Whittaker, J.O. & Lisker, R.(1986) Aldehyde dehydrogenase Polymorphism in North American, South American, and Mexican Indian populations. *Am. J. Hum. Genet.*, 38:395-399.

Greenfield, N.J. & Pietruszko, R. (1977). Two aldehyde dehydrogenases from human liver. isolation via affinity chromatography and characterization of the isozymes. *Biochim. Biophys. Acta*, 483:35-45.

Grunnet, N. & Kondrup, J. (1986). The effect of ethanol on the β-oxidation of fatty acids. *Alcohol. Clin. Exp. Res.*, 10(Suppl):64s-68s.

Guynn, R.W., Veloso, D., Harris, R.L., Lawson, J.W.R. & Veech, R.L. (1973). Ethanol administration and the relationship of malonyl-coenzyme A concentrations to the rate of fatty acid synthesis in rat liver. *Biochem. J.*, 136:639-647.

Hanna, J.M. (1978) Metabolic responses of Chinese, Japanese and Europeans to alcohol. *Alcohol. Clin. Exp. Res.*, 2:89-92.

Higgins, J.H. (1979). Control of ethanol oxidation and its interaction with other metabolic systems. In E. Majchrowitz & E.P. Noble (Eds.), Biochemistry and Pharmacology of Ethanol (pp. 249-351). New York: Plenum Press.

Hoerner, M., Behrens U., Worner, T.M., Blacksberg, I., Braly, L.F., Schaffner, F. & Lieber, C.S. (1988). The role of alcoholism and liver disease in the appearance of serum antibodies against acetaldehyde adducts. *Hepatology*, 8:569-574.

Hurley, T.D., Bosron, W.F., Hamilton, J.A. & Amsel, L.M. (1991) Structure of human $\beta_1\beta_1$ alcohol dehydrogenase: catalytic effects of non-active-site substitutions. *Proc. Natl. Acad. Sci., U. S. A.* 88:8149-8153.

Ikawa, M., Impraim, C.C., Wang, G. & Yoshida, A. (1983). Isolation and characterization of aldehyde dehydrogenase isoenzymes from usual and atypical human livers. *J. Biol. Chem.*, 258:6282-6287.

Impraim, C., Wang, G. & Yoshida, A. (1982). Structural mutation in a major human aldehyde dehydrogenase gene results in loss of enzyme activity. *Am J. Hum. Genet.*, 34:837-841.

Ingelman-Sundberg, M., Johansson, I., Penttila, K.E., Glaumann, H. & Lindros, K.O. (1988) Centrilobular expression of ethanol-inducible cytochrome p-450 (IIE1) in rat liver. *Biochem. Biophys. Res. Commun.*, 157:55-60.

Jörnvall, H., Hempel, J. & Vallee, B.L. (1987a). Structures of human alcohol and aldehyde dehydrogenases. *Enzyme*, 37:5-18.

Jörnvall, H., Höög, J.-O., von Bahr-Lindström, H. & Vallee, B.L. (1987b). Mammalian alcohol dehydrogenase of separate classes: intermediates between different enzymes and intraclass isozymes. *Proc. Natl. Acad. Sci. U.S.A.*, 84:2580-2584.

Julia, P., Farres, J. & Pares, X. (1987). Characterization of three isoenzymes of rat alcohol dehydrogenase. *Eur. J. Biochem.*, 162:179-189.

Kaiser, R., Holmquist, B., Hempel, J., Vallee, B.L. & Jörnvall, H. (1988) Class III human liver alcohol dehydrogenase: a novel structure type equidistantly related to the class I and II enzymes. *Biochemistry*, 27:1132-1140.

Kato, S., Ishii, H., Aiso, S., Yamashita, S., Ito, D. & Tsuchiya, M. (1990) Histochemical and immunohistochemical evidence for hepatic zone 3 distribution of alcohol dehydrogenase in rats. *Hepatology*, 12:66-69.

Koivusalo, M. & Uotila, L. (1990). Glutathione-dependent formaldehyde dehydrogenase (E.C. 1.2.1.1.): Evidence for the identity with class III alcohol dehydrogenase. *Enzymol. Mol. Biol. Carb. Met.*, 3:305-313.

Kurys, G., Ambroziak, W. & Pietruszko, R. (1989) Human aldehyde dehydrogenase. purification of a third isoenzyme with low K_m for γ-aminobutyraldehyde. *J. Biol. Chem.*, 264:4715-4721.

Latipää, P.M., Karki, T.T., Hiltunen, J.K. & Hassinen, I.E. (1986). Regulation of palmitoylcarnitine oxidation in isolated rat liver mitochondria. Role of the redox state of NAD(H). *Biochem. Biophys. Acta*, 875:293-300.

Lellbach, W.K. (1976). Epidemiology in alcoholic liver disease. *Prog. Liv. Dis.*, 5:494-515.

Li, T.-K., Bosron, W.F., Dafeldecker, W.P., Lange, L.G. & Vallee, B.L. (1977). Isolation of π-alcohol dehydrogenase of human liver: is it a determinant of alcoholism? *Proc. Natl. Acad. Sci. U.S.A.*, 74:4378-4381.

Lieber, C.S. & DeCarli, L.M. (1970). Hepatic microsomal ethanol oxidizing system. In vitro characteristics and adaptive properties in Vivo. J. Biol. Chem., 245:2505-2512.

Lieber, C.S. & DeCarli, L.M. (1972). The role of the hepatic microsomal ethanol oxidizing system (MEOS) for ethanol metabolism in vivo. J. Pharmacol. Exp. Ther., 181:279-287.

Lieber, C.S. (1991a) Pathways of ethanol metabolism and related pathology. in T.N. Palmer, Ed. Alcoholism: A Molecular Perspective. Plenum, New York.

Lieber, C.S. (1991b) Alcohol, liver and nutrition. J. Am. College Nutr., 10:602-632.

Lin, R.C., Smith, R.S. & Lumeng, L. (1988). Detection of a protein-acetaldehyde adduct in the liver of rats fed alcohol chronically. J. Clin Invest., 81:615-619.

Lin, R.C. & Lumeng, L. (1989). Further studies on the 37 kD liver protein-acetaldehyde adduct that forms in vivo during chronic alcohol ingestion. Hepatology, 10:807-814.

Lindros, K.O., Vihma, R. & Forsander, A.O. (1972). Utilization and metabolic effects of acetaldehyde and ethanol in the perfused rat liver. Biochem J., 126:945-952.

Lindros, K.O., Stowell, A., Pikkarainen, P. & Salaspuro, M. (1980). Elevated blood acetaldehyde in alcoholics with accelerated ethanol elimination. Pharmacol. Biochem. Behav. 13, Suppl., 1:119-124.

Lumeng, L., Bosron, W.F. & Li, T.-K. (1980). Rate-determining factors for ethanol metabolism in vivo during fasting. In R.G. Thurman (Ed.) Alcohol and Aldehyde Metabolizing Systems-IV (pp.489-496). New York: Plenum Publishing Corporation.

MacKerell, A. D., Blatter, E.E. & Pietriszko, R. (1986). Human aldehyde dehydrogenase: kinetic identification of the isozyme for which biogenic aldehydes and acetaldehyde compete. Alcohol. Clin. Exp. Res., 10:266-270.

Mardh, G., Luehr, C.A. & Vallee, B.L. (1985). Human class I alcohol dehydrogenases catalyze the oxidation of glycols in the metabolism of norepinephrine. Proc. Natl. Acad. Sci., U.S.A. 82:4979-4982.

Mardh, G. & Vallee, B.L. (1986). Human class I alcohol dehydrogenases catalyze the interconversion of alcohols and aldehydes in the metabolism of dopamine. Biochemistry, 25:7279-7282.

Mardh, G., Falchuk, K.H., Auld, D. S. & Vallee, B.L. (1986a) Testosterone allosterically regulates ethanol oxidation by homo- and heterodimeric γ-subunit-containing isoenzymes of human alcohol dehydrogenase. Proc. Natl. Acad. Sci. U.S.A., 83:2836-2840.

Mardh, G., Dingley, A. L., Auld, D. S. & Vallee, B. L. (1986b) Human Class II (π) Alcohol dehydrogenase has a redox-specific function in norepinephrine metabolism. *Proc. Natl. Acad. Sci. U. S. A.*, 83:8908-9812.

McEvily, A.J., Holquist, B., Auld, D.S. & Vallee, B.L. (1988). 3β-hydroxy-5β-steroid dehydrogenase activity of human liver alcohol dehydrogenase is specific to γ subunits. *Biochemistry*, 27:4284-4288.

Mizoi, Y., Tatsuno, Y., Adachi, J., Kogame, M., Fukunaga, T., Fujiwara, S., Hishida, S. & Ijiri, I. (1983). Alcohol sensitivity related to polymorphism of alcohol metabolizing enzymes in Japanese. *Pharm. Biochem. Behav. 18, Suppl.,*1:127-133.

Moreno, A. & Pares, X. (1991). Purification and characterization of a new alcohol dehydrogenase from human stomach. *J. Biol. Chem.*, 266:1128-1133.

Morrison, G.R. & Brock, F.E. (1967) Quantitative measurement of alcohol dehydrogenase in the lobule of normal livers. *J. Lab. Clin. Med.*, 70:116-120.

Moshage, H., Casini, A. & Lieber, C.S. (1990). Acetaldehyde selectively stimulates collagen production in cultured rat liver fat-storing cells but not in hepatocytes. *Hepatology*, 12:511-518.

Niemelä, O., Klajner, F., Orrego, H., Vidins, E., Blendis, L. & Israel, Y. (1987). Antibodies against acetaldehyde-modified protein epitopes in human alcoholics. *Hepatology*, 7:1210-1214.

Niemelä, O., Israel, Y., Mizoi, Y., Fukunaga, T. & Eriksson, C.J. (1990) Hemoglobin-acetaldehyde adducts in human volunteers following acute ethanol ingestion. *Alcohol. Clin. Exp. Res.*, 14:838-841.

Niemelä, O., Juvonen, T. & Parkkila, S. (1991). Immunohistochemical demonstration of acetaldehyde-modified epitopes in human liver after alcohol consumption. *J. Clin. Invest.*, 87:1367-1374.

Nuutinen, H., Lindros, K.O. & Salaspuro, M. (1983). Determinants of blood acetaldehyde. during ethanol oxidation in chronic alcoholics. *Alcohol. Clin. Exp. Res.*, 7:163-168.

Nuutinen, H.U., Salaspuro, M.P., Valle, M. & Lindros, K. (1984). blood acetaldehyde concentration gradient between hepatic and antecubital venous blood in ethanol-intoxicated alcoholics and controls. *Eur. J. Clin. Invest.*, 14:306-311.

O'Dowd, B.F., Rothhammer, F. & Israel, Y. (1990) Genotyping of mitochondrial aldehyde dehydrogenase locus of native American Indians. *Alcohol. Clin. Exp. Res.*, 14:531-533.

Ontko, J.A. (1973). Effects of ethanol on the metabolism of free fatty acids in isolated liver cells. *J. Lipid Res.*, 14:78-86.

Parrilla, R., Ohkawa, K., Lindros, K.O., Zimmerman, U.-J.P., Kobayashi, K. & Williamson, J.R. (1974). Functional compartmentation of acetaldehyde oxidation in rat liver. *J. Biol. Chem.*, 249:4926-4933.

Rex, D.K., Bosron, W.F., Smialek, J.E. & Li, T.-K. (1985) Alcohol aldehyde dehydrogenase isoenzymes in North American Indians. *Alcohol. Clin. Exp. Res.*, 9:147-151.

Segel, I.H. (1975). Enzyme Kinetics (p. 563). New York:John Wiley & Sons.

Shibuya, A. & Yoshida, A. (1988). Genotypes of alcohol metabolizing enzymes in Japanese with alcoholic liver disease: a strong association of the usual Caucasian aldehyde dehydrogenase gene (ALDH2₂) with the disease. *Am. J. Hum. Genet.*, 43:744-748.

Seligson, D., Stone, H.H. & Nemir, P. (1959). The metabolism of ethanol in man. *Surg. Forum, 9*:85.

Sies, H. (1982). Nicotinamide nucleotide compartmentation. In (H. Sies, Ed.) Metabolic Compartmentation (pp.206-231). New York:Academic Press.

Smith, M. (1986). Genetics of human alcohol and aldehyde dehydrogenases. *Adv. Hum. Genet.*, 15:249-290.

Stamatoyannopoulos, G., Chen, S.-H. & Fukui, M. (1975) Liver alcohol dehydrogenase in Japanese. High Population frequency of atypical form and its possible role in alcohol sensitivity. *Am. J. Hum. Genet.*, 27:789-796.

Teng, Y.-S., Jehan, S. & Lie-Injo, L.E. (1979) Human alcohol dehydrogenase ADH₂ and ADH₃ polymorphisms in ethnic Chinese and Indians of West Malaysia. *Hum. Genet.*, 53:87-90.

Teschke, R., Hasumura, Y. & Lieber, C.S. (1975). Hepatic microsomal alcohol oxidizing system. Affinity for methanol, ethanol, propanol and butanol. *J. Biol. Chem.*, 250:7397-7404.

Thomasson, H.R., Li, T.-K. & Crabb, D.W. (1990). Correlation between alcohol-induced flushing, genotypes for alcohol and aldehyde dehydrogenases, and alcohol elimination rates. *Hepatology*, 12:903.

Thomasson, H.R., Edenberg, H.J., Crabb, D.W., Mai, X.-L., Jerome, R.E., Li, T.-K., Wang, S.-P., Lin, Y.-T., Lu, R.B. andYin, S.J. (1991). Alcohol and aldehyde dehydrogenase genotypes and alcoholism in Chinese men. *Am. J. Hum. Genet.*, 48:677-681.

Thieden, H.I.D., Grunnet, N., Damgaard, S.E. & Sestoft, L. (1972). Effect of fructose and glyceraldehyde on ethanol metabolism in human liver and in rat liver. *Eur. J. Biochem.*, 30:250-261.

Tottmar, S.O.C., Pettersson, H. & Kiessling, K.-H. (1973). The subcellular distribution and properties of aldehyde dehydrogenases in rat liver. *Biochem. J.*, 135:577-586.

Tsutsumi, M., Lasker, J., Shimizu, M., Rosman, A.S. & Lieber, C.S. (1989). The intralobular distribution of ethanol-inducible P450IIE1 in rat and human liver. *Hepatology*, 10:437-446.

Tygstrup, N., Winkler, K. & Lundquist, F. (1965). The mechanism of fructose effect on the ethanol metabolism of the human liver. *J. Clin. Invest.*, 44:817-830.

Vaananen, H., Salaspuro, M. & Lindros, K. (1984) The effect of chronic ethanol ingestion on ethanol metabolizing enzymes in isolated periportal and perivenous rat hepatocytes. *Hepatology*, 4:862-866.

vonWartburg, J.-P., Papenberg, J. & Aebi, H. (1965). An atypical human alcohol dehydrogenase. *Canad. J. Biochem.*, 43:889-898.

vonWartburg, J.-P. & Schurch, P.M. (1968). Atypical human liver alcohol dehydrogenase. *Ann. N.Y. Acad. Sci.*, 151:937-946.

Wagner, F.W., Pares, X., Holmquist, B. & Vallee, B.L. (1984). Physical and enzymatic properties of a class III isoenzyme of human liver alcohol dehydrogenase: χ-ADH. *Biochemistry*, 23,2193-2199.

Weiner, H. & Flynn, T.G. (1988). Nomenclature of mammalian aldehyde dehydrogenases. In (H. Weiner & T.G. Flynn, eds.) Enzymology and Molecular Biology of Carbonyl Metabolism (pp. xix-xxi). New York:Alan R. Liss.

Wiebe, T., Lundquist, A. & Belfrage, P. (1971). Time-course of liver fat accumulation in man after a single load of ethanol. *Scand. J. Clin. Lab. Invest.*, 27:33-36.

Williamson, D.H., Lund, P. & Krebs, H. (1967). The redox state of free nicotinamide-adenine dinucleotide in the cytoplasm and mitochondria of rat liver. *Biochem. J.*, 103:514-527.

Williamson, J.R., Scholz, R., Browning, E.T., Thurman, R.G. & Fukami, M.H. (1969). Metabolic effects of ethanol in perfused rat liver. *J. Biol. Chem.*, 244:5044-5054.

Wiseman, M.S., McKay, D., Crow, K.E. & Hardman, M.J. (1991) Rat liver mitochondrial malate dehydrogenase: purification, kinetic properties, and role in ethanol metabolism. *Arch. Biochem. Biophys.*, 290:191-196.

Worrall, S., DeDersey, J., Shanley, B.C. & Wilce, P.A. (1990). Detection of acetaldehyde-modified proteins in the livers of ethanol-fed rats. *Biochem. Soc. Trans.*, 18:678-679.

Xu, Y., Carr, L.G., Bosron, W.F., Li., T.-K. Edenberg, H.J. (1988) Geno-typing of human alcohol dehydrogenase at the ADH_2 and ADH_3 loci following DNA sequence amplification. *Genomics*, 2:209-214.

Yasunami, M., Chen, C.-S. & Yoshida, A. (1991). A human alcohol dehydrogenase gene (ADH6) encoding an additional class of isozyme. *Proc. Natl. Acad. Sci. U.S.A.*, 88:7610-7614.

Yin, S.-J., Bosron, W.F., Magnes, L.J. & Li, T.-K. (1984a). Human liver alcohol dehydrogenase: purification and kinetic characterization of the $\beta_2\beta_2$, $\beta_1\beta_2$, $\alpha\beta_2$ and $\beta_2\gamma_1$ Oriental isoenzymes. *Biochemistry*, 23:5847-5853.

Yin, S.-J., Bosron, W.F., Li, T.-K., Ohnishi, K., Okuda, K., Ishii, H. & Tsuchiya, M. (1984b). Polymorphism of human liver alcohol dehydrogenase: identification of ADH_2 2-1 and ADH_2 2-2 phenotypes in the Japanese by isoelectric focusing. *Biochem Genet.*, 22:169-180.

Yoshida, A., Huang, I.-Y. & Ikawa, M. (1984). Molecular abnormality of an inactive aldehyde dehydrogenase variant commonly found in Orientals. *Proc. Natl. Acad. Sci. U.S.A.*, 81:258-261.

Zeiner, A.R., Girardot, J.M., Nichols, N. & Jones-Saumty, D. (1984) ALDH I isozyme deficiency among North American Indians. *Alcohol. Clin. Exp. Res.*, 9:147-152.

Ethnic Differences in Alcohol Metabolism and Physiological Responses to Alcohol: Implications in Alcohol Abuse

Itaru Yamashita, Tsukasa Koyama, Tetsuro Ohmori
Department of Psychiatry, Hokkaido University School of Medicine
Sapporo, Japan

It has been empirically known for many years that there is an ethnic difference in the sensitivity to alcohol between Asian and European peoples. A considerable number of Japanese adults, for instance, show an inherent intolerence to alcohol. Soon after taking a glass or two of beer, they become markedly red in the face and neck and often have palpitations and tachycardia (flushing syndrome). Their response to alcohol does not change throughout life. They are always excused for not drinking in social gatherings where they are expected to drink. It is a surprise to Japanese to learn that such persons are rarely found among Europeans. This empirical observation was scientifically studied for the first time by Wolff (1972).

In regard to the cause of this difference, Mizoi et al.(1978) found that the blood levels of acetaldehyde are much higher in flushers than in non-flushers. It was then pointed out by Goedde, Harada and Agarwal (1979) that the deficiency of low Km acetaldehyde dehydrogenase (ALDH), quite common in Japanese but not in Germans, may generate a disproportionate elevation of blood acetaldehyde after alcohol intake, which produces marked flushing manifestations in some Asians. Many studies have been done regarding the prevalence rates of low Km ALDH in different ethnic populations. The correlation between low Km ALDH deficiency and drinking habits has also been discussed.

It has been a matter of keen interest whether or not the low incidence of alcohol abuse and dependence among Asian people may have physiological rather than cultural origins. This chapter will deal with this question in terms of ethnic differences in alcohol metabolism and physiologic responses to alcohol and their clinical implications.

Flushing Syndrome

Having observed that many Mongoloids respond with a rapid intense flushing of the face after drinking alcohol in amounts that have no apparent effect on Caucasoids, Wolff (1972) compared systematically the alcohol flushing responses of Caucasoid and various Mongoloid groups. He randomly selected healthy Caucasoid and Mongoloid men and women between 25 and 35 years of age, residing in the United States, Japan, Taiwan, and Korea, respectively. To control for cultural differences in alcohol consumption, diet, and other postnatal environmental influences, he also compared the flushing responses of healthy full-term Caucasoid infants with those of Japanese and Taiwanese infants. All adults were asked to drink beer and infants were given small amounts of port wine in 5 percent glucose solution. Flushing was determined by optical densitometry of the earlobe and inspection of the face. The results indicated that 83 % (68 of 82 cases) of Mongoloid adults responded with a marked visible flush and an increase of optical density greater than 5 mm, whereas only 2 of the 34 Caucasoid adults showed any increase of optical density of the earlobe and only 1 flushed visibly. Population differences were as clear-cut among infants as adults. Of all Mongoloid infants tested, 74 % (26 of 35 cases) indicated a visible flush and an increase of optical density, while only 1 of 20 Caucasoids showed a visible flush and a measurable densitometer response.

In a subsequent study, Wolff (1973) examined alcohol responses of 30 North American Indians, 15 Americans of Japanese or Chinese origin and 50 Americans of European extraction. He again found that Americans of Mongoloid ancestry who were born and reared in the United Stated and raised entirely on Western diet responded in the same way as Mongoloids raised in Asia, and interestingly he also found that the incidence rate (80%) and intensity of flushing after oral alcohol ingestion was as great among American Indians as among native Mongoloids.

Wolff's findings were corroborated by Ewing, Rouse and Pellizzari (1974). Their subjects consisted of 24 Americans of European origin and 25 persons who were at the time of study residing in the United States and whose parents were from Asia. After taking amounts of synthetic ethanol on the basis of body weight, it was found that 17 of the 24 Oriental subjects showed flushing of the face, and sometimes of the chest and palms, while only three of the 24 Occidentals indicated a lesser degree of flushing. The mean heart rates increased significantly in the Oriental compared with the Occidental subjects at 30 and 60 minutes after alcohol ingestion.

Wilson, McClearn and Johnson (1978) also reported findings which are in good agreement with Wolff (1972, 1973). They analyzed the self-report data of the 2418 responders in Hawaii and found that 50 to 60 % of both Oriental and Hapa Haole subjects showed flushing to alcohol, whereas only about 23 % of Caucasians reported such flush responses.

Flushing manifestations among Japanese people will be dealt with later in connection with the development of drinking habits and alcohol abuse.

Blood Acetaldehyde

Concerning the cause of racial differences in flushing after alcohol, Wolff (1972) postulated a specific and probably genetic difference in autonomic nervous system responsivity between the ethnic populations tested. Differences in the rates of absorption and excretion of alcohol, amounts of habitual alcohol consumption, diet, proportion of body fat, etc., had been suggested as possible factors.

Acetaldehyde had been considered as one of the possibilities. It was presaged by the report of Asmussen, Hald and Larsen (1948), who showed that intravenously administered acetaldehyde in humans mimics many of the subjective symptoms and physiological changes observed with disulfiram. Koivula, Koivusalo and Lindros (1975) demonstrated in an animal experiment that the ethanol-avoiding rat strain has lower acetaldehyde dehydrogenase activity in the liver than rats of the ethanol-preferring strain.

Ewing et al. (1974) estimated the blood acetaldehyde levels from breath samples of the tested subjects. They found that the overall blood acetaldehyde levels of the Oriental subjects after ingesting ethanol did exceed those of the Occidental subjects, although the differences did not reach statistical significance.

Reed et al.,(1976) carried out examinations of alcohol and acetal-dehyde metabolism in 58 Caucasians, 20 Chinese and 24 Ojibwa Indians in Ontario. The blood alcohol levels after oral ethanol inges-tion did not differ significantly among the groups. However,the most striking finding was the approximately 50 % higher mean value of blood acetaldehyde in Ojibwa (14.6 %μg/ml) compared with Chi-nese (10.0 %μg/ml) and Caucasian (9.4 %μg/ml) subjects. It was also stated in the report that "An incidental and as yet unexplained finding is that one subject, excluded because of vomiting,showed remarkably high acetaldehyde values, including a value of 72.1 %μg/ml at 120 minutes." This finding seems by no means just inci-dental, but very meaningful in view of later reports.

Zeiner, Paredes and Christensen (1979) also studied the role of acetaldehyde in mediating reactivity to alcohol among different ra-cial groups. They monitored physiologic changes in 10 white and 7 Chinese volunteers, including facial flush, heart rate, blood pressure, alcohol absorption time, and blood alcohol and acetaldehyde con-centrations. Chinese and white subjects did not differ significantly in peak blood alcohol concentration. However, both peak and mean acetaldehyde values for Chinese were three times higher than for whites. It was also commented here that "Not all of the Chinese subjects showed the sensitivity to ethanol. Those who showed the sensitivity were characterized by rapid ethanol absorption, rapid and high acetaldehyde peaks, large increases in heart rate, and large decreases in both systolic and diastolic blood pressure. It is interest-ing to note that the heaviest flushers had the largest heart rate increases and highest acetaldehyde concentrations".

Meanwhile, the most detailed study was reported by Mizoi et al.(1979). They examined, in Experiment 1, degrees of facial flushing, blood alcohol level and alcohol elimination time in 75 Japanese subjects after ingestion of 200 ml of sake (Japanese rice wine, with 16% v/v ethanol content). The subjects were classified into three groups: 28 high flushers (marked facial flushing and sometimes flushing of the neck, anterior chest, upper and lower extremities), 16 slight flushers (flushing only around the eyelids) and 31 non-flushers (no flushing). The maximum blood alcohol levels were 0.47 mg/ml in the highly flushing group, 0.45 mg/ml in the slightly flushing group and 0.44 mg/ml in the non-flushing group. Alcohol disap-peared from the blood in all three groups in 5 hr post-drink. In Experiment 2, they studied the relationship between physiologic responses to alcohol, blood alcohol and acetaldehyde levels and urinary excretion of catecholeamines in the highly flushing group (11 subjects) and non-flushing group (15 subjects). It was found that there was no difference in the blood alcohol levels between the two groups. In contrast, the blood acetaldehyde levels of the highly flushing group were markedly increased and reached to the maxima 0.48 - 0.95 %μg/ml between 0.5 and 2 hr post-drink, while those of the non-flushing group scarcely increased and remained 0 - 0.31 %μg/ml. Pulse rate in the former group strikingly increased 30-60 minutes after drinking, whereas the rate in the latter group virtually showed no change. The excretion of both epinephrine and no-repinephrine was significantly increased in the flushing group, but no increase occurred in the non-flushing group.

Deficiency of Low Km Acetaldehyde Dehydrogenase (ALDH)

The reports cited above clearly demonstrate the correlation between increased blood acetaldehyde concentration and manifest physi-ologic responses to alcohol in some racial groups, and particularly in highly flushing individuals. Regarding the possible basis for produc-ing such a sustained increase of acetaldehyde, two hypotheses have been presented in terms of polymorphic enzymes of alcohol dehy-drogenase (ADH) and acetaldehyde dehydrogenase (ALDH).

Many years earlier, von Wartburg, Papenberg and Aebi (1965) found in two human livers an atypical enzyme variant of ADH possessing a three-to-five-fold higher activity than the typical ADH. It was later reported that this active ADH variant occurs in 20 % of Swiss and 4 % of British subjects (von Wartburg and Schurch, 1968), while in as much as 85 % of the Japanese population (Stamatoyan-nopoulos, Chen & Fukui, 1975). Stamatoyannopoulos et al.(1975) speculated that this atypical ADH, with higher catalytic activity at physiological pH, could oxidize ethanol to acetaldehyde faster than the typical ADH and may produce adverse reactions to alcohol observed often in the Japanese subjects.

On the other hand, however, since most of the acetaldehyde formed in the liver is immediately further oxidized by ALDH, any change in ALDH isozymes may result in an altered concentration of blood acetaldehyde. Harada, Misawa, Agarwal and Goedde (1980) identified in human livers two ALDH isozymes; a low Km ALDH migrating faster on electrophoresis and a high Km ALDH migrating slower, both of which had been characterized earlier by Greenfield and Pietruzko (1977). They also found in 40 autopsy liver specimens from Japanese individuals that the faster migrating low Km ALDH was missing in 52 %, while no such polymorphism was observed in 68 liver specimens from German individuals. Agarwal, Harada and Goedde (1981) found that, in 11 Japanese subjects, all of the 6 persons with deficiency of low Km ALDH flushed, but the remaining 5 did not flush, while the 9 persons with atypical ADH responded variably to alcohol intake. Accordingly, a new hypothesis regarding the racial differences in alcohol sensitivity was presented (Goedde, Harada & Agarwal, 1979), suggesting that the high sensitivity to alcohol in a large number of Japanese subjects may be due to their inability to metabolize acetaldehyde quickly and effectively in the absence of the faster migrating, low Km isozyme of ALDH. Thus, delayed oxidation of acetaldehyde, rather than its higher-than-normal production through atypical ADH, may be responsible for the marked flushing manifestations following alcohol intake in the Japanese and other Mongoloid populations. The findings by Mizoi el al. (1979) mentioned above are also in support of this assumption.

The next topic of interest was the prevalence rates of low Km ALDH deficiency among different racial groups, who are either sensitive or non-sensitive to alcohol. Teng (1981) examined a total of 101 autopsy liver specimens from Chinese and 53 specimens from Indian subjects obtained in Kuala Lumpur, Malaysia, in terms of ALDH bands in starch gel electrophoresis, and found that the band for low Km ALDH isozyme was missing in 50 of 101 Chinese specimens, yet only in 2 of the Indian specimens.

After developing new micro-methods with isoelectric focusing, which allows the detection of ALDH isozymes from hair root cell extracts (Goedde, Agarwal & Harada,1980), Goedde et al.(1983) carried out extensive studies. They found a deficiency of low Km ALDH in 57 % of 82 Vietnamese, 44 % of 184 Japanese, 39 % of 30 Indonesians, 35 % of 196 Chinese, 8 % of 110 Thais in the northern part of Thailand, 69 % of 33 Highland Indians from Ecuador, and no deficiency in 160 Egyptians and Sudanese, 169 Liberians, 15 Kenyans and 224 Europeans. Four population subgroups residing in mainland China were also studied by Goedde et al (1984), with the result that the low Km ALDH isozyme was deficient in 25 % of 209 Korean, 30 % of 198 Mongolian, 45 % of 106 Zhuang and 50 % of Han subjects.

We had performed a similar study as a WHO collaborative multicenter project in a number of different ethnic groups (Yamashita et al., 1990). Hair root samples were collected from normal and schizophrenic volunteers and examined for ALDH isozymes using the same method as Goedde el al.(1980). It was found that in Japan the low Km ALDH was missing in 43 % of 117 normal subjects and in 33

% of 82 schizophrenic patients (the difference was not significant), while no case with the deficiency was detected in 146 samples collected from countries outside of Asia; Europe (Basel 7 cases, Moscow 26, Zagreb 24), Australia (Nedlands 12; European descents), India (Lucknow 26), Morocco (Casablanca 31) and Mexico (Mexico City 20). Our group also found that low Km ALDH was deficient in 35 % of 40 Taiwanese and 10 % of 34 filipinos (Ohmori et al.,1986).

Flushing Syndrome, Low Km ALDH Deficiency, Drinking Habits and Alcoholism

All the findings mentioned above may be implicated in biological aspects of alcoholism. Flushing manifestations of individual subjects were therefore reexamined in correlation with the absence or presence of the low Km ALDH isozyme and with the liability to develop a drinking habit and alcohol dependence. Our data in Sapporo, Japan, (Ohmori, Koyama & Yamashita, 1985, Yamashita et al.,1990) are shown in Tables 1, 2 and 3. Table 1 demonstrates that out of 117 normal subjects, mainly hospital staff members, 50 persons (43 %) are deficient in low Km ALDH, as mentioned before, while 67 (57 %) are not deficient. On a questionnaire about their usual experiences of somatic manifestations after alcohol ingestion, the former group of subjects indicated flushing, tachycardia, palpitations, headache and nausea of higher degree and in much higher frequency than the latter group. It is shown in Table 2 that psychic experiences after alcohol intake are much the same between the two groups in terms of happy, talkative, relaxed and confident moods. Table 3 indicates the drinking habits of these normal male and female subjects. Those who drink every day or almost every day were classified as having a drinking habit and those who do not drink, or drink only on special occasions, as without such a habit. It is interesting and clinically meaningful that only 18 % (9 of 50 cases) of low Km ALDH-deficient persons, most of whom have physical discomfort of various degrees after alcohol ingestion, reported that they have a drinking habit, while 46 % (31 of 67 cases) of low Km ALDH-positive individuals are habitual drinkers. The difference is highly significant (P<0.01). It seems also that some social factors are involved in the formation of a drinking habit, since only 4 % (1/27) of women with low Km ALDH deficiency drink habitually, while 35 % (8/23) of men with ALDH deficiency are habitual drinkers. In Japan, women have many fewer chances for social drinking than men.

Table 1

*Self-reports of experiences about somatic symptoms after alcohol inges-
tion by 50 low Km ALDH-deficient (-) and 67 ALDH-positive (+) persons.
(From itemized questionnaires filled in before enzyme examination was
performed)*

Symptoms	ALDH	No. of Subjects			
(Degrees)		++	+	±	−
Flushing *	(−)	23	22	4	1
	(+)	0	6	27	34
Tachycaldia *	(−)	14	17	6	13
	(+)	1	2	16	48
Palpitations *	(−)	8	12	9	21
	(+)	1	5	10	51
Headache *	(−)	9	15	12	14
	(+)	2	6	14	45
Nausea *	(−)	4	16	17	13
	(+)	0	8	24	35
Sleepiness	(−)	10	23	10	7
	(+)	17	20	13	17
* P < .001 (Mann-Whitney's U test)					

Table 2

*Mood changes after alcohol ingestion in 50 low Km ALDH-deficient and 67
ALDH-positive persons.*

Moods	ALDH	No. of Subjects		
(Degrees)		++	+	−
Happy	(−)	10	33	7
	(+)	20	39	8
Talkative	(−)	5	29	16
	(+)	23	33	11
Relaxed	(−)	8	34	8
	(+)	15	37	15
Confident	(−)	1	16	33
	(+)	4	25	38

All these observations seem to suggest a protective role for the
genetically derived deficiency of the low Km ALDH in developing a

drinking habit and alcoholism. In fact, Harada et al.(1982) examined the frequency of low Km ALDH isozyme in normal, alcoholic, schizophrenic and drug dependent subjects in Japan. The results were striking; low Km ALDH was deficient in only 2.3 % (4 of 175 cases) of alcoholic patients, in sharp contrast to 41.0 % (43 of 105) of normal controls, 41.9 % (36 of 86) of schizophrenic and 48.9 % (23 of 47) of drug dependent subjects.

Table 3
Drinking habits observed in 50 low Km ALDH-deficient persons (23 males and 27 females) and 67 ALDH-positive persons (29 males and 38 females).

	ALDH	No. of Subjects (#): %	
		Drinking Habit	No Drinking Habit
Total	(−)	9 (18)	41 (82)
	(+)	31 (46)	35 (54)***
Male	(−)	8 (35)	15 (65)
	(+)	20 (69)	9 (31)*
Female	(−)	1 (4)	26 (96)
	(+)	11 (29)	27 (71)**

* $P < .05$, ** $P < .025$, *** $P < .01$ (χ^2 test)

We performed a similar study and found the incidence of low Km ALDH deficiency in only 4 % (5 of 113 cases) of alcoholic volunteers, but in 43 % of normal and 33 % of schizophrenic subjects (Ohmori, Koyama & Yamashita, 1985, Ohmori et al., 1986, Yamashita et al., 1990). Of the alcoholics with deficiency of low Km ALDH, one had a history of marked withdrawal symptoms, including delirium tremens, and the remaining four were diagnosed as nondependent abuse of alcohol according to the ICD-9 classification (Ohmori et al.,1986).

It has been clearly demonstrated that low Km ALDH deficient individuals, who are very common among Mongoloid peoples but are not or at least only exceptionally found among non-Mongoloid populations, usually present a manifest flushing syndrome soon after alcohol ingestion and consequently tend to avoid drinking and hence have much less possibility to develop alcoholism. However, the cause of alcoholism is certainly not as simple as the presence or absence of the inherent low Km ALDH isozyme deficiency. Alcoholism is a socio-psycho-biological disorder and should be dealt with as such. Tables 1, 2 and 3 indicate that low Km ALDH-deficient persons suffer from marked physical discomfort after drinking. However, both ALDH deficient and positive individuals share the same happy, relaxed and talkative feelings following alcohol ingestion. It appears that in low Km-ALDH deficient individuals, "comfortable" effects of alcohol are counterbalanced by "uncomfortable" effects of acetalde-hyde to various degrees. Some ALDH-deficient subjects cannot drink even a little because of severe physical responses to alcohol, while others enjoy happy and relaxed moods from alcohol, even while suffering from flushing manifestations. Some other individuals with certain personality traits and under certain pressures of life may drink excessively despite considerable flushing phenomena, in order to alleviate their emotional turmoil.

It seems appropriate to quote here a comment of Wolff (1973); "One must draw the obvious conclusion that the incidence of alco-holism is determined by more complex factors than variations in vasomotor sensitivity to alcohol. Such a biological variation could, however, exercise its effect through interaction with sociocultural forces. Conceivably, the prevalence of the highly visible flushing response will inhibit Mongoloid groups from drinking as long as their social structure is intact and exercises sanctions against intoxi-cation."

Summary

Inherent deficiency of a low Km acetaldehyde dehydrogenase (ALDH) isozyme is observed in nearly half (30 to 70 %) of Mongoloid populations, but usually not in other racial groups.

The prevalence of ALDH deficiency corresponds closely to the higher frequency of flushing manifestations of Asians following al-cohol ingestion, compared to non-Asians. Drinking habits and alco-hol abuse are significantly less in flushing, low Km ALDH-deficient Asian individuals than in non-flushing, ALDH-positive Asian indi-viduals. Alcoholism should be dealt with as a socio-psycho-biologi-cal disorder and the ALDH isozyme variation is to be considered as one protective factor against alcoholism.

References

Agarwal, D.P., Harada, S. & Goedde, H.W. (1981). Racial differences in biological sensitivity to ethanol: The role of alcohol dehydro-genase and aldehyde dehydrogenase isozymes. *Alcoholism: Clini-cal and Experimental Research*, 5:12-16.

Asmussen, E., Hald,J. & Larsen,V. (1948). The pharmacological action of acetaldehyde on the human organism. *Acta Pharmacologica,* 4:311-320.

Ewing, J.A., Rouse, B.A. & Pellizzari, E.D. (1974). Alcohol sensitivity and ethnic background. *American Journal of Psychiatry,* 131:206-210.

Goedde, H.W., Harada, S. & Agarwal, D.P. (1979). Racial differences in alcohol sensitivity: A new hypothesis. *Human Genetics,* 51:331-334.

Goedde, H.W., Agarwal, D.P. & Harada, S. (1980). Genetic studies on alcohol-metabolizing enzymes: Detection of isozymes in human hair roots. *Enzyme,* 25:281-286.

Goedde, H.W., Agarwal,D.P.,Harada, S.,Meier-Tackmann, D., Ruofu.D., Bienzle, U., Kroeger, A. & Hussein, L. (1983). Population genetic studies on aldehyde dehydrogenase isozyme deficiency and alcohol sensitivity. *American Journal of Human Genetics,* 35:769-772.

Goedde, H.W., Benkmann, H.G., Kriese, L., Bogdanski, P., Agarwal, D.P., Ruofu, D., Chen, L., Cui, M., Yuan, Y., Xu, J., Li, S. & Wang, Y. (1984). Aldehyde dehydrogenase isozyme deficiency and alcohol sensitivity in four different Chinese populations. *Human Heredity,* 34:183-186.

Greenfield, N.J. & Pietruszko, R. (1977). Two aldehyde dehydrogenases from human liver: Isolation via affinity chromatography and characterization of the enzyme. *Biochemica et Biophysica Acta,* 483:35-45.

Harada, S., Misawa, S., Agarwal, D.P., Goedde, H.W. (1980). Liver alcohol dehydrogenase and aldehyde dehydrogenase in the Japanese: Isozyme variation and its possible role in alcohol intoxication. *American Journal of Human Genetics,* 32:8-15.

Harada, S., Agarwal, D.P., Goedde, H.W., Tagaki, S. & Ishikawa,B. (1982). Possible protective role against alcoholism for aldehyde dehydrogenase isozyme deficiency in Japan. *The Lancet,* October 9, p827.

Koivula, T., Koivusalo, M. & Lindros, K.O. (1975). Liver aldehyde and alcohol dehydrogenase activities in rat strains genetically selected for their ethanol preference. *Biochemical Pharmacology,* 24:1807-1811.

Mizoi, Y., Ijiri, I., Tatuno, Y., Kijima, T., Fujiwara, S. & Adachi, J. (1979). Relationship between facial flushing and blood acetaldehyde levels after alcohol intake. *Pharmacology, Biochemistry and Behavior,* 10:303-311.

Ohmori, T., Koyama.T. & Yamashita, I. (1985). WHO collaborative studies on biological basis of alcoholism: Regional experience. *Biological Psychiatry,* 20:1516-1518.

Ohmori, T., Koyama, T., Chen, C., Yeh, E., Reyes, B.V. & Yamashita, I. (1986). The role of aldehyde dehydrogenase isozyme variation in alcohol sensitivity, drinking habits formation and the development of alcoholism in Japan, Taiwan and the Philippines. *Progress in Neuro-Psychopharmacology and Biological Psychiatry,* 10:229-235.

Reed, T.E., Kalant, H., Gibbins, R.J.,Kapur, B.M. & Rankin, J.G. (1976). Alcohol and acetaldehyde metabolism in Caucasians, Chinese and Amerinds. *Canadian Medical Journal,* 115:851-855.

Stamatoyannopoulos, G., Chen, S. & Fukui, M. (1975). Liver alcohol dehydrogenase in Japanese: High population frequency of atypical form and its possible role in alcohol sensitivity. *American Journal of Human Genetics,* 27:789-796.

Teng, Y. (1981). Human liver aldehyde dehydrogenase in Chinese and Asiatic Indians: Gene deletion and its possible implications in alcohol metabolism. *Biochemical Genetics,* 19:107-114.

von Wartburg, J.P., Papenberg, J. & Aebi, H. (1965). An atypical human alcohol dehydrogenase. *Canadian Journal of Biochemistry,* 43:889-898.

von Wartburg, J.P. & Schurch, P.M. (1968). Atypical human liver alcohol dehydrogenase. *Annals of New York Academy of Science.* 151:936-946.

Wilson, J.R., McClearn, G.E. & Johnson, R.C. (1978). Ethnic variation in use and effects of alcohol. *Drug and Alcohol Dependence,* 3:147-151.

Wolff, P.H. (1972). Ethnic differences in alcohol sensitivity. *Science* 175:449-450.

Wolff, P.H. (1973). Vasomotor sensitivity to alcohol in diverse mongoloid populations. *American Journal of Human Genetics,* 25:193-199.

Yamashita, I., Ohmori, T., Koyama, T., Mori, H., Boyadjive, S., Kielholz, P., Gastpar, M., Moussaoui, D.,Bouzekraoui, M.,Sethi, B.B., Reyes, B.V., Vartanian, M.E., de la Fuente,J. ,German, G.A., Bohacek, N., Sartorius, N., Morozov, P. & Prilipko, L.L. (1990). Biological study of alcohol dependence syndrome with reference to ethnic difference:Report of a WHO collaborative study. *Japanese Journal of Psychiatry and Neurology,* 44:79-84.

Zeiner, A.R., Paredes, A., Christensen, H.D. (1979). The role of acetaldehyde in mediating reactivity to an acute dose of ethanol among different racial groups. *Alcoholism: Clinical and Experimental Research,* 3:11-18.

Genetic Components of Alcoholism and Subtypes of Alcoholism

Abbas Parsian and C. Robert Cloninger
Departments of Psychiatry and Genetics
Washington University School of Medicine
St. Louis, Missouri, USA

The term "alcoholism" was first used by a Swedish public health official in 1849. The notion that alcoholism is a disease and not simply a "weakness" has its roots in the writings of 19th century physicians such as Benjamin Rush and Thomas Trotter. Hospitals dedicated to the treatment of alcoholics were opened in the United States beginning in the 1840s, and alcoholism became a subject of serious medical study in the latter half of the 19th century. Systematic studies of the relatives of alcoholics began with the pioneering work of Long. He reported that of all the "inherited disease" observed in the offspring of alcoholics, 21% was due directly to alcoholism in the parents. Other similar studies suggested that alcoholism was a major cause of mentally defective offspring. Shuttleworth and Beach noted that 19% of the "idiots" in a paupers' home, and 13% in a charity house had at least one alcoholic parent. The largest study of its kind was done by McNicholl who found that 53% of 6624 children of alcoholics were retarded to some degree compared with only 10% of 13000 children of abstainers (Goodwin, 1987; Goodwin & Guze, 1989).

Crothers (1909) in his classic and early study of familiality found that over 70% of the more than 4000 alcoholics whom he had treated over a 35-year period had a positive family history of alcoholism. Over the past 80 years this result has been replicated over and over again. There is only one negative report, by Elderton and Pearson (1910), which has detracted from this basic observation. Dahlberg and Stenberg (1934) noted that 25% of the alcoholics they studied had a positive family history. Among first-degree male relatives of alcoholics the risk was 20-25% and among first-degree female relatives it was only 5%. These risks were four to five times greater than those in the general population at that time. It should be noted that "familial" does not necessarily mean "hereditary." Jellinek and Joliffe (1940) were the first to suggest that alcoholism was a heterogeneous disease, having both familial and non-familial forms. They also reported that there was no evidence for a genetic component in either form. The research over the past 30 years or so has confirmed that alcoholism is heterogeneous and there are both familial and nonfamilial cases. These newer studies also suggest a prominent genetic component in the familial forms of alcoholism.

Genetic Studies of Alcoholism

The genetics of complex disorders (e.g. alcoholism) is usually studied through twin, family, and adoption research. The genetic predisposition, if it exists, will be found by twin and adoption studies. The characteristics and mode of inheritance of such a predisposition will be determined by family studies.

Twin studies

Twin studies provide a meaningful and powerful method to search for environmental and genetic factors in relation to phenotypic differences in any particular complex disorder. Monozygotic (MZ) twins are genetically identical and dizygotic (DZ) twins share only one half of their genes on average. For a genetic trait or disorder a greater concordance among MZ than DZ twins is expected. From these differences in concordance between MZ and DZ the heritability can be estimated.

The earliest twin study was carried out by Kaij in the 1950s. A sample of 174 Swedish male twins was ascertained by searching County Temperance Board records. It was reported that there was greater MZ (0.71) than DZ (0.32) concordance for chronic alcoholism as diagnosed using a combination of information from official records and personal interviews. The focus of this study was on alcohol abuse. The derived heritability estimate suggested that most of the variance in alcohol related traits is under direct genetic control.

Partenan et al. (1966) studied a sample of 902 young adult male Finnish twins (who were not selected for drinking history). Although alcoholism or alcohol abuse was not directly diagnosed, twin correlations and heritability estimates were reported for several relevant quantitative drinking scales. Significant heritabilities were reported for the two scales that assessed quantity-frequency of alcohol use (i.e., density and amount) but not for the two scales that assessed problematic patterns of abuse (i.e., lack of control and social complications). The main findings were moderate heritabilities for frequency and amount of drinking.

In 1981 Hrubec and Omenn reported on the results of a sample of 715 male twins ascertained from the National Academy of Sciences - National Research Council register of U.S. Armed Services veterans. Diagnosis of alcoholism based on Department of Veterans Affairs medical records resulted in significantly greater MZ (0.26) than DZ (0.12) concordances. Further, MZ twins were significantly more concordant for secondary effects such as alcoholic psychosis and liver cirrhosis.

Gurling et al. (1981) ascertained a sample of twins from the Maudsley Hospital, London, England, Psychiatric Twin Register. Both female and male alcoholic twins were included in the study. Diagnoses were based on personal interview and followed by criteria for the World Health Organization Alcohol Dependence Syndrome. No difference in MZ/DZ concordance was found, either in male (MZ=0.33, n=15; DZ=0.30, n=20) or female (MZ=0.08, n=13; DZ=0.13, n=8) samples. The observed MZ and DZ concordances were nearly equal and suggested little if any underlying genetic influence. Failure to find significant differences in this small study however, may be due to lack of statistical power or the type of registry.

The latest twin study in alcoholism which included both male and female subjects was reported by Pickens et al. (1990). The sample consisted of clients admitted to alcohol and drug abuse treatment and follow-up programs during 1974-1988 in Minnesota. From a sample of 392 pairs, 169 same-sex twin pairs were used in this study. Both members of pairs participated in the interview portion of the study, pair zygosity was accurately determined, and the proband met DSM-III criteria for alcohol abuse and/or dependence. Zygosity was determined using serologic markers for 159 pairs and by questionnaire for 10 pairs. The sample included 50 MZ and 64 DZ male pairs and 31 MZ and 24 DZ female pairs. Except for MZ male subjects being younger than DZ male subjects and male MZ co-twins being more likely to be married or cohabitating than male DZ co-twins, none of the other MZ/DZ differences in demographic characteristics were statistically significant for either male or female subjects. There were several important findings in Pickens et al. (1990) study, some of which will be presented here. Sex differences were evident in the overall level of twin concordance for alcohol diagnoses, with male subjects having higher concordance rates than female subjects in each of the diagnostic categories. For male subjects, significantly higher concordance was found in MZ than in DZ twins for diagnoses of alcohol abuse, alcohol dependence, and alcohol abuse and/or dependence. For female twins, MZ showed significantly higher concordance than DZ twins only for alcohol dependence. For the composite of alcohol abuse and/or dependence, genetic factors appear to have a modest influence on risk in both sexes. This genetic influence appears, however, to be differently distributed between the two alcohol diagnoses. For alcohol abuse, liability in male subjects was largely attributed to genetic and shared environmental factors; however, in female subjects, liability was largely attributed to shared and nonshared environmental factors with no evidence of a genetic influence. For alcohol dependence, liability variance in male subjects was associated largely with genetic factors and in female subjects it was associated largely with genetic and nonshared environmental factors. Both alcohol abuse and alcohol dependence evidenced significant familial aggregation. The relative contribution of genetic and shared environmental factors to this familial aggregation appears, however, to differ. For alcohol abuse, which reflects a pattern of pathologic alcohol use and impairment of social or occupational functioning, familial risk appears to be due largely to shared environmental factors. For both male and female subjects, approximately 50% of the liability variance was attributed to shared environmental factors. In contrast, for alcohol dependence, which reflects either pathologic use or impairment as well as evidence of tolerance and/or withdrawal, familial risk appears to be due largely to the influence of genetic factors. The estimated heritability was 0.595 for male subjects and 0.420 for female subjects.

In summary, the results of the majority of twin studies are consistent with the existence of significant genetic factors which predispose individuals to develop alcoholism.

Family studies

Family studies will provide knowledge about structure and inheritance of predisposition to alcoholism from one generation to the next. There have been several important family studies on alcoholism. The basis for the classification of alcoholism into familial and nonfamilial (sporadic or environmental) types is from observation of alcoholics and their families. The alcoholics who have a positive family history of alcohol abuse almost invariably had a poorer prognosis than did alcoholics who had negative family histories.

Jellinek and Jolliffe (1940) were first to suggest that there was a familial and a nonfamilial form of alcoholism. As mentioned earlier, they also reported the heterogeneity of the disorder and found no evidence for a genetic component in either form.

Penick et al reported in 1978 the results of a large study of alcoholics in Veterans Administration hospital treatment programs. Among 568 male alcoholics selected for the study, 65% reported a positive family history of alcoholism involving first-degree relatives. These patients demonstrated a significantly lower age-of-onset, had more severe symptoms, had more frequent but less successful treatment and had more general medical problems, such as liver complaints, and pancreatitis. These alcoholic patients also had a greater number of legal problems due to alcohol-related arrests. The alcoholics with a positive family history of alcoholism not only had increased risk to psychiatric illness, in particular, depression, obsessive-compulsive disorder, and antisocial personality themselves, but also increased risk among their family members. The most striking increases in nonalcoholic psychiatric illnesses among their family members were seen for depression and antisocial personality. Based on these findings, Penick et al. suggested that the term "familial alcoholism" may embrace a suite of allied psychiatric disorders among the first-degree relatives of alcoholics.

In 1984, Frances et al. reported the results of their very large family studies of alcoholism. The sample consisted of 2215 male alcoholics treated in the United States Navy alcohol rehabilitation centers. The alcoholics who had at least one first-degree alcoholic relative (n=1203) did significantly worse at follow-up than did those who had no family history of alcoholism. The male alcoholics who had positive family history and had two or more alcoholic first-degree relatives (n=643) had significantly poorer follow-up results than those with positive family history and one first-degree alcoholic relative (n=560).

Schuckit et al. (1972) studied 164 half-sibs of 69 alcoholics. Sixty of these probands were male and remaining 9 were female. The half-sibs who became alcoholic were most often male. Concordance was highest if the shared parent was the alcoholic regardless of whether or not they shared an alcoholic home environment. So, the best predictor of alcoholism among half-sibs was the existence of a shared alcoholic parent.

To study the effects of changes in alcohol use between generations on the inheritance of alcohol abuse, Cloninger et al. (1987) took into account temporal trends in per capita alcohol consumption in addition to proband sex. The sample included 286 hospitalized alcoholics (male and female), 157 convicted felons with a high frequency of alcohol abuse, and 60 control subjects. They observed that as alcohol consumption in the community as a whole increased, there was an exponential increase in familial alcoholism and not simply an increase in sporadic cases. Social and temporal trends in the consumption of alcohol will influence the observed inheritance of alcoholism. This is true for secular trends in any common illness. However, when risk is not vertically transmitted, the effect of a secular trend similar to that seen in the recent past in alcohol use will manifest itself in a general increase in sporadic cases and not in the familial forms. Thus, for alcoholism, the effect of social or temporal trends is to strengthen the case for vertical transmission rather than to weaken it. Moreover, the clinical characteristics of nonfamilial alcoholics have proved to be less reliable on follow-up than are those among familial alcoholics. Indeed, the so-called sporadic cases are often diagnosed as not alcoholic at follow-up.

Since 1977, pedigrees have been ascertained in the St. Louis Family Interview Study of Alcoholism, a longitudinal, multi-dimensional project which is part of the Washington University Alcohol Research Center (ARC). The sample consisted of 503 Caucasian probands born within 100 miles of the St. Louis metropolitan area. Two hundred eighty-six of these individuals were hospitalized alcoholics drawn from four St. Louis hospitals, 157 convicted felons from local probation and parole offices, and 60 medically ill controls with no history of psychiatric illness or substance abuse. Feighner criteria were used for hospitalized alcoholics' diagnosis. Gilligan et al. (1987) analyzed the data for the Caucasian hospitalized alcoholics and their first-degree relatives, spouses, step-relatives, and half-siblings. From the 286 hospitalized alcoholics ascertained in the index study, direct interview data regarding the classes of relatives of interest were available for 195 probands, including 140 male and 55 female subjects. The 195 extended pedigrees comprised 288 nuclear families.

Complex segregation analysis of alcoholism has been carried out in these families considering variation in risk according to age and sex (Gilligan et al., 1987). Several models were used as criteria to evaluate possible etiologic heterogeneity. The principal feature of a comparison of the models was that the subsample of families of female probands was described by a multifactorial-polygenic model, with unequal adult and offspring heritability and no significant evidence of a major gene effect. In contrast, the subsample of families of male probands incorporated a transmissible major effect in addition to a multifactorial-polygenic background that differs between adult and offspring. There was no statistical evidence for heterogeneity in the seemingly distinct models of transmission between families of male and female probands. Of course, the patterns of transmission of liability to alcoholism appeared markedly dissimilar.

From the results of segregation analyses in St. Louis (Fig. 1) and other data Cloninger (1990) concluded that the risks of alcoholism in different classes of relatives of alcoholics indicate that alcoholism has a complex mode of inheritance. No single Mendelian gene with complete penetrance can explain its pattern of familial transmission. Segregation analyses were compatible with either of two possible modes of inheritance: (1) Genetic heterogeneity, in which there are two distinct subtypes, including Type 1 with moderate multifactorial inheritance and no major gene locus and Type 2 with both a major dominant gene locus and high polygenic heritability. (2) A mixed model comprising the effects of a major gene with a multi-factorial background. These are not practically different from each other, because under the mixed model the effects of the major gene will vary in its importance.

Adoption studies

The most objective means of evaluating gene-environment interaction for non-Mendelian disorders is to study the biological and adoptive families of adoptees who have been separated from their biological parents at an early age. The first published adoption study of alcoholism which failed to observe alcohol-related problems in adopted-away children of heavy drinkers was carried out by Roe and Burks in 1940s. Their small sample consisted of 27 children of alcoholic biological parents and 22 children of normal biological parents. They found that good foster placement was associated with no alcohol abuse in 26 out of 27 children of alcoholic biological parents and 21 of 22 children of normal biological parents. It was reported that none of the 21 adopted-out sons of alcoholics had drinking problems as adults.

Goodwin et al. (1973) conducted larger adoption studies in Denmark. Observations made on 55 males born to an alcoholic biologic parent (usually the father) and 78 control adoptees strongly supported the hypothesis that genetic factors are important in determining alcohol abuse in males. No clear statements regarding the inheritance of alcoholism in women could be made because of the small sample size, the low rate of alcoholism in Danish women, and the small number of alcoholic mothers in their adoptive population. Only two of the 49 family history positive adopted females and two of 47 control females became alcoholic. Overall, 5% of the control adoptees developed alcoholism later in life, compared to 18% of the adoptees with a positive biological family history. The alcoholic males also exhibited symptoms such as loss of control, hallucinations, and morning drinking which could not be seen in female adoptees.

Cadoret and Garth (1978) studied 127 male and 87 female adoptees in the United States. They suggested separate genetic influences on antisocial personality and alcoholism and found no evidence for gene-environment interaction in these two disorders. However, the demonstration of no gene-environment interaction must be tempered by the relatively small sample of adoptees, particularly the small sizes obtained when they were separated into gene by environment interaction cells.

These different findings were difficult to compare because of differences in the clinical characteristics of alcohol abuse in the parents and differences in the adoptive placements. Goodwin et al. (1973) studied children whose biological parents had been hospitalized for alcoholism, but none of the parents studied by Roe and Burks had been treated. Also the children of alcoholics studied by Roe and Burks were more often placed in rural areas (where drinking was infrequent) than were the children of alcoholics in Goodwin's study.

Because of these discrepancies, Bohman, Cloninger and coworkers undertook a large-scale adoption study of alcoholism in Sweden. The sample included 862 men and 913 women of known paternity who were born to single women in Stockholm, Sweden, from 1930 to 1949. Most of the subjects were separated from their biological relatives in the first months of life (average, 4 months), and all had their final placement in the adoptive home before the age of three years (average, 8 months). Of course, it is important to notice that all of these subjects were adopted by nonrelatives. Information about alcohol abuse, psychopathology, and medical treatment was available for the entire lifetimes of the adoptees and their parents from hospitals, clinics, and several registers that are systematically maintained in Sweden. Identification of alcohol abuse from these sources could identify about 70% of alcoholics; those so identified were representative of alcoholics in general, with no appreciable bias for either Type 1 or Type 2 alcoholics (see Table 1). Such detailed information permitted a population-based study large enough that the adoptees could be divided into subgroups related to Type 1 and Type 2 alcoholism.

Table 1.
Distinguishing characteristics of two types of alcoholism.

	Type of alcoholism	
Characteristic features	**Type 1**	**Type 2**
Alcohol-related problems		
Usual age of onset (years)	After 25	Before 25
Spontaneous alcohol-seeking (inability to abstain)	Infrequent	Frequent
Fighting and arrests when drinking	Infrequent	Frequent
Psychological dependence (loss of control)	Frequent	Infrequent
Guilt and fear about alcohol dependence	Frequent	Infrequent
Personality traits		
Novelty seeking	Low	High
Harm avoidance	High	Low
Reward dependence	High	Low

Subtypes of Alcoholism

One of the important findings of The Stockholm Adoption Study was the distinction of two types of alcoholics (Cloninger et al., 1981). The two types of alcohol abuse were distinguished on the basis of the pattern of alcohol abuse in the biological parents of the adoptees. If the biological fathers or mothers had an adult onset of alcohol abuse and no criminality requiring prolonged incarceration, the adoptees were classified as Type 1 genetic background. If the biological fathers had extensive treatment for alcohol abuse and serious criminality beginning in their adolescence or early adulthood, the adoptees were considered as Type 2 genetic background (Table 1). There were few biological mothers with Type 2 characteristics for separate analysis. Alcohol abuse in the adoptive parents was not associated with an increased risk of abuse in the children they reared, so there was no evidence that alcoholism is familial because children imitate their rearing parents. It was found that both genetic predisposition and postnatal provocation were necessary if the adopted-away sons were to express susceptibility to loss of control (Type 1) alcoholism. More specifically, if there was either a genetic predisposition or a provocative postnatal environment, but not both, the risk of alcohol abuse was lower than in the general population. However, if both occurred in the same person, the risk of severe alcohol abuse was more than doubled. Consequently, Type 1 alcoholism has been described as "milieu-limited." In contrast, in adopted-away sons of fathers with spontaneous alcohol-seeking (Type 2), the risk of alcoholism increased regardless of environmental background. In these families the risk of alcohol abuse in the adopted-away sons of Type 2 alcoholic fathers was nine times that in the sons of all other fathers.

To evaluate this apparent genetic heterogeneity further, Cloninger and colleagues (1985) tested the predictions in the adopted-away daughters of Type 1 and Type 2 alcoholics. The background of the daughter's biological parent was classified as it was in the study of the men. The daughters of Type 1 alcoholics were predicted to be at increased risk for alcohol abuse because the mothers in these families were often alcohol abusers; the daughters at high risk for Type 1 alcoholism were three times as likely to abuse alcohol as those at low risk. In contrast, the adopted-away daughters of Type 2 alcoholic fathers were found to be at higher risk only for somatic anxiety (that is, somatization or frequent disabling physical complaints), which is associated with high novelty seeking. Consequently Type 2 alcoholism has been called "male-limited."

The hypothesis that the families of male probands are composed of two etiologically heterogeneous subtypes was tested by Gilligan et al. (1987). This hypothesis, which had been generated by the Stockholm Adoption Study, was supported by the finding that the two subtypes explained the segregation significantly better than did the assumption of homogeneity. Heritability estimates were 88% for Type 2 families of male probands compared to 21% for Type 1 families of male probands. This fits the data significantly better than the composite heritability of 69% under the assumption of homogeneity (heterogeneity $\chi^2=14.22$ with one degree of freedom, $p<0.01$). The segregation analyses of the Type 2 families indicated significant evidence of a major gene effect, with maximum likelihood estimates of allele frequency $q=0.11$, displacement between homozygotes $t=2.30$, dominance parameter $d=1.0$, and multifactorial background $H=0.15$. Compatibility to Mendelian transmission was tested by estimating the transmission probability of the susceptibility allele from parent to child, which was found to be close to the value of 0.5 expected under Mendelian transmission. In contrast, there was no evidence for any effect of a major locus in Type 1 families (Figure 1).

Figure 1.
Summary of segregation analysis in St. Louis Family Study of Alcoholism.

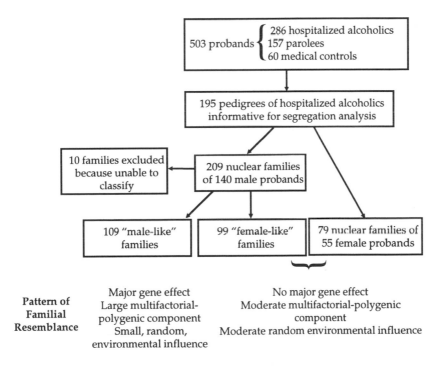

Molecular Genetic Studies in Alcoholism

With advancements in biotechnology, especially in recombinant DNA, it is possible to systematically search for genes involved in alcoholism. These techniques include a variety of approaches such as DNA sequencing and genotyping. These techniques and discoveries are now being applied to the study of alcoholism and its complications. The hope is that through molecular cloning we can identify genes involved in alcohol abuse, or genes that may serve as markers of risk for alcoholism/alcohol dependence. There are two strategies for identifying and cloning gene(s) for predisposition to alcoholism. Namely, candidate gene(s) and systematic screening.

Candidate gene approach

Numerous candidate genes have been proposed to account for the increased familial risk of alcoholism. A detailed discussion of this approach is included in the chapter by Sherman et al. (this volume), and only two types will be discussed here. The first group of candidate genes are the ones which code for the enzymes responsible for the oxidative pathway in ethanol metabolism. These are alcohol dehydrogenases (ADHs) and aldehyde dehydrogenases (ALDHs). Three of these genes, αADH, βADH and γADH that code for ADH1, ADH2 and ADH3, respectively, are classified as class I enzymes. The human ALDHs are coded for by four independent loci. These four loci are ALDH1, or cytosolic ALDH, which is constitutively expressed. The mitochondrial ALDH (ALDH2) is expressed in liver, kidney and heart. ALDH3 and ALDH4 expressed in stomach and liver respectively (Smith, 1986). As Gilligan and Cloninger (1987) have noted and as our own molecular genetic studies have shown, there has not been any relation between these enzymes and alcoholism. In other words, the activity of any of the known ADH or ALDH isozymes variants does not in any way influence the risk of developing alcoholism. On the other hand, the possible protective effects of particular phenotypes and genotypes of ADH and ALDH in alcoholism are described by Ehrig and Li (this volume).

The second group of candidate genes are neurotransmitter genes like dopamine and serotonin receptor genes. The human dopamine D2 receptor gene (DRD2) recently has become one of the most interesting and important candidates for alcoholism. There have been several reports regarding the association of the 3′ Taq I minor allele of DRD2 with alcoholism. Blum et al. (1990) reported an association between alcoholism and the minor allele (A1) in a group of 35 alcoholics versus 35 controls. The alcoholic group studied had a severe form of the illness since all had repeated treatment failures and many died from medical complications of their drinking. The A1 allele was present in 64% of 22 white alcoholics and only 17% of 24 white controls, and in 77% of 13 black alcoholics and 27% of 11 black controls. The differences in allele frequency were not due to sex differences between the two groups.

Bolos et al. (1990) studied 40 unrelated white alcoholics admitted to the National Institutes of Heath Clinical Research Center. The control populations included 62 unrelated white patients who had cystic fibrosis and 65 unrelated white individuals from CEPH reference families. The sex and age of this heterogeneous control panel was not described, and psychiatric interviews were not available to exclude alcoholism. They found that the A1 allele was present in 38% of 40 alcoholics compared to 30% of 127 controls. It is important to note that alcoholics with acutely active medical disorders of functional impairment from drug abuse were excluded. Given the differences in ascertainment and assessment procedures for both alcoholics and controls, it is difficult to interpret the discrepancies with certainty.

In order to evaluate the possible association of alleles of DRD2 with alcoholism, Parsian et al. (1991) have studied the DRD2 allele types in a group of probands from multiple incidence, alcoholic families and a group of unrelated, non-alcoholic controls. 41% of 32 white alcoholics carried the A1 allele compared with 12% of 25 white controls. The association with the A1 allele was significant when controls were compared with a subset of 10 alcoholics with severe medical problems (60% vs 12%), but not less severe cases. There was no evidence of linkage of the A1 allele and increased susceptibility to alcoholism in 17 nuclear families. We have two explanations for this possible association in the general population without linkage in families. First, it could be due to chance variation in small samples; second, it might be due to a modifying effect of the A1 allele that increases severity among alcoholics.

Comings et al. (1991) reported several samples in which the A1 allele may have a modifying effect on a wide spectrum of behavioral disorders characterized by their familial association with alcoholism or possible involvement with dopaminergic neurotransmission. They found the A1 allele was significantly increased in 104 alcoholics (42%). It was suggested that the A1 allele is likely to modify the expression of alcoholism, rather than to be a necessary or sufficient cause. The reason was that most of alcoholics do not carry the A1 allele, the A1 allele does not cosegregate with alcoholism in pedigrees, and it is associated with other behavioral disorders that do not cosegregate with alcoholism.

Gelernter et al. (1991) described results like those of Bolos et al. (1990). They suggested that earlier positive observations were based on falsely low estimates of the prevalence of the A1 allele in controls. The alternative hypothesis is that the estimate of the prevalence in controls by Gelernter et al. (1991) and by Bolos et al. (1990) was falsely high as a result of sampling variation and/or failure to exclude alcoholism and other psychopathology (Cloninger, 1991). Ongoing studies are designed to control for these potentially confounding factors. We have developed three new RFLPs within the human D2 gene (Parsian et al., 1991b; Suarez et al., 1994) and genotyped larger alcoholic and normal control samples. We determined that all of these markers (Taq IA, B and C, phD2-248, and phD2 249) were in linkage disequilibrium. There was no significant difference in the frequency of any polymorphism between alcoholics and normal controls. However, for marker phD2-244 (taqI C) the alcoholic sample showed a significant departure from Hardy-Weinberg equilibrium. The pattern of pairwise composite disequilibrium coefficients was broadly similar in the two groups, although when five-marker haplotype frequencies were compared, a significant difference was revealed. This difference appears to be due to greater linkage disequilibrium of the control sample (Suarez et al., 1994). Hence, our expanded study does not support the hypothesis that mutant forms of the DRD2 gene are associated with alcoholism. Further information on published studies on DRD2 association with alcoholism is included in the chapter by Sherman et al. (this volume).

Systematic genome screening

The complexity of alcoholism and the rather limited evidence for any candidate gene is such that a systematic search of the genome is necessary. The entire human genome is approximately 3300 centimorgans (cM, one cM is one million base pairs). To cover this genome with markers that are spaced every 10 cM will therefore require about 300 DNA markers. The use of genetic maps should be a powerful strategy for testing linkage of traits that might be heterogenous (Lander & Botstein, 1986).

To date, a number of genetic diseases have been mapped in this way, beginning with Huntington disease (Gusella et al., 1983); the list is increasing rapidly. Several genes initially localized in this way have since been isolated, allowing detailed studies of their functions, e.g. Duchenne muscular dystrophy (Monaco et al., 1986); retinoblastoma (Lee et al., 1987); chronic granulomatous disease (Royer-Pokora et al., 1986); cystic fibrosis (Rommens et al., 1989; Riodan et al, 1989; Bat-Sheva et al., 1989). All of these successes have been for disorders which follow Mendelian patterns of inheritance (autosomal recessive, autosomal dominant, etc.).

Linkage and association studies

Although the susceptibility to alcoholism is strongly familial, its mode of inheritance cannot be explained by simple Mendelian patterns of inheritance, such as the effect of a single autosomal gene with complete penetrance. In addition, there have been large group differences in the prevalence of alcoholism because of sociocultural influences. Both consumption and complications have varied widely from country to country, between social classes, between persons of different occupation, and between men and women (Cloninger, 1981). The observations show that the mode of inheritance of alcoholism is developmentally complex and affected by incomplete penetrance, variable expressivity, and gene/environment interaction demonstrated in studies of twins, adoptees, and multigenerational pedigrees. Therefore, alcoholism is considered a non-Mendelian trait.

The methodology for mapping Mendelian disorders is relatively straightforward (Conneally & Rivas, 1980; Ott, 1985). The strategy begins with selection of appropriate families, large multigeneration families with high density of affected individuals. Such families are critical to an optimal linkage study. The primary assumption under lying lod score analysis is that the traits being analyzed are single-locus, Mendelian traits, with known mode of inheritance, which is correctly specified in the analysis. Risch (1992) believes that violation of the Mendelian assumption in lod score analysis may have serious consequences. If the genetic mechanism underlying a disease is complex, possibly involving several loci, successful detection of linkage may be more difficult than in the simple Mendelian case. The reason is that, unlike the Mendelian one-to-one correspondence between genotype and phenotype, the correspondence between phenotype (affected, unaffected) and genotype may be weak. Disease status alone does not allow clear discrimination among genotypes at a disease susceptibility locus. Therefore, for the non-Mendelian disorders, accurate specification of the mode of inheritance in lod score analysis is generally not possible.

In the case of alcoholism, an alternative to the classical method of linkage is the sib-pair method. This method was used in the early days of linkage analysis for Mendelian disorders (Penrose, 1935). It has recently been adopted for linkage analysis as a non-parametric method. Suarez et al. (1978) refined the method to include disease susceptibility loci closely linked to a marker locus and also included parental information. The sib-pair method can be very useful in finding a linked marker. Its major advantage is that no genetic mechanism needs to be postulated, since affected sibs can be assumed to have the same underlying genotype for the disorder. It is reported that the method results in consistent estimates of the recombination fraction if the disease susceptibility is due to an incompletely penetrant simple Mendelian locus (Suarez et al., 1978). Weeks and Lange (1988) have developed a method called the affected-pedigree-member method of linkage analysis. It is a compromise between the two methods mentioned above because they use only affected members in the family. The use of this method in linkage analysis of complex disorders requires further testing to know the circumstances in which its conclusions are robust.

At the present time, the difficulties in conducting linkage analyses with disorders of unknown mode of inheritance have encouraged further consideration of studies of candidate genes and of association with genetic markers in the general population. The a priori odds of detecting a true association are low (simply because of the size of the genome). However, when the result of association studies are positive and replicable (e.g., when a polymorphic gene difference between alcoholics and non-alcoholics is statistically significant), the next step to clarify the nature of the genetic influence might be DNA sequencing. For example, the exon(s) of the related gene will be sequenced from genomic DNA samples from alcoholics and normal controls who carry the specific allele. If there are sequence variation(s) in any of the genes under study between alcoholics and controls, then the position of the variations will be determined. The segregation of these sequence variations within family pedigrees can be studied. Of course, it is important to determine the frequency of any sequence variations in alcoholic and normal groups. Finally, the role of amino acid substitutions in altering the gene's activity or regulation can be studied. These results may provide evidence for the role of any of candidate enzymes or receptors genes in development of susceptibility to alcoholism. Further discussion of methodology used to search for genetic loci predisposing alcoholism can be found in the chapter by Sherman et al. (this volume).

Conclusion

These studies show that the mode of inheritance of alcoholism is developmentally complex and affected by incomplete penetrance. The twin, family and adoption studies have demonstrated variability in clinical expression and gene-environment interaction. The Stockholm adoption studies showed that childhood personality traits account for most of the predictable risk of adult alcoholism. The clinical subtypes that have been described in the Stockholm adoption study are prototypes of two developmental pathways (Type 1 and Type 2 alcoholism).

It seems unlikely that one or two genes will account for a large proportion of the variance in risk for alcoholism. It is more likely that there are several genes that are detectable with current methods for detecting and mapping genes in the human genome. The prolonged developmental course of risk and abuse will afford opportunities for joint studies of biogenetic and sociocultural influences on risk. Such collaborative efforts are likely to be critical as a result of the gene-environment interaction on risk of alcoholism.

References

Blum, K., Noble, E.P., Sheridan, P.J., et al. (1990). Allelic association of human dopamine D2 receptor gene in alcoholism. *Journal of the American Medical Association*, 263(15): 2055-2060.

Bohman, M., Cloninger, C.R., Sigvardson, S., et al. (1987). The genetics of alcoholism and related disorders. *Journal of Psychiatric Research*, 21: 447-452.

Bolos, A.M., Dean, M., Lucas-Derse, S., et al. (1990). Population and pedigree studies reveal a lack of association between the dopamine D2 receptor gene and alcoholism. *Journal of the American Medical Association*, 264: 3156-3160.

Cadoret, R.J. & A. Gath. (1978). Inheritance of alcoholism in adoptees. *British Journal of Psychiatry*, 132: 252-258.

Cloninger, C.R., Bohman, M., Sigvardson, S., et al. (1985). Psychopathology in adopted-out children of alcoholics: The Stockholm Adoption Study. *Recent Development on Alcoholism*, 3: 37-51.

Cloninger, C.R., Reich, T., Sigvardson, S., et al. (1987). The effects of changes in alcohol use between generations on the inheritance of alcohol abuse. In R. Rose (Ed.), *Alcoholism: A Medical Disorder.* New York: Raven Press.

Cloninger, C.R., Bohman, M., & Sigvardson, S. (1981). Inheritance of alcohol abuse: Cross-fostering analysis of adopted men. *Archives of General Psychiatry,* 38: 861-868.

Cloninger, C.R. (1990). Genetic epidemiology of alcoholism: observations critical in the design and analysis of linkage studies. In C.R. Cloninger and H. Begleiter (Eds.), *Genetics and Biology of Alcoholism* (pp. 105-133). Banbury Report 33. New York: Cold Spring Harbor Laboratory Press.

Cloninger, C.R. (1991). D2 dopamine receptor gene is associated but not linked with alcoholism. *Journal of the American Medical Association,* 266: 1833-1834.

Comings, D.E., Comings, B.G., Muhlman, D., et al. (1991). The dopamine D2 receptor locus as a modifying gene in neuropsychiatric disorder. *Journal of the American Medical Association,* 266: 1793-1800.

Conneally, P.M. & Rivas, M.L. (1980). Linkage analysis in man. In H. Harris and K. Hirschhorn (Eds.), *Advances in Human Genetics* (pp. 209-266). New York: Plenum Publishing Corp.

Conneally, P.M. (1989). Criteria for optimal linkage studies in alcoholism. In K. Küanmaa, B. Tabakoff, and T. Saito (Eds.), *Genetic Aspects of Alcoholism* (pp. 259-264). Helsinki: Finn Foundation on Alcohol Studies.

Crothers, T.D. (1909). Heredity in the causation of inebriety. *Br. Med. J.* 2:659-661.

Dahlberg, G. & Stenberg, S. (1934). *Alkoholism som Samhalls problems.* Stockholm: Oskar Eklunds.

Elderton, E. & Pearson, K. (1910). A first study of the influence of parent's alcoholism on the physique and ability of the offspring. *Eugenics Laboratory Memoir X.* London: Cambridge University Press.

Feighner, J.P., Robins, E., Guze, S. B., et al. (1972). Diagnosis criteria for use in psychiatric research. *Archives of General Psychiatry,* 26: 57-63.

Frances, R.J., Bucky, S., Alexopoulos, G. S. (1984). Outcome study of familial and nonfamilial alcoholism. *American Journal of Psychiatry,* 141: 1469-1471.

Gelernter, J., O'Malley, S., Risch, N., et al. (1991). No association between an allele at the D2 dopamine receptor gene (DRD2) and alcoholism regardless of severity. *Journal of American Medical Association,* 266: 1801-1807.

Gilligan, S.B., Reich, T., & Cloninger, C.R. (1987). Etiologic heterogeneity in alcoholism. *Genetic Epidemiology*, 4: 395-414.

Goodwin, D.W., Schulsinger, F., Hermansen, L., et al. (1973). Alcohol problems in adoptees raised apart from alcoholic biological parents. *Archives of General Psychiatry*, 18: 238-243.

Goodwin, D.W. (1987). Genetic influence in alcoholism. *Advances in Internal Medicine*, 32: 283-298.

Goodwin, D.W. & Guze, S.B. (1989). *Psychiatric Diagnosis*, 4th Ed. Oxford: Oxford University Press.

Gurling, H.M.D., Murray, R.M., & Clifford, C.A. (1981). Investigations into the genetics of alcohol dependence and into its effects on brain function. *Twin Research 3: Epidemiology and Clinical Studies*. New York: Alan R. Liss.

Gusella, J.F., Wexler, N. S., Conneally, P.M., et al. (1983). A polymorphic DNA marker genetically linked to Huntington's disease. *Nature*, 306: 234 238.

Hrubec, Z. and Omenn, G.S. (1981). Evidence of genetic predisposition to alcoholic cirrhosis and psychosis: Twin concordance for alcoholism and its end points by zygosity among male veterans. *Alcoholism: Clinical and Experimental Research*, 5: 207-215.

Hsu, L.C., Yoshida, A., & Mohandas, T. (1986). Chromosomal assignment of the genes for human aldehyde dehydrogenase-1 and aldehyde dehydrogenase-2. *American Journal of Human Genetics*, 38: 641-648.

Jellinek, E.M. & Jolliffe, N. (1940). Effect of alcohol on the individual: Review of the literature of 1939. *Quarterly Journal on the Studies of Alcoholism*, 1: 110-181.

Kaij, L. (1960). *Studies of the Etiology and Sequels of Abuse of Alcohol*. Sweden: University. of Lund Press.

Kerem, B.T., Rommens, J.M., Buchanan, J. A., et al. (1989). Identification of the cystic fibrosis gene: Genetic analysis. *Science*, 245: 1073-1080.

Lander, E.S. & Botstein, D. (1986). Strategies for studying heterogeneous genetic traits in humans by using a linkage map of restriction fragment length polymorphisms. *Proceedings of the Nationl Academy of Science, USA*, 83: 7353-7357.

Lee, W.H., Bookstein, R., Hong, F., et al. (1987). Human retinoblastoma susceptibility gene: Cloning, identification and sequence. *Science*, 235: 1394-1399.

Ott, J. (1991). *Analysis of Human Genetic Linkage* (Rev. ed.). Baltimore: The Johns Hopkins University Press.

Parsian, A., Todd, R.D., Devor, E.J., et al. (1991a). Alcoholism and alleles of the human dopamine D2 receptor locus: Studies of association and linkage. *Archives of General Psychiatry,* 48: 654-660.

Parsian, A., Fisher, L., O'Malley, K.L., Todd, R.D. (1991b). A new TaqI RFLP within intron 2 of human dopamine D2 receptor gene (DRD2). *Nucleic Acids Res,* 19: 6977.

Partanen, J., Bruun, K., Markanen, T. (1966). *Inheritance of drinking behavior.* Helsinki: Finn Foundation on Alcohol Studies.

Penick, E.C., Read, M.R., Crowley, P.A., et al. (1978). Differentiation of alcoholics by family history. *Journal on Studies of Alcoholism,* 39: 1944-1948.

Penrose, L.S. (1935). The detection of autosomal linkage in data which consists of pairs of brothers and sisters of unspecified parentage. *Annal of Eugenics,* 6: 133-138.

Pickens, R.W., Svikis, D.S., McGue, M., et al. (1990). Heterogeneity in the inheritance of alcoholism. *Archives of General Psychiatry,* 48: 19-28.

Riordan, J.R., Rommens, J.M., Kerem, B.- T., et al. (1989). Identification of the cystic fibrosis gene: Cloning and characterization of complementary DNA. *Science,* 245: 1066-1072.

Risch, N. (1992). Genetic linkage: Interpreting lod scores. *Science,* 255: 803-804.

Roe, A. and Burks, B. (1945). *Memoirs of Section on Alcohol Studies.* New Haven: Yale University Press.

Rommens, J.M., Jannuzzi, M.C., Kerem, B.- S., et al. (1989). Identification of the cystic fibrosis gene: Chromosome walking and jumping. *Science,* 245: 1059-1065.

Royer-Pokora, B., Kunkel, L.M., Monoca, A.P., et al. (1986). Cloning the gene for an inherited human disorder—chronic granulomatous disease—on the basis of its chromosomal location. *Nature,* 322: 32-38.

Santisteban, J., Povey, S., West, L., et al. (1985). Chromosome assignment, biochemical and immunological studies on a human aldehyde dehydrogenase, ALDH3. *American Journal of Human Genetics,* 49: 87-100.

Schuckit, M.A., Goodwin, D. W., & Winokur, G. A. (1972). A study of alcoholism in half-siblings. *American Journal of Psychiatry,* 128: 1132-1136.

Smith, M. (1986). Genetics of human alcohol and aldehyde dehydrogenases. In H. Harris and K. Hirschhorn (Eds.), Advances in Human Genetics (pp. 249-290). New York: Plenum Publishing Corp.

Smith, M. (1989). Practical implications of gene mapping and cloning. In K. Kiianmaa, B. Tabakoff, and T. Saito (Eds.), *Genetic Aspects of Alcoholism*. Helsinki: Finnish Foundation on Alcohol Studies.

Suarez, B.K., Rice, J.P., & Reich, T. (1978). The generalized sib-pair IBD distribution: Its use in the detection of linkage. *American Journal of Human Genetics*, 42: 87-94.

Suarez, B.K., Parsian, A., Hampe, C.L., et al. (1994). Linkage disequilibrium at the D2 dopamine receptor locus (DRD2) in alcoholics and controls. *Genomics*, 19: 12-20.

Tsukahara, M., & Yoshida, A. (1989). Chromosomal assignment of the alcohol dehydrogenase cluster locus to human chromosome 4q21-23 by in situ hybridization. *Genomics*, 4: 218-220.

Weeks, D.E. & Lange, K. (1988). The affected-pedigree-member method of linkage analysis. *American Journal of Human Genetics*, 42: 315-326.

Emerging Markers of Predisposition to Alcoholism

D.I.N. Sherman, R.J. Ward, Roger Williams and T.J. Peters.
Department of Clinical Biochemistry and Institute of Liver Studies,
King's College School of Medicine and Dentistry, London, UK

Over the past twenty years there have been important advances in our understanding of the biochemistry and molecular genetics of alcoholism and its consequences. In Western societies alcohol abuse has a prevalence of between 10 to 15 %, and yet within this group there is striking variability in individual response to the chronic effects of ethanol. There is now widespread acceptance that genetic influences account for up to one quarter of this variation between individuals. The resulting search for the "gene(s)" for alcoholism and other markers of susceptibility has involved not only basic scientists such as molecular geneticists, biochemists and neuroscientists but also psychiatrists, physicians and members of other disciplines. During a period in which the molecular basis of many single gene disorders has been elucidated, researchers into alcoholism have, in contrast, become increasingly aware of the difficulties involved in investigating the genetic background to such a complex, heterogeneous disorder.

At present, there are no specific laboratory tests that can be used by clinicians to advise individual patients on their risk of becoming an alcoholic in the same way that, for example, serum lipoproteins are used to define the risk of coronary heart disease. However, recent studies of gene markers suggest that our understanding of the genetic basis for individual susceptibility to the effects of alcohol is likely to increase considerably over the next few years. This review will concentrate, therefore, on the application of the techniques of molecular genetics in studies of alcoholics and normal subjects.

The evidence that individuals may be rendered susceptible to alcoholism by inherited factors has been mostly derived from family studies (Goodwin, 1987). The findings of increased concordance for alcoholism amongst monozygotic in comparison with dizygotic twins in some studies (Hrubec & Omenn,1981; Kaij, 1960) but not in others (Gurling, Murray & Clifford,1984), and adoption studies showing inheritance of alcoholism in sons of alcoholic fathers despite adoption into a non-alcoholic environment (Bohman, 1978; Bohman, Sigvardsson & Cloninger, 1981; Cadoret & Gath, 1978; Cadoret, O'Gorman, Troughton and Haywood,1985; Goodwin et al., 1973) suggested that environmental influences were not of overriding importance (see chapter by Parsian and Cloninger, this volume, for more detail). Furthermore, attempts to subtype alcoholics into phenotypes according to age of onset, sex, clinical course, personality characteristics and the influence of heredity and environment (Cloninger, Bohmann & Sigvardsson, 1981), has provided a useful model to relate to putative biochemical and genetic markers. Analysis of a recent sophisticated twin study by Pickens et al. (1990) has also suggested that heterogeneity may exist in the inheritance of different subtypes of alcoholism.

Part of the difficulty in studying alcoholism lies in the fact that the pathogenesis of the various clinical syndromes has not been clearly elucidated. However, it is likely that the main pathway of alcohol metabolism via alcohol and aldehyde dehydrogenases plays a central role. Martin et al. (1984) studied ethanol metabolism in over 200 twin pairs and concluded that genetic factors accounted for much of the repeatable variation in ethanol metabolism between individuals. Heritabilities of 0.62 for peak blood alcohol concentration and 0.49 for ethanol elimination rate were demonstrated, and similar results were obtained by Kopun and Propping (1977). Biochemical studies of ethanol and acetaldehyde metabolism in alcoholics admitted to hospital for detoxification provided further evidence by demonstrating increased rates of ethanol elimination and peak acetaldehyde levels in alcoholics with features of dependency in comparison to non-dependent alcohol abusers and controls (Peters, Ward, Rideout and Lim, 1987).

Racial differences in susceptibility to the effects of ethanol are well known (Mendenhall et al., 1989), and it is likely that this is explained by inter-racial genetic polymorphism as well as cross-cultural differences in drinking behaviour. The molecular basis for the marked aversion to ethanol exhibited by 40 - 50 % of Japanese resulting in protection against alcoholic liver disease is described below.

The clinical heterogeneity of individual responses is seen not only in alcoholism, but also in the resulting organ damage. Surveys of liver histology amongst alcoholics who have drunk in excess of 80 g daily for a minimum of ten years reveal that 90 to 100 % have fatty liver, but only 30 % have alcoholic hepatitis and 10 to 20 % cirrhosis (Lelbach, 1976; Lieber, 1982). Although other environmental factors such as nutritional status, autoimmunity, etc., may be operating, it seems likely that a genetic effect may confer increased susceptibility to alcoholic liver damage, possibly via genes quite distinct from those connected with alcoholism. Arria, Tarter, Williams & Van Thiel (1991) recently suggested that a family history of alcoholism, particularly in females, may be associated with an earlier age of onset of autoimmune chronic active hepatitis as well as of alcoholic liver disease. This raises the possibility that the genetics of alcoholism and certain chronic liver diseases may be related. Differential organ toxicity, for example the low incidence of severe alcoholic cardiomyopathy in patients with severe alcoholic cirrhosis (Hassanein, Wright, Follansbee & Van Thiel, 1991), may also be influenced by genetic as well as environmental factors.

Genetic approaches

There is, therefore, strong evidence for genetic involvement in the wide variation in individual susceptibility to the multiple effects of ethanol abuse. This has led to alcoholism being labelled as " a pharmacogenetic disorder caused by ethyl alcohol" (Omenn, 1975). Any proposed genetic model for alcoholism must take into account the multifactorial nature of the disease process. Clinical manifestations differ between body systems *ie.* there are several different possible phenotypes. Cloninger's classification goes some way towards resolving this issue for alcohol dependency, but it is likely that the picture is even more complex than this. A simple Mendelian autosomal dominant or recessive model has been rejected, suggesting that multiple polymorphic gene loci are involved (Cloninger, 1990).

Each of these may show varying degrees of penetrance, and non-inherited influences may produce similar phenotypes or phenocopies (see Gordis, Tabakoff, Goldman & Berg, 1990). Even if genes are fully penetrant, interactions with external factors may vary expressivity in individuals (Cloninger, 1991). It seems likely that a small number of allelic "major" loci account for most of the heritability observed in phenotypic studies, with additional effects attributed to a few "minor" loci.

As there is no precise pathophysiological model for alcoholism and organ damage, we can postulate the role of genetic factors at different levels in the progression from social drinker to alcoholic (Omenn, 1975). Genes contributing to predisposing cognitive and behavioural factors that result in certain forms of drinking behaviour are likely to be unrelated to those influencing cirrhosis or cardiomyopathy. The loci responsible for ethanol metabolism may be implicated at several levels: acute response, adaptation to chronic intake and organ damage. Susceptibility genes for CNS tolerance to ethanol, psychological dependence (and perhaps even the Wernicke-Korsakoff syndrome) may be shared with other psychiatric disorders, particularly other forms of drug abuse.

In the search for genetic loci implicated in any disorder, there are in general two possible lines of approach. If family studies indicate that a condition is likely to be inherited in a simple Mendelian manner, but there is little knowledge of its biochemical basis at the protein level, random gene probes may be used in studies of family pedigrees informative for the disorder, to look for a linkage effect between a marker probe and the unknown gene(s). The rationale is based on the fact that during meiosis, the frequency of recombination of alleles at two loci is directly proportional to the distance between them along the chromosome, and can therefore be used as a measure of genetic closeness. Thus, the proximity of the marker probe to the index gene can be calculated by examining cosegregation (usually of one of its alleles and the disease phenotype) in families. The strength of linkage is expressed as a logarithmic probability function known as a LOD score (Morton, 1962), and linkage is said to definitely exist at a score of 3 (indicating a probability level of 1 in 1000). Usually a particular model of inheritance, eg. autosomal dominance with 99% penetrance, has to be assumed. The use of such an approach to localize a gene, if necessary with multiple random probes covering large portions of the genome, then allows its more formal isolation and definition.

A second approach is to look for "candidate" genes with probes specific for genes that have already been isolated. Usually these are derived from loci that encode proteins that are known to play a role in the disorder.This is more suitable for research into alcoholism since linkage effects of random probes to a single locus may be weak, and therefore difficult to detect in small numbers of families, in which definition of the phenotype may be problematical.

The molecular biological techniques required to perform such studies are well established. Direct genotyping is possible when the cDNA (which is complementary to the exons or coding regions) of the gene in question has been cloned and detailed sequencing performed. This knowledge is used to design specific oligonucleotide primers for use in the Polymerase Chain Reaction, the primers acting as templates so that the polymorphic region of the sequence may be amplified. Differences between allelic forms that are distinguished by a single base mutation are then detected by hybridisation (or binding) with specific probes after utilising appropriate restriction enzymes which cut DNA at the mutation site.

Alternatively, larger probes for putative candidate genes may be generated for Restriction Fragment Length Polymorphism (RFLP) analysis (Botstein, White, Skolnick & Davis, 1980). These can be derived from screening DNA libraries and therefore do not necessarily depend on detailed sequencing information being avaliable. They can therefore be used in linkage studies of random probes or candidate genes. Here the specificity lies in the ability of restriction endonucleases to cut DNA at sites of specific base sequences. Variations in DNA sequence, or polymorphisms, at identical sites on a pair of homologous chromosomes may prevent the recognition of a cutting site, resulting in differences in the length of fragments produced after digestion. With this technique different allelic forms are recognised by the hybridisation of the probe to these restriction fragments. The technique of Southern blotting (Southern, 1975) allows immobilisation of these fragments on filters, so that several different probes may be used on the same sample. Thus, RFLPs may serve as markers for allelic forms of a particular genetic locus, allowing them to be traced in population or family studies. Furthermore, if genomic rather than cDNA probes are used, polymorphisms in intronic (noncoding) parts of the gene may be detected, possibly reflecting differences in gene regulation.

If linkage is shown between a particular disorder and a candidate gene in family studies, it is highly likely that the gene is implicated in that disorder.

If linkage studies are negative, or families are unavailable, studies have to be limited to the population at large. An association is said to exist if the frequency of a particular allele is significantly increased in affected subjects compared with controls. The presence of association without linkage does not necessarily imply that a candidate gene is implicated causally in a disorder as there are other possible explanations (see Parsian *et al.*,1990): 1) this may occur by chance in small samples; 2) related individuals may be sampled as opposed to a true cross-section of the population; 3) population stratification may occur; 4) the sample population may be racially heterogenous, with differing gene frequencies in each group; 5) epistasis, or inter-action between multiple genes may be operating. Given the difficulties of collecting well-characterised families of alcoholics, this is a frequent problem.

Problems with clinical genetic studies

Clinical studies of genetic markers for alcoholism in populations (or families) have encountered certain difficulties. If a polygenic model accounts for most of the susceptibility, large numbers of subjects need to be included as the effects of a single locus may be weak or masked, and to lessen the chance of population stratification or disproportionate sampling of inter-breeding groups. Ideally such studies should be prospective to allow optimum collection of clinical data. DNA for study can be obtained from peripheral blood leuco-coytes, so that collection of other tissue is unnecessary.

In order to maximise the chance of detecting a true genetic effect, the selection of controls and definition of alcoholics is crucial. Both should obviously be drawn from identical racial groups and have similar sex distribution, age being of less importance although large differences should be avoided as this would affect the expected frequency of alcoholism in the sample. Although some workers have argued that a random population sample is adequate as a control group (Gelertner et al., 1991), it seems likely that screening controls to exclude alcoholism would increase the chance of detecting a difference, especially as the average population frequency of alcoholism in the Western countries is of the order of 10%. Banks of DNA compiled for the investigation of another disorder should not be used if their racial make-up is uncertain or if they are affected by a disease directly or indirectly related to alcoholism or the marker gene being used. It is equally important to document alcoholic patients for the full range of alcohol related disorders, as if they were separate entities. Thus medical complications such as cirrhosis, peripheral neuropathy, pancreatitis, etc. should be screened for with the same detail as that used in psychiatric interviews to detect dependency. This can only be done with co-operation between disciplines, and by using standardised protocols so that data from several studies can be pooled.

Other techniques

Other indirect evidence of predisposition may be obtained from studies of phenotypes in sons of alcoholics who have not developed alcoholism. This approach has been used for a number of neuro-physiological and biochemical markers (Ehlers & Schukit, 1988; Polick and Bloom, 1988; Von Knorring, Halmann, Von Knorring & Oreland, 1991). Animal studies of, for example, strains of rats bred to express preferences for alcohol may reveal physiological, biochemical and genetic information. These are alluded to elsewhere in this volume.

Genetic Markers

Alcohol dehydrogenase

The alcohol dehydrogenase (ADH) genes are obvious choices for candidate genes for both alcoholism and alcohol induced organ damage. ADH (E.C. 1.1.1.1) plays a central and rate-limiting role in ethanol metabolism, accounting for approximately 90% of ethanol elimination by the liver (Crabb, Bosron & Li, 1987) as well as contributing to gastric first pass metabolism (Frezza *et al.*, 1990). In addition, it has been directly implicated in the pathogenesis of alcoholism and alcoholic liver disease, particularly in relation to the properties of its highly toxic metabolite, acetaldehyde (Peters & Ward, 1988). For example, the ability of acetaldehyde to form adducts with some proteins in the liver *in vitro* and *in vivo* resulting in the formation of neoantigens, which contribute to autoimmune damage in alcoholic hepatitis, has been shown to be dependent upon ADH activity (Lin *et al.*,1988; Lin & Lumeng, 1990). Similarly tetrahydroisoquinolones (THIQs), produced by the condensation of acetaldehyde and biogenic amines, have been implicated in dependency (Collins, Rom, Borge, Teas & Goldfarb, 1979). Thus , variations in ADH activity may relate to both alcoholism and varying susceptibility to organ damage.

In the last 10 years, the biochemistry and molecular genetics of the 20 or more ADH isoenzymes have been elucidated (Bosron & Li, 1986; Hittle & Crabb, 1988; Yoshida, 1990). Five major gene loci, ADH_{1-5}, encoding 5 different polypeptide subunits α, β, γ, χ, and π, have been isolated so far. There are three classes of ADH isoenzymes. Class I enzymes, which are encoded by ADH_{1-3} genes, are the more important for ethanol metabolism in man in terms of enzyme kinetics (Bosron, Magnes & Li, 1983). ADH_1, ADH_2 and ADH_3 have been mapped to the long arm of chromosome 4, where they lie adjacent to each other (Smith, 1986,1988; Yasunami, Kikuchi, Sarapata & Yoshida, 1990). The ADH_2 and ADH_3 loci are polymorphic, consisting of 3 and 2 allelic forms, respectively. Cloning and sequencing of the cDNAs for each of these 3 genes has revealed that the 3 alleles of ADH_2 ($ADH_2{}^1$,$ADH_2{}^2$ and $ADH_2{}^3$) have a high degree of conservation (Duester, Smith, Bilanchone & Hatfield, 1986; Ikuta, Szeto & Yoshida, 1986). In fact, the polypeptides encoded by these alleles (β_1, β_2 and β_3) differ only by a single amino acid substitution encoded by a single base difference in the DNA sequence (Matsuo, Yokoyama & Yokoyama, 1989). In their active forms, ADH isoenzymes consist of homo- or hetero-dimers of two polypeptide subunits. Only β and γ subunits have the ability to form homo- or heterodimers with other α, β and γ subunits. Comparisons of the *in vitro* catalytic properties of β_1, β_2 and β_3 homodimers reveal marked differences (Bosron and Li, 1986) suggesting that the variation in ethanol elimination observed *in vivo* is genetically determined at this locus in some individuals. Data from starch gel electrophoresis of liver tissue has shown that there is marked inter-racial variation in the frequency of the β subunits, with β_1 predominant in Caucasians, β_2 in Orientals and β_3 occuring only in Afro-Caribbeans (Agarwal, Harada & Goedde, 1981; Bosron, Li & Vallee, 1980). The ADH_3 locus also shows inter-racial variation (Harada, Misawa, Agarwal & Goedde, 1980). However, such techniques are unable to demonstrate the heterozygous state of any locus with any certainty.

The first studies of ADH genotyping in alcoholics were performed by Shibuya and Yoshida (1988) in Japanese. Forty nine non-alcoholic controls and 23 patients with histologically proven alcoholic liver disease (ALD) were studied. Genotyping was performed by double digestion of leucocyte DNA with EcoR1 and PvuII restriction enzymes, followed by electrophoresis and in-gel hybridisation with oligonucleotide probes specific for the $ADH_2{}^1$ and $ADH_2{}^2$ alleles. The control subjects showed allele frequencies of 0.29 for $ADH_2{}^1$ and 0.71 for $ADH_2{}^2$, which did not significantly differ from the ALD group. Not surprisingly, the predominant genetic effect in this population was the aversive effect of the mutant allele for the acetaldehyde dehydrogenase ($ALDH_2$) gene (see below).

Further information on Orientals was provided by a study of genotyping in male Taiwanese by Thomasson *et al.* (1991). Forty nine non-alcoholic controls and 47 patients diagnosed as having alcohol dependency by DSM-III criteria were studied. Methodology was

similar to that used by Xu *et al.*, (1988), employing PCR and oligonucleotide probe hybridisation. When ADH_2 and ADH_3 allele frequencies were examined independent of the effects of $ALDH_2$ genotype,
by looking at homozygotes for the wild type of $ALDH_2$ only, the
alcoholics were found to have reduced frequencies of both $ADH_2{}^2$
and $ADH_3{}^1$. Since the isoenzymes encoded by these two alleles cause
an increased rate of acetaldehyde formation, it was postulated that
they may have contributed to aversion to ethanol intake. Although
this appears to be a significant finding in an Oriental population, no
information was given as to the severity of the alcohol dependency
in the patient sample, or the presence of medical complications.

Only three studies have been performed to date in Caucasians. In
the first, Couzigou *et al.* (1990) studied 46 alcoholic patients judged
to have cirrhosis by clinical criteria (AC) and 39 medical students
with low alcohol intakes . All controls were male, as opposed to 31
out of 46 of the AC group, who were of a much higher median age
than the students (57 *vs* 23 yrs). Genotyping was performed by PCR
amplification and restriction enzyme digestion. Overall, the frequency of the $ADH_2{}^2$ allele was less than 2.5% in controls and alcoholics, with no homozygotes being detected in this population. This
was much lower than the frequency inferred from previous phenotypic isoenzyme studies, which suggested that the β_2 isoform was
present in 5 to 20% of Caucasians (Bosron & Li, 1986; Coutelle *et al.*,
1989). No significant differences were seen in the frequencies of the
$ADH_3{}^1$ and $ADH_3{}^2$ alleles between the two groups. It is not therefore
possible to comment on the significance of the ADH_2 gene from this
study, although it can be concluded that coding diferences in the
ADH_3 gene do not appear to confer susceptibility to ALD in French
Caucasians.

In a comprehensive study looking at ADH_2, ADH_3 and $ALDH_2$
genotypes in a relatively homogenous population derived from the
northeast of England, Day *et al.* (1991) studied 59 patients with
alcohol-related cirrhosis, 13 with alcoholic chronic pancreatitis and
79 randomly selected control subjects. Not surprisingly, all subjects
were homozygous for the wild type of $ALDH_2$. The incidence of the
$ADH_2{}^2$ genotype was virtually nil, with only one of the controls
heterozygous for this allele. Although an increase in $ADH_3{}^1$ allele
frequency was seen in the patients with alcoholic cirrhosis and pancreatitis, this was of only borderline statistical significance. No other
information, such as sex, age, degree of alcohol dependence etc.,
which could have aided interpretation of these results, was mentioned. Taken together with data from Couzigou *et al.*, and our recent

studies on British Caucasians (Sherman *et al.*, 1992, in preparation), it can be concluded that there is currently no evidence for an association of an allele of the ADH_3 locus with alcoholic liver disease in Caucasian populations.

There is clearly a need for large studies of ADH genotyping in various racial groups and well characterised alcoholics to establish accurate allele frequencies and to determine their role in susceptibility. Demonstration of a relationship between such a marker and clinical severity would provide strong evidence. However, in the case of Orientals it is possible that genetic susceptibility for aversion to ethanol overrides any other influence, whereas outcome in Caucasians is determined by susceptibility genes for addiction and/or organ damage.

A number of RFLPs for the ADH_2 and ADH_3 genes have been detected (Pandolfo & Smith, 1988; Smith, 1988; Shah, McPherson, Ward, Peters & Yoshida, 1989), but until recently there have been no studies of these polymorphisms in alcoholism. We have recently demonstrated a two allele polymorphism to a 1.3 Kb genomic probe for the ADH_2 gene (denoted ADH36) in Caucasians (Smith, 1986; Peters *et al.*, 1991). We proceeded to study this RFLP in 23 non-alcoholic controls and 46 alcoholic patients. All subjects were Caucasian and unrelated. Sex distribution was similar in the two groups (56% male in the controls, 58% in the alcoholics), but the control group was younger (36 vs. 54 years). Liver histology was available in 39 patients: 26 had cirrhosis (16 with co-existent alcoholic hepatitis), 5 alcoholic hepatitis alone and 8 fatty liver. Twenty one patients were diagnosed as having alcohol dependency on the basis of appropriate clinical features and/or a positive postal questionnaire. In this respect all but two patients conformed to Cloninger Type 1 alcoholics. A positive family history for alcoholism (at least one first degree relative affected) was obtained in 19 patients.

The two alleles, A and B, were denoted by a 5.1 Kb band and a 3.1/2.9 Kb doublet, respectively, on Southern hybridisation. Overall comparison between the two groups showed a highly significant increase in the frequency of the B allele in the alcoholics (0.63) versus controls (0.15), ($X^2 = 25.8$, $p < 0.001$). The degree of significance was maintained if the alcoholic group was compared to the controls with respect to liver histology, dependency and family history. In addition, there was an association of the B allele with severity of liver diseasea greater proportion of those with cirrhosis and/or alcoholic hepatitis had the B allele than those with fatty liver alone ($X^2 = 10.76$, $p < 0.05$).

This study has therefore demonstrated a strong association of an ADH36 RFLP marker for the ADH_2 gene with both alcoholism and alcoholic liver disease in a Caucasian population. The correlation between the frequency of the B allele and severity of liver involvement suggests that this may be the strongest effect operating. These findings raise the possibility that inherited variations in ethanol metabolism resulting from polymorphism of the ADH_2 gene may confer an increased susceptibility to alcoholic liver disease and alcohol dependency on the individual. It remains to be seen whether the mutation responsible for this RFLP is derived from a coding or non-coding sequence. However, if further work confirms these results, it is likely to be a most informative marker, and possibly provide further insight into the pathogenesis of some alcohol related disorders.

Aldehyde dehydrogenase

There is extensive heterogeneity of the aldehyde dehydrogenase enzyme. Based on their separation by physical techniques, tissue subcellular distributions and enzymatic properties, at least nine isoenzymes of aldehyde dehydrogenase (EC 1.2.1.3) have so far been distinguished. The aldehyde dehydrogenase enzymes in the cytosol ($ALDH_1$) and mitochondria ($ALDH_2$) of liver have been isolated, the amino acid sequences determined (Hempel, Kaiser & Jornvall, 1985) and the genes cloned and sequenced (Hsu, Bendel & Yoshida , 1988; Hsu, Chang & Yoshida, 1989). The two forms are closely related, there being 68% sequence homology between the subunits. Mitochondrial aldehyde dehydrogenase is considered to play the major role in acetaldehyde oxidation in the liver, its K_m for acetaldehyde being approximately 100 fold lower (1 μmol/l) than that of the cytosolic $ALDH_1$ (approximately 100 μmol/l). A third isoenzyme, $ALDH_x$, has also been cloned and sequenced (Hsu and Chang, 1991). The degree of resemblance between the deduced amino acid sequence of $ALDH_x$ and those of $ALDH_1$ and $ALDH_2$ are 67.8% and 72.5%, respectively. These three isoenzymes all show the presence of amino acids: *Cys-162, Cys-302, Glu-268, Glu-487, Gly-223, Gly-225, Gly-229, Gly-245,* and *Gly-250,* which have been implicated in both the structural and functional importance of the enzyme activity. However, the substrate specificity and physiological role of $ALDH_x$ remain to be elucidated.

The isoenzymes $ALDH_3$ and $ALDH_4$ have been identified in the liver. $ALDH_3$ exhibits optimal activity for both benzaldehyde and long chain aliphatic aldehydes while $ALDH_4$ oxidises short chain aliphatic aldehydes. Both of these isoenzymes have a high K_m for acetaldehyde (in the mmolar range). γ-ALDH, also found in the liver, has a low K_m for acetaldehyde (μmolar range) but is most active for oxidation of γ-aminobutyraldehyde. Brain $ALDH_1$ is thought to be similar in its activity to the liver cytosolic $ALDH_1$ isoenzyme and to play an important role in the metabolism of neurotransmitters. Two other brain mitochondrial ALDH isoenzymes, ($ALDH_{2a}$ and $ALDH_{2b}$) both oxidise acetaldehyde and 3,4,-dihydroxyphenyl-acet-aldehyde (DOPAL) (Yoshida, Hsu and Yasunami, 1990). A further ALDH isoenzyme, which shows a relatively low Km for acetalde-hyde (106 μmol/l), has been identified in saliva although little is known as yet of its amino acid sequence (Yoshida et al., 1990).

Acetaldehyde

Acetaldehyde is the primary oxidative metabolite of ethanol in vivo and is considered to participate in the toxicity of ethanol . It has been implicated in liver disorders, cardiac abnormalities, the foetal alco-hol syndrome, changes in membrane composition, membrane trans-port disorders, aversive behaviour towards ethanol, tolerance accompanied by alterations in various membrane components, changes in membrane fluidity; reinforcement, tolerance and physical dependence; and in the antabuse effect (Latge, Lamboeuf, Roumec & de Saint Blanquat, 1987). Acetaldehyde will also bind to free amino groups of proteins, including a 37 kilodalton hepatic protein, the acetaldehyde adduct of which may elicit an antibody response (Lin, Smith & Lumeng, 1988; Lin & Lumeng, 1990).

Such effects have been attributed to the physico-chemical proper-ties of acetaldehyde, particularly its ability to bind to reactive groups of proteins (Lucas et al.,1986); and its reactivity towards cysteine and glutathione, coenzyme A, biogenic amines, haemoglobin, membrane phospholipids; and damage to mitochondria (either by reducing the aldehyde dehydrogenase activity or changing the intracellular redox potential), thus causing profound metabolic consequences. Never-theless it is difficult to isolate the specific participation of acetalde-hyde in the numerous effects of chronic alcoholism (Peters & Ward, 1988).

This diversity of action for acetaldehyde may relate in part to its distribution and concentration within certain tissues and in part to the presence of specific acetaldehyde dehydrogenases for its oxida-tion to acetate. Tissue and blood acetaldehyde concentration will principally be determined by the rate of elimination of ethanol by alcohol dehydrogenase and secondly the rate of oxidation of acetaldehyde to acetate by acetaldehyde dehydrogenase.

Increased blood concentrations of acetaldehyde have been demonstrated in alcoholics (Korsten, Matsuzaki, Feinman, & Leiber, 1975), although other investigators, including Eriksson and Peachey (1980) could not identify a difference in blood acetaldehyde concentration in comparison with controls. These diverse results must reflect a multitude of variables in such studies e.g: the methodology for acetaldehyde determination (Eriksson & Peachey, 1980; Peters, Ward, Rideout & Lim, 1987), the mode of administration of ethanol, in addition to the heterogeneity of the alcoholic subjects investigated with regard to end organ damage and time of withdrawal from ethanol. Indeed, in a well controlled study where the tolerance of alcoholic subjects to an alcohol challenge was tested one week after admission for detoxification, there were marked differences in blood acetaldehyde levels only between those alcoholic subjects defined as dependent by questionnaire, clinical features and biochemical criteria compared to non-dependent alcohol abusers (Peters & Ward, 1988).

The increased blood acetaldehyde found in alcoholics would be influenced by a variety of factors including ADH genotype and activity of cytochrome P450 IIE1 of the Microsomal Ethanol Oxidising System (MEOS) , both of which will influence the ethanol elimination rate (high elimination rates could lead to more frequent alcohol consumption while slower rates of ethanol degradation would prolong the length of the drug effect, both of which may ultimately influence physical dependence), and the activities of both the erythrocyte and hepatic aldehyde dehydrogenase isoenzymes. It is clear that in order to assess such influences it is important to identify both biochemical and genetic changes that may occur, which will determine both protective and predisposing factors to alcohol drinking behaviour.

Mutant ALDH$_2$

In the past decade a mutant form of ALDH$_2$ (ALDH$_2{}^2$) has been detected (Goedde, Harada, & Agarwal, 1979). The mutation in the ALDH$_2$ enzyme has been identified by its amino acid substitution of a glutamic acid for a lysine residue at the 14th position from the C-terminus (487th position from the amino terminus) (Hempel et al., 1987), and in the gene by a point mutation with a substitution of GC for AT in exon 12 (Yoshida, Wang& Dave, 1983). Homozygotes for the genotype $ALDH_2^2$ exhibit markedly reduced activity of the $ALDH_2$ enzyme, and a significant effect on the enzyme is also seen in heterozygotes.

Studies of limited pedigrees have shown an autosomal co-dominant mode of inheritance (Goedde & Agarwal, 1987). A study of 85 individuals from 2 extended and 18 nuclear families from China (12), Japan (6) and South Korea (2) showed a linear transmission of the normal and mutant alleles, with the mutant allele $ALDH_2^2$ showing dominance over the $ALDH_2^1$ allele (Singh et al., 1989). The presence of this genetic variant $ALDH_2^2$ has been shown in many studies to be a deterrent to alcohol consumption. The administration of a small amount of ethanol to affected individuals will cause extremely unpleasant symptoms which include facial flushing, dysphoria, tachycardia, nausea and hypertension, all of which are caused by high blood concentrations of acetaldehyde. In the Oriental population the presence of the normal Caucasian $ALDH_2^1$ gene is associated with a much higher prevalence of alcoholism. Orientals with the mutant isoenzyme show reduced ethanol consumption (Ohmori *et al.*,1986). A significantly lower incidence of the mutant $ALDH_2^2$ genotype was observed in a group of alcoholic Japanese patients compared to schizophrenic patients, drug dependents and healthy controls (Harada, Agarwal, Goedde, Tagaki & Ishikawa, 1982). Only 2% of 175 alcoholics were found to have this mutant gene, whereas in drug dependents, schizophrenics and healthy controls the incidence was more than 40% (Goedde & Agarwal, 1990), suggesting an aversive effect specific to ethanol. Similarly, Shibuya and Yoshida (1988) genotyped healthy subjects and patients with alcoholic liver disease. They showed that of the 49 control subjects 21 were homozygous for wild type $ALDH_2$ (*i.e.* $ALDH_2^1$ / $ALDH_2^1$), 22 were heterozygous ($ALDH_2^1$ / $ALDH_2^2$), and 6 were homozygous for the mutant $ALDH_2$ ($ALDH_2^2$ / $ALDH_2^2$). In contrast, in the patients with alcoholic liver disease, 20 were of the wild type $ALDH_2^1$, 3 were heterozygous but none showed the homozygous mutant genotype, thus confirming the advantage that the inheritance of this mutant isoenzyme confers against the development of alcoholism. More recently, Thomasson *et al.* (1991) determined the genotypes of the $ALDH_2$ loci in the leucocyte DNA of alcoholics and non-alcoholic Chinese men and similarly showed a lower frequency of the $ALDH_2^2$ allele in the alcoholics compared to the non-alcoholics.

Recently, Enomoto, Takase, Takada and Takada (1991) attempted to correlate estimated alcohol consumption and histological severity of alcoholic liver disease with $ALDH_2$ genotype. Of the 47 patients studied, 40 were heterozygotes for the wild type $ALDH_2{}^1$, the remaining seven were heterozygotes for the mutant $ALDH_2{}^2$, and no homozygotes for $ALDH_2{}^2$ were found. In this small sample, the mean daily alcohol intake was lower in the heterozygotes compared to those homozygous for $ALDH_2{}^1$, and despite this they had more severe liver histology. Since heterozygotes show significant lowering of $ALDH_2$ activity and increases of blood acetaldehyde (Enomoto, Takase, Yasukara & Takada, 1991), the implications of this study are that acetaldehyde must be involved in the pathogenesis of alcoholic liver disease, and that heterozygotes are susceptible to liver damage at lower cumulative doses of ethanol than $ALDH_2{}^1$ homozygotes. It also demonstrates that phenotypic studies (Takase, Takada, Yasukara & Tsutsumi, 1989) may have underestimated the allele frequency of $ALDH_2$ in alcoholic liver disease.

Numerous epidemiological studies have identified the phenotypes and genotypes of the mutant $ALDH_2$ in certain populations. Phenotyping studies have shown a high prevalence of this mutant $ALDH_2$ isoenzyme, approximately 50%, in the livers of Japanese and Chinese populations (Goedde, Harada & Agarwal, 1979), while studies of hair root lysates have shown a prevalence of 30-50% for the inactive mutant ALDH isoenzyme in both Oriental populations of Mongoloid descent and South American Mapuche Indians from Southern Chile (Goedde et al., 1986). Only a small percentage of North American Indians, particularly Sioux, Navajo and Mexican Indians (Agarwal & Goedde, 1989) show the presence of this mutant. Since it is not possible to differentiate between homozygous and heterozygous ALDH-deficient phenotypes by the starch or iso-electric focusing gel methods, it is essential to determine gene frequences by enzymatic amplification of DNA with the polymerase chain reaction using allele-specific oligonucleotides. Such studies have shown $ALDH_2{}^2$ allele frequencies in the blood of Korean, Chinese and Japanese populations to be 0.15, 0.20 and 0.35, respectively (Goedde et al., 1989). Other workers measuring $ALDH_2{}^2$ frequencies in Japanese found similar values of 0.35 (Shibuya & Yoshida, 1988) and 0.40 (Shibuya, Yasunami & Yoshida, 1989) in leucocyte DNA, whilst Crabb, Edenberg, Bosron and Li (1989) found an allele frequency of 0.23 in liver DNA samples taken from 24 Japanese individuals.

However, there are some discrepancies between phenotypic and genotypic findings. For example, although it was reported that 40% of South American Indians are deficient in $ALDH_2$ activity (Goedde et al., 1986), the presence of the Oriental mutant $ALDH_2$ allele was not demonstrated by genotyping (O'Dowd, Rothhammer & Israel, 1990). As yet, this mutant $ALDH_2$ gene has not been identified in the Caucasian or Negroid population (Goedde et al., 1986).

Mutant $ALDH_1$

Polymorphism of the isoenzyme of $ALDH_1$ activity had been previously reported in two isolated individuals, one in the liver extract of a Chinese subject who showed four minor bands on electrophoresis in addition to the normal $ALDH_1$ isoenzyme band (Yoshida, Wang & Dave, 1983). Similar additional bands were observed in the red cell lysate of a healthy Thai blood donor (Eckey, Agarwal, Saha & Goedde, 1986). More recently, other variants of $ALDH_1$ have been identified, (Peters, McPherson Ward & Yoshida, 1990; Ward et al.,1991; Yoshida, Dave, Ward & Peters, 1989). Furthermore, we have shown that the low $ALDH_1$ erythrocyte activity in Caucasian subjects is related to an alcohol-induced flush, causing an aversion to ethanol especially in female subjects (Ward, Macpherson, Chow & Peters, 1991). The nature of the flush appears to be different from that of the Orientals , being of shorter duration with no associated increase in pulse rate or decrease in blood pressure, and no increase in blood acetaldehyde. In the families studied, this mutant cytosolic ALDH is inherited in an autosomal dominant fashion (Ward, McPherson, Chow& Peters, 1991).

Hsu , Chang and Yoshida (1989) correlated functional domains with the thirteen exons of the $ALDH_1$ gene, and identified a possible coenzyme-binding region, as judged by *Gly* distribution, β-sheet pattern and residue conservation in part of exons 7 and 8. Exon 9 encodes a feasible active site segment which included the active *Cys* 302 residue which has been impicated as the disulphiram-reactive site (Hempel et al., 1985). Exon 10 and part of exon 9 encode a presumed subunit interaction segment.

Despite extensive studies only exons 7 and 10 have been amplified and sequenced, and these show complete homology to the published sequence of $ALDH_1$ (Hsu, Chang & Yoshida, 1989). Both exons 8 and exon 9 show the correct base pair size after amplification by PCR indicating no major deletion or insertion. Since it is presumed that the active site of the enzyme is attributable to this part of the ALDH gene, the existence of a point mutation in this region in $ALDH_1$ deficient Caucasian subjects who exhibit this alcohol-induced flushing remains a distinct possibility .

Molecular studies of the ALDH₁ and ALDH₂ genes

Two cDNA probes have been used to screen genomic DNA from both Caucasians and Orientals for informative RFLPs (Hsu, Tani, Fujiyoshi, Kurachi, & Yoshida, 1985): a 1.6 Kb $ALDH_1$ clone , which includes a coding sequence for 340 amino acid residues and a 3' noncoding sequence of 538 Kb, and a 1.2 Kb $ALDH_2$[1] clone, which includes a coding sequence for 399 amino acid residues and a short 3' noncoding sequence. Msp1 restriction enzyme shows polymorphism in both Caucasian and Oriental controls for both $ALDH_1$ and $ALDH_2$ cDNA probes (Yoshida & Chen, 1989).

In a further association study Shripakash, Abbott and Mathews (1989) used a 1.8 Kb $ALDH_1$ cDNA probe to study placental DNA extracted from aboriginals and non-aboriginals. After EcoR1 digestion, a 4.2 Kb band was absent in all non-aboriginals and present in 47% of the aboriginals, while a 3.1 Kb band was absent in all aboriginals and present in 20% of non-aboriginals. It was concluded that such genetic polymorphism may be involved in the predisposition of aboriginals to the development of alcoholism, although no information was obtained on the drinking histories or development of alcoholism in the group investigated.

Dopamine receptor genes

The recent cloning of the rat dopamine D_2 receptor gene (Bunzow et al.,1988), subsequent chromosomal mapping and demonstration of a 2 allele Taq 1 RFLP for a genomic D_2 receptor probe (Grandy et al.,1989) have had a profound effect on the clinical genetics of alcoholism. The dopamine receptor genes are clearly plausible candidate genes for alcoholism, in view of their important neuromodulatory role in addictive behaviour, as well as other physiological functions.

A total of eight studies have been published to date examining the role of the D_2 receptor polymorphism in alcoholism. All have utilised the λhD2G1 genomic probe with which Grandy et al. (1989) demonstrated a 2 allele RFLP in Taq 1 digests of human genomic DNA. Using the full length 18 Kb clone, containing 16.4 Kb of non-coding sequence as well as the 3' coding exon, the allele frequencies in 43 unrelated Caucasians were 0.24 for the A1 allele and 0.76 for the A2 allele. Examination of 3 family pedigrees revealed codominant Mendelian inheritance for the 2 alleles.

In the first study in alcoholism Blum et al. (1990) obtained genomic DNA from post mortem brain bank tissue from 35 alcoholics and 35 controls of mixed racial origin. A full length λhD2G1 clone was then hybridised to Taq 1 digests. The subjects were matched for age and gender, but were of mixed racial origin consisting of Negroes as well as Caucasians. All clinical data were analysed retrospectively by 2 psychiatrists. Although full details were not given, the alcoholic subjects were said to have had repeated failure of rehabilitation treatments and to have died of severe medical complications related to their chronic alcoholism. The controls were screened to exclude alcoholism. In this relatively small sample the frequency of the A1 allele was significantly increased in the alcoholics compared with the controls (0.37 and 0.13 respectively, p = 0.002), and the findings for the Caucasian alcoholics and controls (n = 22 and 24 respectively) reached a similar level of significance (p = 0.003). It was therefore concluded that the the D_2 receptor gene may confer "susceptibility to at least one form of alcoholism."

In the same study a number of other probes for likely candidate genes for alcoholism including tyrosine hydroxylase, monoamine oxidase and an alcohol dehydrogenase clone (pADH 13) were analysed for polymorphism to Msp 1 , Eco R1, Taq 1 and Pst 1 restriction endonucleases. None of these probes demonstrated an RFLP associated with alcoholism, although pADH 13 was polymorphic to Msp 1.

The demonstration of such a significant association between a genetic marker and alcoholism was an exciting finding, but also slightly surprising in view of the complex genetic background and heterogenous clinical picture of alcoholism. Bolos et al. (1990) attempted to replicate these findings in a prospective study of 40 well-documented alcoholics and 127 unscreened controls consisting of 62 unrelated cystic fibrosis patients and 65 subjects derived from pedigrees compiled by the Centre D'Etude du Polymorphism Humaine (Dausset et al., 1990). All subjects were Caucasian, 10 of the latter sample originating from France. The alcoholic subjects all required hospitalisation, met DSM-III-R criteria for alcohol dependence, were interviewed according to both SADS-L (Endicott & Spitzer, 1978) and MAST

(Selzer, 1976) schedules, and were excluded if they had co-existent psychiatric conditions and/or drug abuse. It is of note that the presence of any acute medical disorder was also considered to be a reason for exclusion, suggesting that overall this was a less severe group of alcoholics than in Blum's study.

The frequency of the A1 allele was not significantly increased in the alcoholic group compared with controls (0.22 vs 0.18, respectively), even when the former were subtyped according to Cloninger types 1 and 2 (Cloninger *et al.* 1981). The A1 allele frequencies in both groups therefore differed markedly from Blum's study. Two family pedigrees informative for alcoholism according to RDC criteria (Spitzer et al., !978) were also examined for the D_2 alleles, using a model assuming autosomal dominant inheritance and a high level of penetrance. This yielded negative LOD scores, suggesting the absence of linkage of the D_2 gene with alcoholism as defined in this study. In addition, Bolos's group examined a separate polymorphism detected by amplifying a portion of the 3' noncoding region of the D_2 gene by PCR, followed by single strand conformation polymorphism (SSCP) analysis. This also failed to detect any difference between the two groups.

The results from these two apparently conflicting studies must, however, be interpreted in the light of the rather different groups of both alcoholics and controls that they examined. Blum *et al.* excluded alcoholism from their control population, whereas those studied by Bolos *et al.* were randomly selected from reference pedigrees and a group of cystic fibrotics, which were of a younger mean age and were not screened for alcoholism. Similarly, whereas both Blum and Bolos selected alcoholics with severe alcohol dependence syndrome, the former group died of alcohol-related medical complications. Such differences in the characteristics of study groups appear in subsequent studies that have been performed.

Parsian et al. (1991) performed a case-control study of 25 controls and 32 alcoholics derived in part from 21 family pedigrees informative for alcoholism. Some of the controls were non-alcoholic spouses from these families, resulting in a lower incidence of men in the control group (36% compared with 81%), although allele frequency did not differ between the sexes. Although the results obtained in the control group were comparable to Blum et al., with a low A1 allele frequency of 0.06 , the frequency in the alcoholics was more comparable to that of Bolos at 0.20. When Cloninger subtyping of alcohol dependence was performed, A1 allele frequency did not significantly differ between types 1 and 2. However, in agreement with Blum's finding, alcoholics classified as "severe" according to the presence of medical complications or marked physical symptoms of withdrawal had a significantly higher incidence of the A1 allele.

Further study of 12 family pedigrees which showed segregation for the A1 allele did not show any evidence of linkage with susceptibility to alcoholism. The authors discounted population stratification as a cause of association of the D_2 gene with a disorder without linkage, and suggested that it may be acting as a modifying gene in the predisposition to severe physical complications arising from alcoholism.

Noble's group (Noble, Blum, Ritchie, Montgomery & Sheridan, 1991) were meanwhile pursuing the relationship between the D_2 polymorphism and the binding characteristics of the receptor in the caudate nuclei of brain samples from their previous study. Based on a ligand binding assay, the number of receptor binding sites (B_{max}) was found to be decreased in A1 compared with A2 homozygotes, with intermediate values for heterozygotes, in both alcoholic and control groups. Binding affinity (K_d) was reduced in alcoholics but showed no correlation with the A1 allele.

A study by Schwab et al. (1991) investigated a racially homogenous sample from the German population of Upper Bavaria consisting of 69 controls and 45 alcoholic patients admitted for detoxification. The finding of a lower A1 allele frequency of in the alcoholic group compared with controls (0.12 and 0.22 respectively) may reflect characteristics of this racial group, but also illustrates the problems associated with analysis of a racially heterogenous sample such as most North American Caucasian populations.

Comings et al. (1991) broadened the area of study by looking at patients not only with alcoholism but also with other psychiatric disorders in which alterations in dopaminergic transmission have been implicated. These included antisocial personality disorder, depression and drug abuse, all of which have been associated with alcoholism and therefore may have been responsible for the increased incidence of the A1 allele in previous studies. Twenty controls were screened to exclude alcoholism. Analysis of 108 controls from 4 different sources in conjunction with 206 controls from 4 other studies revealed an A1 allele frequency of 0.13 in the total sample and of 0.07 in the 69 subjects in whom alcoholism had been excluded. Patients with Tourette's syndrome (0.26), attention deficit hyperactivity disorder (0.32), autism (0.32) and post traumatic stress disorder (0.26) all showed significantly increased A1 allele frequencies, whereas there was no significant association with depression, Parkinson's disease or panic attacks. The prevalence of alcoholism was not examined in these groups. 104 patients with alcoholism from this study had a highly significant increase of A1 frequency of 0.23, although no information was given on medical complications. Drug abuse and schizophrenia showed increased A1 prevalence only when compared to controls in which alcoholism had been excluded. Examination of family pedigrees informative for Tourette's syndrome failed to show evidence of linkage.

The authors therefore concluded that alcoholism was merely one of a number of disorders in which the presence of the A1 allele exerted a modifying effect. The wide range of conditions implicated and the lack of evidence of genetic linkage simply confirmed that the D_2 receptor probably does not play a primary role in any of these disorders, and that the interplay of genetics and pathophysiology is far more complex. It was also clear that

future studies in alcoholics should attempt to exclude other psychiatric conditions from both patient and control groups.

Another negative study, originating from a group which had also investigated the role of the D_2 receptor in Tourette's syndrome and schizophrenia, was reported by Gelernter et al. (1991). A random population sample from reference families (including pedigrees of Tourette's syndrome and Multiple Endocrine Neoplasia Type 1) was used as a control group , the authors arguing that this did not detract from the power of the study. The alcoholics were derived from patients participating in therapeutic drug trials for alcoholism, and as such were excluded if they had a history of liver disease, abnormal liver function tests or any other coexisistent medical condition. In this respect the selection of subjects loosely resembled that of Bolos et al. (1991), and interestingly the A1 frequencies were similar with 0.20 in the controls and 0.23 in the alcoholics. The lack of an association was upheld when the alcoholics were classified with respect to family history, age of onset and presence of withdrawal symptoms. It was therefore claimed that the original findings of Blum, confirmed to some extent by Parsian and Comings, had been refuted. In response to this Blum et al. (1991) have confirmed their previous findings in 96 alcoholics of varying severity and 43 non-alcoholic controls, demonstrating a higher A1 frequency in severe alcoholics.

In summary, a total of eight studies have been performed in the last 2 years, four of which have shown a significant association between alcoholism and the dopamine D_2 A1 allele. In general, the control groups in the positive studies have attempted to exclude alcoholism, resulting in lower A1 allele frequencies. The use of random population samples from varying sources resulted in higher A1 frequencies and negative results, although in fact the highest A1 frequencies in controls occurred in samples from a) racially homogenous Bavarians (Schwab et al., 1991); b) cystic fibrotics (Bolos et al., 1990); and c) reference families with either Tourette's syndrome or M.E.N. Type 1. There has been considerable debate as to the relative merits of these differing approaches to the ascertainment of control subjects (Holden, 1991).

The relative contribution of increased A1 frequency in alcoholic subjects is also difficult to discern. For example, the results in alcoholics in the studies of Bolos, Parsian, Comings and Gelernter all lie between 0.20 and 0.23. Only those of Blum and Noble's group show much higher allele frequencies. As to whether this is due to the inclusion of patients with medical complications, a conclusion cannot be reached on the data so far. However, given the potential importance of the dopamine D_2 receptor in alcohol dependency, and of Comings' finding of an association with other psychiatric syndromes, it is surprising that no study has shown correlation of A1 frequency with phenotypes such as Cloninger's subtypes or severity of dependence. Future studies will need to document end organ damage, e.g. liver disease, more carefully.

In two recent authoritative reviews Cloninger (1991) and Conneally (1991) have concluded that there was sufficient evidence for association of the A1 allele with alcoholism in the general population (referring to Caucasians), but that there is no linkage of the allele with any variant of the disorder in families. Whether this finding is in fact due to the presence of a psychological factor, itself associated with the A1 allele, that has a high prevalence in alcoholism (or one of its subtypes) remains to be seen.

Other possible markers

A number of phenotypic polymorphisms have been investigated in man in an attempt to find genetic association or linkage between such markers and alcoholism. However, when an association is identified the relationship between the chosen marker and alcoholism is often tenuous. For example, in one study, (Tanna, Wilson, Ainokur & Elston, 1988) a wide range of "random" polymorphic genetic markers (using DNA probes for 30 loci)were investigated in 42 families, some of which contained alcoholic probands. The only marker showing linkage with alcoholism was Esterase-D.

HLA antigens. Histocompatibility antigens, which are encoded by five allelic gene loci on chromosome 6, are associated with a number of diseases, particularly those of an autoimmune origin. Prompted by evidence for autoimune mechanisms in the pathogenesis of alcoholic liver disease, numerous studies have searched for an association between HLA antigens and alcoholic hepatitis and cirrhosis. The majority examined Caucasian populations. It is clear from an analysis of the individual studies that there is no striking association between alcoholic cirrhosis and any single HLA antigen. Some studies failed to correct for the number of antigens tested. The frequencies of Aw32, B8, B13, B27 and B37 were significantly higher amongst patients with alcoholic cirrhosis than in matched controls in a combined analysis performed by Eddleston and Davis (1982), with no evidence of heterogeneity.

In a more detailed study that included questioning on lifetime alcohol consumption, Saunders et al. (1982) compared British Caucasian men and women with similar degrees of alcoholic liver disease, and showed a lower mean duration of alcohol intake in those with HLA B8, suggesting an effect on susceptibility. However, there was no association with mean daily intake. Although these results would imply that a weak association exists between particular HLA antigens and alcoholic cirrhosis, such findings must be interpreted with care, as (i) the prevalence of HLA types will vary between populations; (ii) the effects of alcoholism and cirrhosis were not distinguished; (iii) chance variations could not be excluded. Thus, despite the problems inherent in association studies, the possibility remains that genetic loci encoding certain HLA antigens may be weakly linked to genes involved in alcoholic liver disease.

Blood group antigens. Before the era of molecular genetics, blood groups and other genetically determined serum proteins were used for genetic studies. Serological markers, including 6 blood group antigens and 5 genetically determined serum proteins were analysed by Hill, Goodwin, Cadoret, Osterland and Doner (1975). Deficiency of the S antigen showed an association with protection from alcoholism, although linkage analysis failed to show any relationship between the S antigen and alcoholism. The blood groups Kell, Duffy and Xg did not show any significant association with alcoholism, while the Rh system suggested linkage in repulsion between the D gene and alcoholism. In the same study, the three main types of haptoglobin, Hp_{1-1}, Hp_{2-1} and Hp_{2-2}, showed similar distributions between alcoholics and non-alcoholics, whilst the three common phenotypes of group-specific component, Gc_{1-1}, Gc_{2-2} and Gc_{2-1}, the G_m (a+) or G_m (a-) gamma globulin system, and α_1-antitrypsin failed to yeild any interesting associations with alcoholism. All of the alcoholics and their non-alcoholic relatives had an SS phenotype for complement C3, which was higher than the expected prevelance rate of 50%.

More recent work by Feizi, Wallace, Haines and Peters (1991) confirmed the lack of association of blood group or secretor status with alcoholism in a racially and clinically well-defined population.

The only positive association found was seen with changes in glycosylation of salivary proteins, probably due to effects of alcohol on parotid gland function.

Peripheral markers for central nervous system enzymes. Activities of certain enzymes that are involved in neurotransmission in the brain may be reflected in platelets and lymphocytes. These readily accessible peripheral markers have been studied extensively in alcoholism. Platelet monoamine oxidase (MAO) levels have been shown in many studies to be significantly reduced in alcoholic patients. This may be attributable to ethanol or acetaldehyde-induced metabolic effects, or may signify a genetic vulnerability for the development of alcoholism (Lykouras, Markianos and Moussas, 1989). Other studies have shown correlations with a wide diversity of psychological problems and there is recent evidence for an association with type II alcoholism as defined by Cloninger (Sullivan et al., 1990). There is, however, little evidence at present to suggest that this phenotypic marker may reflect any genetic predisposition that results in altered monoamine metabolism in the brain: *i.e.* it is more likely to be a "state" rather than a "trait" marker. Further molecular evidence resulting from the recent cloning of the genes for MAO-A and MAO-B will help to confirm or refute this.

Adenylate cyclase (AC) is an adenosine receptor-coupled enzyme present in blood lymphocytes and platelets which has been implicated in ethanol-induced CNS damage. AC is activated by receptor stimulation, leading to increased production of the intracellular messenger cyclic AMP (cAMP). In a small initial study, freshly isolated lymphocytes from 10 alcoholic patients showed a significant reduction in basal and adenosine receptor-stimulated cAMP levels in comparison with matched groups controlled for alcoholism and liver disease (Diamond, Wrubel, Estrin & Gordon, 1987). The alcoholics also showed a reduction in the accumulation of cAMP normally seen on lymphocyte incubation with ethanol. In contrast, lymphocytes from alcoholics showed higher basal cAMP levels and increased sensitivity to ethanol exposure after prolongued culture in the abscence of ethanol (Nagy, Diamond, & Gordon, 1988). Although genetic factors may have contributed to the differences in lymphocyte cAMP signal transduction after prolongued culture in comparison with the freshly isolated state, further studies were clearly required.

In a larger study, Tabakoff et al. (1988) found no differences in basal activity of AC or MAO in platelet membranes of alcoholics or controls. However, AC responses after stimulation with fluoride (and other agents) were significantly lower in platelets from alcoholics, including those who had abstained from alcohol for up to 4 years. A recent genetic study using complex segregational analysis of fluoride-stimulated AC activity in families has suggested that this effect can be attributed to a single major locus with a modest multifactorial background (Devor, Cloninger, Hoffman & Tabakoff, 1991). Taken together, these results have raised the possibility that signal transduction by the AC - cAMP system may provide a trait marker informative for alcoholism. Further studies will be required to confirm these interesting findings.

Plasma levels of dopamine β-hydroxylase activity have been shown to correlate inversely with the presence of dementia in alcoholics (Lykouras, Markianos & Moussas, 1989). Since the circulating levels of dopamine β-hydoxylase are in part genetically determined, studies of this gene in patients with alcohol-induced dementia may yield informative results.

Type I collagen gene in cirrhosis. Weiner, Eskreis, Compton, Orrego and Zern (1988) investigated the hypothesis that part of the variation in individual susceptibility to liver disease in alcoholics was due to polymorphism in the collagen genes. This followed from the observation that increased synthesis of Type I collagen occurs in alcoholic cirrhosis. RFLPs at two regions of the pro-α-2(1) collagen gene were demonstrated using EcoRI and Msp I restriction enzymes. Analysis of haplotype frequencies showed that a specific haplotype was increased in alcoholic cirrhotics when compared with alcoholics without cirrhosis and controls. Subsequent studies using other probes have not found a similar correlation, but the possibility remains that a genetic predisposition contributes to some forms of alcoholic liver disease. For example, loci encoding proteins that control collagen metabolism may show more promise as candidate genes than those encoding collagen structure.

Cytochrome P450 enzyme systems. The Microsomal Ethanol Oxidising System (MEOS), which is highly inducible and plays a significant role in ethanol metabolism, exhibits genetic polymorphism and therefore provides suitable candidate genes for study. The gene for the ethanol-inducible cytochrome P450IIE1 has been localized to chromosome 10 and the cDNA cloned (Song, Gelboin, Park, Yang & Gonzalez, 1986). A Taq I polymorphism was found in DNA from North American Caucasians (McBride, Umeno, Gelboin and Gonzalez, 1987).

A related P450 enzyme, Debrisoquine 4-hydroxylase, is also polymorphic and has been studied in a group of patients with alcoholic liver disease (Lauthier et al., 1984). Five to ten percent of caucasians show the poor metabolizer (PM) phenotype, which is inherited in an autosomal recessive manor. Oxidation phenotyping, measured by analysis of urinary metabolites after an oral dose of Debrisoquine, was compared in 100 chronic alcoholic patients with liver disease (30 with fatty liver only, 70 with alcoholic hepatitis and/or cirrhosis) and 100 patients with non-alcoholic liver disease. There was no association between the presence of the PM phenotype and alcoholic liver disease or the severity of liver damage. However the CYP2D6 gene, which encodes this enzyme, has recently been completely sequenced and the PM phenotype attributed to the presence of at least 2 mutant alleles (Kimura, Umeno, Skoda, Meyer, & Gonzalez, 1989). Heim and Meyer (1991) have recently developed a technique for allele-specific amplification of these mutant alleles by PCR, thus opening the way for direct genotyping studies.

Other markers. Alterations in the renin-angiotensin system occur in genetically-selected alcohol-preferring Dahl rats. Increased consumption of ethanol in such rat lines was shown to correlate with a double dose of the "S" allele of the renin gene (O'Dowd & Grupp, 1991), although it remains to be seen whether this allele cosegregates with alcohol preference in breeding experiments. The relevance of phenotypic or genotypic changes in the renin-angiotensin system in man to the pathophysiology of alcoholism is unclear. Brain cyclic AMP-dependent kinase activity has also been proposed as a biochemical parameter associated with the molecular expression of phenotypic alcohol preference (Beeker, Lee, Phung, Smith & Pennington, 1990).

Directions for Future Research and Clinical Implications

It is now widely accepted that alcoholism results from a combination of environmental and genetic factors. The varying responses to ethanol seen among racial groups suggests that their relative contributions may differ between individuals. Despite the enormous strides that have been achieved in this field in a relatively short space of time, we still do not have sufficient information on the number of "major" gene loci that determine an individual's predisposition to alcoholism and its asociated problems, nor on the way that the various genes interact. The difficulties involved in performing linkage studies in families and in interpreting association studies suggest that the way forward lies in large multicentre studies using common clinical criteria, such as that set up by the N.I.A.A.A. (Gordis, 1990). Many of the genes that encode the major neurotransmitters and their corresponding receptors have now been cloned, allowing a large number of genetic polymorphisms to be correlated with clinical, biochemical and neurophysiological variables. Rapidly increasing knowledge of the entire human genome may yield other important genes, in addition to those determining neurophysiological responses and ethanol metabolism. Conversely, genetic studies are likely to provide valuable insights into pathogenic mechanisms involved in alcohol-related disorders.

The pharmacogenetic nature of alcoholism implies that these advances will not yield a pharmacological "cure" for alcoholism *per se,* nor should they be used to diminish an individual's responsibility for his/her drinking problem. However, screening of individuals, particularly in affected families, may be a useful preventative measure. Accumulated evidence for hereditary factors in alcoholism may provide a useful tool to persuade governments to provide increased resources for alcoholism prevention and treatment. The prospect of gene therapy seems unlikely given the multifactorial nature of the condition, and probably undesirable, except perhaps in the case of well documented single gene effects such as the Oriental acetaldehyde flush.

References

Agarwal, D.P. & Goedde, H.W. (1989). Human aldehyde dehydrogenases: their role in alcoholism. *Alcohol,* 6: 517-523.

Agarwal, D.P., Harada, S., & Goedde, H.W. (1981). Racial differences in biological sensitivity to ethanol: the role alcohol dehydrogenase and aldehyde dehydrogenase isoenzymes. *Alcoholism: Clinical and Experimental Research,* 5: 12-16.

Arria, A.M., Tarter R.E., Williams R.T., & Van Thiel, D.H.(1990). Early onset of nonalcoholic cirrhosis in patients with familial alcoholism. *Alcoholism: Clinical and Experimental Research,* 14: 1-5.

Beeker, K.R., Lee, R.C., Phung, H.M., Smith, C.P., & Pennington, S.N. (1990). Genetically determined alcohol preference and cyclic AMP binding proteins in mouse brain. *Alcoholism: Clinical and Experimental Research,* 14: 158-164.

Blum, K., Noble, E.P., Sheridan, P.J., Finley, O., Montgomery, A., Ritchie, T., Ozkaragoz, T., Fitch, R.J., Sadlack, F., Sheffield, D., Dahlmann, T., Habardier, S. and Nogami, H. (1991). Association of the A1 allele of the D2 dopamine receptor gene with severe alcoholism. *Alcohol*, 8:409-416.

Blum, K., Noble, E.P., Sheridan, P.J., Montgomery, A., Ritchie, T., Jagadeeswaran, P., Nogami, H., Briggs, A.H. & Cohn, J.B. (1990). Allelic association of human dopamine D2 receptor gene in alcoholism. *Journal of the American Medical Association*, 263: 2055-2060.

Bohman, M. (1978). Some genetic aspects of alcoholism and criminality: A population of adoptees. *Archives of General Psychiatry*, 35: 269-276.

Bohman, M., Sigvardsson, S., & Cloninger, C.R. (1981). Maternal inheritance of alcohol abuse. *Archives of General Psychiatry*, 38: 965-969.

Bolos, A.M., Dean, S., Lucas-Derse, S.,Ramsburg, M., Brown, G.L. & Goldman, D. (1990). Population and pedigree studies reveal a lack of association between the dopamine D2 receptor gene and alcoholism. *Journal of the American Medical Association*, 264: 3156-3160.

Bosron, W.F., Li, T-K., & Vallee, B.L. (1980). new molecular forms of liver alcohol dehydrogenase: isolation and characterization of ADH_Indianapolis. *Proceedings of the National Academy of Sciences U.S.A.*, 77: 5784-5788.

Bosron, W.F., Magnes, L.J., & Li, T-K. (1983). Kinetic and electrophoretic properties of native and recombined isoenzymes of human liver alcohol dehydrogenase. *Biochemistry*, 22: 1852-1857.

Bosron, W.F., & Li, T-K. (1986). Genetic polymorphism of human liver alcohol and aldehyde dehydrogenases and their relationship to alcohol metabolism and alcoholism. *Hepatology*, 6: 502-510.

Botstein, D., White, R.L., Skolnick, M., & Davis, R.W. (1980). Construction of a genetic linkage map in man using restriction fragment length polymorphisms. *American Journal of Human Genetics*, 32: 314-331.

Bunzow, R.J., Van Tol, H.H.M., Grandy, D.K., Albert, P.,.Salon, J., Christie, M., Machida, C.A., Neve, K.A., & Civelli, O. (1988). Cloning and expresion of a rat D2 dopamine receptor cDNA. *Nature*, 336: 783-787.

Cadoret, R., & Gath, A. (1978). Inheritance of alcoholism in adoptees. *British Journal of Psychiatry*, 132: 252-258.

Cadoret, R.J., O'Gorman, T.W., Troughton, E., & Haywood, E. (1985). Alcoholism and antisocial personality: interrelationships, genetic and environmental factors. *Archives of General Psychiatry*, 42: 161-167.

Cloninger, C.R. (1991). D$_2$ dopamine receptor gene is associated but not linked with alcoholism. *Journal of the American Medical Association*, 266: 1833-1834.

Cloninger, C.R., Bohman, M. & Sigvardsson, S. (1981). Inheritance of alcohol abuse: Cross-fostering analysis of adopted men. *Archives of General Psychiatry*, 38: 861-868.

Cloninger, C.R. (1990). Genetic epidemiology of alcoholism: Observations critical in the design and analysis of linkage studies. In H. Beigleter & C.R. Cloninger (Eds.), *Banbury Report Series (No. 33): Genetics and Biology of Alcoholism* (pp. 105-133). New York: Cold Spring Harbor Laboratory Press.

Collins, M.A., Rom, W.P., Borge, G.F., Teas, G., & Goldfarb, C. (1979). Dopamine-related tetrahydroisoquinolines: significant urinary excretion by alcoholics after alcohol consumption. *Science*, 206: 1184-1186.

Comings, D.E., Comings, B.G., Muhleman, D., Dietz, G., Shahbahrami, B., Tast , D., Knell, E., Kocsis, P., Baumgarten, R., Kovacs, B., Levy, D., Smith,M., Borison, R., Durrell Evans, D., Klein, D.N., Macmurray, J., Tosk, J., Sverd, J., Gysin, R. & Flanagan, S.D. (1991). The dopamine D$_2$ receptor locus as a modifying gene in neuropsychiatric disorders. *Journal of the American Medical Association*, 266: 1793-1800.

Conneally, P.M. (1991). Association between the D$_2$ dopamine receptor gene and alcoholism. *Archives of General Psychiatry*, 48: 664-666.

Coutelle, C., Fleury, B., Couzigou, P., Poupon, R.E., Nalpas, B., Iron, A., Higueret, D., Seric, J., Masson, B., Beraud, C., & Cassaigne, A. (1989). Distribution of β and γ_isoenzymes of hepatic alcohol dehydrogenases (ADH) in France (Abstract). *Alcohol and Alcoholism*, 24: 369.

Couzigou, P., Fleury, B., Groppi, A., Cassaigne, A., Begueret, J., Iron, A., and The French Group for Research on Alcohol and Liver. (1990). genotyping study of alcohol dehydrogenase class I polymorphism in french patients with alcoholic cirrhosis. *Alcohol and Alcoholism*, 25: 623-626.

Crabb, D.W., Bosron, W.F., & Li Ti-K. (1987). Ethanol metabolism. *Pharmacology and Therapeutics*, 34: 59-73.

Crabb, D.W., Edenberg, H.J., .Bosron, W.F.&

Li , T-K. (1989). Genotypes for aldehyde dehydrogenase deficiency and alcohol sensitivity: the inactive ALDH$_2^2$ allele is dominant. *Journal of Clinical Investigation*, 83: 314-316.

Dausset , J., Cann, H., Cohen, D., Lathrop, M., Lalouel, J.M. & White, R. (1990). Centre d'Etude du Polymorphisme Humain (CEPH): collaborative genetic mapping of the human genome. *Genomics*, 6: 676-677.

Day, C.P., Bashir, R., James, O.F.W., Bassendine, M., Crabb, D.W., Thomasson, H.R., Li, T-K., & Edenberg, H. (1991). Investigation of the role of polymorphisms at the alcohol and aldehyde dehydrogenase loci in genetic predisposition to alcohol-related-end organ damage. *Hepatology*, 14: 798-801.

Devor, E.J., Cloninger, C.R., Hoffman, P.L., Tabakoff, B. (1991). A genetic study of platelet adenylate cyclase activity: evidence for a single major locus effect in fluoride-stimulated activity. *American Journal of Human Genetics*, 49: 372-377.

Diamond, I., Wrubel, B., Estrin, W., Gordon, A. (1987). Basal and adenosine receptor-stimulated levels of cAMP are reduced in lymphocytes from alcoholic patients. *Proc. Natl. Acad. Sci. USA*, 84: 1413-1416.

Duester, G., Smith, M., Bilanchone, V., & Hatfield, G.W. (1986). Molecular analysis of the human class 1 alcohol dehydrogenase gene family and nucleotide sequence of the gene coding the β subunit. *Journal of Biological Chemistry*, 162: 2027-2033.

Eckey, R., Agarwal, D.P., Saha, N., & Goedde, H.W. (1986). Detection and partial characterisation of a variant form of cytosolic aldehyde dehydrogenase isoenzyme. *Human Genetics*, 72: 95-97.

Eddleston, A.W.L.F., & Davis, M. (1982). Histocompatibility antigens in alcoholic liver disease. *British Medical Bulletin*, 38: 13-16.

Ehlers, C.L., & Schukit, M.A. (1988). EEG response to ethanol in sons of alcoholics. *Psychopharmacology Bulletin*, 24: 434.

Endicott, J. & Spitzer, R.L. (1978). A diagnostic interview: the Schedule for Affective Disorders and Schizophrenia. *Archives of General Psychiatry*, 35: 837-844.

Enomoto, N., Takase, S., Takada, N., & Takada, A. (1991). Alcoholic liver disease in heterozygotes of mutant and normal aldehyde dehydrogenase-2 genes. *Hepatology*, 13: 1071-1075.

Enomoto, N., Takase, S., Yasukara, M., & Takada, A. (1991). Acetaldehyde metabolism in different aldehyde dehydrogenase-2 genotypes. *Alcoholism: Clinical and Experimental Research*, 15: 141-144.

Eriksson, C.J.P., & Peachey, J.E. (1980). Lack of difference in blood acetaldehyde of alcoholics and controls after ethanol ingestion. *Pharmacology, Biochemistry and Behaviour*, 13 (suppl.): 101-105.

Feizi, T., Wallace, P., Haines, A., & Peters, T.J. (1991). Blood groups, secretor status and salivary Lewis[a], Lewis[b] and 19.9 antigen levels in alcoholics and ethnic origin-matched controls. *Alcohol and Alcoholism*, 26: 535-539.

Frezza, M., Di Padova, C., Pozzato, G., Terpin, M., Baraona, E., & Leiber, C.S. (1990). High blood alcohol levels in women: The role of decreased gastric alcohol dehydrogenase activity and first pass metabolism. *New England Journal of Medicine*, 322: 95-99.

Gelertner, J., O'Malley, S., Risch, N., Kranzler, H.R., Krystal, K., Merikangas, K., Kennedy, J.L. & Kidd, K. (1991). No association between an allele at the D2 dopamine receptor gene (DRD2) and alcoholism. *Journal of the American Medical Association*, 266: 1801-1807.

Goedde, H.W., Agarwal, D.P., Harada, S., Rothammer, F., Whittaker, J.O., & Lisker, R. (1986). Aldehyde dehydrogenase polymorphisms in North American, South American and Mexican Indian Population. *American Journal of Human Genetics*, 38: 395-399.

Goedde, H.W., & Agarwal, D.P. (1987). Polymorphism of aldehyde dehydrogenase and alcohol sensitivity. *Enzyme*, 37: 29-44.

Goedde, H.W., & Agarwal, D.P. (1990). Pharmacogenetics of aldehyde dehydrogenase (ALDH). *Pharmacology and Therapeutics*, 45: 345-371.

Goedde, H.W., Harada, S., & Agarwal, D.P. (1979). Racial differences in alcohol sensitivity: a new hypothesis. *Human Genetics*, 51: 331-34.

Goedde, H.W., Singh, S., Agarwal, D.P., Fritze, G., Stapel, K., & Paik, Y.K. Genotyping of mitochondrial aldehyde dehydrogenase in blood samples using allele-specific oligonucleotides: comparison with phenotyping in hair roots. *Human Genetics*, 81: 305-307.

Goodwin, D.W., Schulsinger, F., Hermansen, L., Guze, S.D., & Winokur, G. (1973). Alcohol problems in adoptees raised apart from alcoholic biological parents. *Archives of General Psychiatry*, 28: 238-243.

Goodwin, D.W. (1987). Genetic influences in alcoholism. *Advances in Internal Medicine*, 32: 283-298.

Gordis, E. (1990). Comments: the NIAAA consortium on the genetics of alcoholism. In C.R. Cloninger & H. Begleiter (Eds.), *Banbury Report Series (No.33): Genetics and Biology of Alcoholism* (pp.213-214). New York: Cold Spring Harbor Laboratory Press.

Gordis, E., Tabakoff, B., Goldman, D., & Berg, K. Finding the gene(s) for alcoholism. *JAMA*, 263: 2094-2095.

Grandy, D.K., Litt, M., Allen, L., Bunzow, J.R., Marchionni, M., Makam, H., Reed, L., Magenis, E. & Civelli, O. (1989). The human dopamine D2 receptor gene is located on chromosome 11 at q22-

q23 and identifies a Taq 1 RFLP. *American Journal of Human Genetics*, 45: 778-785.

Gurling, H.M.D., Murray, R.M., & Clifford, C.A. (1984). Investigations into the genetics of alcohol dependence and its effect on brain function. *Twin Research 3: Epidemiologic Clinical studies*, (pp. 77-87). New York: Alan R. Liss.

Harada, S., Agarwal, D.P., Goedde, H.W., Tagaki, S., & Ishikawa, B. (1982). Possible protective role against alcoholism for aldehyde dehydrogenase isoenzyme deficiency in Japan. *Lancet*, (ii): 827.

Harada, S., Misawa, S., Agarwal, D.P., & Goedde, H.W. (1980). Liver alcohol and aldehyde dehydrogenases in the Japanese: isozyme variation and its possible role in alcohol intoxication. *American Journal of Human Genetics*, 32: 8-15.

Hassanein, T., Wright, H.I., Follansbee, W., & Van Thiel, D.H. (1991). Alcoholic cardiomyopathy in patients with alcoholic end stage liver disease (ESLD). *Hepatology*, 14 (Supplement): 239A. (Abstract).

Heim, M.H., Meyer, U.A. (1991). Genetic polymorphism of debrisoquine oxidation: restriction fragment analysis and allele-specific amplification of mutant alleles of CYP2D6. *Methods in Enzymology*, 206: 173-183.

Hempel, J., Kaiser, R., & Jornvall, H. (1985). Mitochondrial Aldehyde Dehydrogenase from human liver: Primary structure, differences in relation to the cytosolic enzyme and functional correlations. *European Journal of Biochemistry*, 153: 13-28.

Hill, S.Y., Goodwin, D.W., Cadoret, R., Osterland, K., & Doner, S.M. (1975) Association and linkage between alcoholism and eleven serological markers. *Journal of Studies on Alcohol*, 36: 981-992.

Hittle, J.B., & Crabb, D.W. (1988). The molecular biology of alcohol dehydrogenase: implications for the control of alcohol metabolism. *Journal of Laboratory and Clinical Medicine*, 112: 7-15.

Holden, C. (1991). Alcoholism gene: coming or going?. *Science*, 254: 200.

Hrubec, Z., & Omenn, G.S. (1981). Evidence of genetic predisposition to alcoholic cirrhosis and psychosis: twin concordances for alcoholism and its biological end points by zygosity among male veterans. *Alcoholism: Clinical and Experimental Research*, 5: 207-215.

Hsu, L.C., Bendel, R.E., & Yoshida, A. (1988). Genomic structure of the human mitochondrial aldehyde dehydrogenase gene. *Genomics*, 2: 57-65.

Hsu, L.C., & Chang, W-C. (1991) Cloning and characterisation of a new functional human aldehyde dehydrogenase gene. *Journal of Biological Chemistry*, 266: 12257-12265.

Hsu, L.C., Chang, W-C, & Yoshida, A. (1989). Genomic structure of the human cytosolic aldehyde dehydrogenase gene. *Genomics*, 5: 865-887.

Hsu, L.C., Tani, K., Fujiyoshi, T., Kurachi, K., & Yoshida, A. (1985). Cloning of cDNAs for human aldehyde dehydrogenase 1 and 2. *Procedings of the National Academy of Science, USA*, 82: 3771-3775.

Ikuta, T., Szeto, S., & Yoshida, A. (1986). Three human alcohol dehydrogenase subunits : cDNA structure and molecular and evolutionary divergence. *Proceedings of the National Academy of Sciences U.S.A.*, 83: 634-638.

Kaij, L. (1960). *Alcoholism in Twins*. Stockholm: Almqvist & Wiksell.

Kimura, S., Umeno, M., Skoda, R.C., Meyer, U.A., & Gonzalez, F.J. (1989). The human debrisoquine 4-hydroxylase (CYP2D) locus: sequence and identification of the the polymorphic CYP2D6 gene, a related gene, and a pseudogene. *American Journal of Human Genetics*, 45: 889-904.

Kopun, M. & Propping, P. (1977). The kinetics of ethanol absorbtion and elimination in twins and supplementary repetitive experiments in singleton subjects. *European Journal of Clinical Pharmacology*, 11: 337-344.

Korsten, M.A., Matsuzaki, L., Feinman, L., & Lieber, C.S. (1975). High blood acetaldehyde levels in alcoholics. *New England Journal of Medicine*, 292: 386-389.

Latge, C., Lamboeuf, Y., Roumec, C., & de Saint Blanquat. (1987). Effect of chronic acetaldehyde intoxication on ethanol tolerance and membrane fatty acids. *Drug and Alcohol Dependence*, 20: 47-55.

Leiber, C.S. (1982). *Medical Disorders of Alcoholism: Pathogenesis and Treatment*. Philadelphia: W.B. Saunders.

Lelbach, W.K. (1976). Epidemiology of Alcoholic Liver Disease. *Progress in Liver Disease*, 5: 494 -513.

Lin, R.C., Lumeng, L., Kelly, T., Pound, D. (1988). Protein-acetaldehyde adducts in serum of alcoholic patients. In K. Kuriyama, A. Takada, H. Ishito (Eds.), *Excerpta Medica International Congress Series* (pp. 541 -544). Amsterdam.

Lin, R.C., Smith, R.S., & Lumeng, L. (1988). Detection of a protein -acetaldehyde adduct in the liver of rats fed alcohol chronically. *Journal of Clinical Investigation*, 81: 615-619.

Lin, R.C. & Lumeng, L. (1990). Formation of the 37KD protein-acetaldehyde adduct in liver during alcohol treatment is dependent on alcohol dehydrogenase activity. *Alcoholism: Clinical and Experimental Research*, 14: 766 -770.

Lucas, D., *et al.* (1986). Elevated blood acetaldehyde in alcoholics with accelerated ethanol elimination. *Pharmacology*, 32: 134.

Lykouras,E., Markianos, M., & Moussas, G. (1989). Platelet monoamine oxidase, plasma dopamine β-hydroxylase activity, dementia and family history of alcoholism in chronic alcoholics. *Acta Psychiatric Scandanavia*, 80: 487-491.

Martin, N.G., Perl, J , Oakeshott, J.G., Gibson, J.B., Starmer, G.A., & Wilks, A.V. (1984). A twin study of ethanol metabolism. *Behavioural Genetics*, 15: 93-109.

Matsuo, Y., Yokoyama, R., & Yokoyama, S. (1989). Human alcohol dehydrogenase β_1 and β_2 differ by only one nucleotide. *European Journal of Biochemistry*, 183: 317-320.

McBride, O.W., Umeno, M., Gelboin, H.V., & Gonzalez, F.J. (1987). A Taq I polymorphism in the human P450 IIE1 gene on chromosome 10 (CYP2E). *Nucleic Acids Research*, 15: 10071.

Mendenhall, C L., Gartside, P.S., Roselle, G.A., Grossman, C.J., Weesner, R.E., Chedid, A., and the V.A. Cooperative Study Group. (1989). Longevity among ethnic groups in alcoholic liver disease. *Alcohol and Alcoholism*, 24: 11-19.

Morton, N.E. (1962). Segregation and linkage. In W.J. Burdette (Ed.), *Methodology in human genetics* (pp.17-52). San Francisco: Holden Day.

Nagy, L.E., Diamond I., Gordon, A. (1988). Cultured lymphocytes from alcoholic subjects have altered cAMP signal transduction. *Proc. Natl. Acad. Sci. USA*, 85: 6973-6976.

Noble, E.P., Blum, K., Ritchie, T., Montgomery, A. & Sheridan, P.J. (1991). Allelic association of the D2 dopamine receptor gene with receptor binding characterisitics in alcoholism. *Archives of General Psychiatry*, 48: 648-654.

O'Dowd, B.F., & Grupp, L.A. (1991). The influence of the renin gene on alcohol consumption in Dahl rats. *Alcoholism: Clinical and Experimental Research* , 15: 145-149.

O'Dowd, B.F.,Rothhammer, F., & Israel, Y. (1990). Genotyping of mitochondrial aldehyde dehydrogenase locus of native American Indians. *Alcohol: Clinical and Experimental Research*, 14: 531.

Ohmori, T., Koyama, T., Chen, C., Yeh, E., Reyes Jr, B.V., & Yamashita, I. (1986) The role of aldehyde dehydrogenase isoenzyme variance in alcohol sensitivity, drinking habits formation and the development of alcoholism in Japan, Taiwan and the Philippines. *Progress in Neuro Psychopharmacology Biol. Psychiat*, 10: 229-235.

Omenn, G.S., (1975). Alcoholism: A pharmacogenetic disorder. In J. Mendelwicz (Ed)," *Genetics and Psychopharmacology"* (pp. 12-22).New York: S. Karger.

Pandolfo, M., & Smith, M. (1988). A PvuII RFLP in the human ADH3 gene. *Nucleic Acids Research,* 16: 11857.

Parsian, A. & Todd, R.D., Devor, E.J., O'Malley, K.L., Suarez, B.K., Reich, T. and Cloninger, C.R. (1991). Alcoholism and alleles of the human D$_2$ dopamine receptor locus: studies of association and linkage. *Arch Gen Psychiatry,* 48: 655-663.

Peters, T.J., MacPherson, A.J.S., Ward, R.J., & Yoshida, A. (1990). Aquired and genetic deficiences of cytosolic acetaldehyde dehydrogenase; in C.R. C.R. Cloninger and H. Begleiter (Eds.), *Banbury report (33): Genetics and Biology of Alcoholism* (pp. 265-276). New York: Cold Spring Harbor Laboratory Press.

Peters, T.J., Ward, R.J., Rideout, J., & Lim C.K. (1987). Blood acetaldehyde and ethanol levels in alcoholism. *Progress in Clinical and Biological Research,* 241: 215-230.

Peters, T.J. & Ward, R.J. (1988). Role of acetaldehyde in the pathogenesis of alcoholic liver disease. *Molecular Aspects of Medicine,* 10: 179-190.

Peters, T.J., Sherman, D., MacPherson, A.J.S., Ward, R.J., Cook, C., & Gurling, H. (1991). Molecular studies of alcohol-metabolising enzymes by RFLPs (Abstract). *Alcohol and Alcoholism,* 26: 256.

Pickens, R.W., Svikis, D.S., McGue, M., Lykken, D.T., Heston, L.L., & Clayton, P.J. (1991). Heterogeneity in the inheritance of alcoholism: a study of male and female twins. *Archives of General Psychiatry,* 48: 19-28.

Polick, J. & Bloom, F.E. (1988). Event-related brain potentials in individuals at high and low risk for developing alcoholism: Failure to replicate. *Alcoholism: Clinical and Experimental Research,* 12: 368.

Saunders, J.B., Haines, A., Portmann, B., Wodak, A.D., Powell-Jackson, P.R., Davis, M., & Williams, Roger. (1982). Accelerated development of alcoholic cirrhosis in patients with HLA-B8. Lancet, (i): 1381-1384.

Schwab, S., Soyka, M, Niederecker, M, Ackenhill, M., Scherer, J.& Wildenaur, D.B. (1991). Allelic association of human dopamine D2 receptor DNA polymorphism ruled out in 45 alcoholics. *American Journal of Human Genetics,* 49 (suppl): 203.

Selzer, M. (1976). The Michigan Alcohol Screening Test: the quest for a new diagnostic instrument. *American Journal of Psychiatry,* 127: 1653-1655.

Shah, T., MacPherson, A.J.S., Ward, R.J., Peters, T.J., & Yoshida, A. (1989). A PvuII RFLP in the ADH$_2$ gene. *Nucleic Acids Research*, 17: 7549.

Shibuya, A., Yasunami, M., & Yoshida, A. (1989). Genotypes of alcohol dehydrogenase and aldehyde dehydrogenase loci in Japanese alcohol flushers and non-flushers. *Human Genetics*, 82: 14-16.

Shibuya, A., & Yoshida, A. (1988). Frequency of the atypical aldehyde dehydrogenase-2-gene (ALDH$_2^2$) in Japanese and Caucasians. *American Journal of .Human.Genetics*, 43: 741-743.

Shibuya, A., & Yoshida, A. (1988). Genotypes of alcohol-metabolising enzymes in japanese with alcohol liver disease: a strong association of the usual caucasian-type aldehyde dehydrogenase gene (ALDH$_2^1$) with the disease. *American Journal of Human Genetics*, 43: 744-748.

Shriprakash, K.S., Abbott, C., & Mathews, J. (1989). Aldehyde dehydrogenase (ALDH$_1$) polymorphism in the aboriginal population. *Menzies School of Health. Annual Report*, 119.

Singh, S., Fritz, G., Fang, B.,Harada, S.,Paik, Y.,Eckey, R., Agarwal, D.P., & Goedde, H.W. (1989). Inheritance of mitochondrial aldehyde dehydrogenase: genotyping in Chinese, Japanese and South Korean families reveals dominance of the mutant allele. *Human Genetics*, 83: 119 -121.

Smith, M. (1986). Genetics of human alcohol and aldehye dehydrogenases. In H. Harris & K. Hirschorn (Eds.), *Advances in Human Genetics* (pp. 249-290). New York: Plenum Press.

Smith, M. (1988). Molecular genetic studies on alcohol and aldehyde dehydrogenase: individual variation, gene mapping and analysis of regulation. *Biochemical Society Transactions*, 16: 227-230.

Song, B-J., Gelboin, H.V., Park, S-S., Yang, C-S., & Gonzalez, F.J. (1986). Complementary DNA and protein sequences of ethanolinducible rat and human cytochrome P-450s. *Journal of Biological Chemistry*, 261: 16689-16697.

Southern, E.M. (1975). Detection of specific sequences among DNA fragments separated by gel electrophoresis. *Journal of Molecular Biology*, 98: 503-517.

Spitzer, R.L., Endicott, J. & Robins, E. (1978). Research Diagnostic Criteria. *Arch Gen Psychiatry*, 35: 773-782.

Sullivan, J.L., Baenziger, J.C., Wagner, D.L., Rauscher, F.P., Nurnberger, J.I., & Holmes, J.S. (1990). Platelet MAO in subtypes of alcoholism. *Journal of Biological Psychiatry*, 27: 911-922.

Tabakoff, B., Hoffman, P.L., Lee, J.M., Saito, T., Willard, B., de Leon-Jones, F. (1988). Differences in platelet enzyme activity between alcoholics and nonalcoholics. *New England Journal of Medicine*, 318: 134-139.

Takase, S., Takada, A., Yasukara, M., & Tsutsumi, M. (1989). Hepatic aldehyde dehydrogenase activity in liver diseases, with particular emphasis on alcoholic liver disease. *Hepatology*, 9: 704-709.

Tanna, V.L., Wilson, A.F., Winokur, G., & Elston, R.C. (1988). Possible linkage between alcoholism and esterase-D. *Journal of Studies on Alcohol*, 49: 472-476.

Thomasson, H.R., Edenberg, H.J., Crabb, D.W., Mai, X-L., Jerome, R.E., Li, T-K., Wang, S-P., Lin, Y-T., Lu, R-B., & Yin, S-J. (1991). Alcohol and aldehyde dehydrogenase genotypes and alcoholism in chinese men. *American Journal of Human Genetics*, 48: 677-681.

Von Knorring, A-L., Halmann, J., Von Knorring, L., & Oreland, L. (1991). Platelet momoamine oxidase activity in type I and type 2 alcoholism. *Alcohol and Alcoholism*, 26: 409 -416.

Ward, R.J., MacPherson, A.J.S., Chow, C., & Peters, T.J. (1991). $ALDH_1$ deficiency in caucasian subjects. *Alcohol and Alcoholism*, 26: 264.

Ward R.J., McPherson, A.J.S., Warren-Perry, M., Dave, V., Hsu, L., Yoshida, A., & Peters, T.J. (1991). Biochemical and genetic studies in ALDH1-deficient subjects. In T.N. Palmer (Ed.), *Alcohol: A Molecular Perspective* (pp. 139-143). New York: Plenum Press.

Weiner, F.R., Eskreis, D.S., Compton, K.V., Orrego, H., & Zern, M.A. (1988). Haplotype analysis of a type I collagen gene and its association with alcoholic cirrhosis in man. *Molecular Aspects of Medicine*, 10: 159-168.

Xu, Y., Carr, L., Bosron, W.F., Li, T-K., & Edenberg, H. (1988). Genotyping of human alcohol dehydrogenases at the ADH_2 and ADH_3 loci following DNA sequence amplification. *Genomics*, 2: 209-214.

Yasunami, M., Kikuchi, I., Sarapata, D., & Yoshida, A. (1990). The human class 1 alcohol dehydrogenase gene cluster: three genes are tandemly organised in an 80-Kb-long segment of the genome. *Genomics*, 7: 152-158.

Yoshida, A., & Chen, S-H. (1989). Restriction fragment length polymorphism of human aldehyde dehydrogenase 1 and aldehyde dehydrogenase 2 loci. *Human Genetics*, 83: 204.

Yoshida, A., Dave, V., Ward, R.J., & Peters, T.J. (1989). Cytosolic aldehyde dehydrogenase ($ALDH_1$) variants found in alcohlc flushers. *Annals of Human Genetics*, 53: 1-7.

Yoshida, H., Hsu, L.C., & Yasunami, M. (1990). Genetics of human alcohol-metabolising enzymes. In W. Cohn & K. Moldave (Eds.), *Progress in Nucleic Acid Research and Molecular Biology*. Orlando: Academic Press.

Yoshida, A., Wang, G., & Dave, V. (1983). Determination of genotypes of human liver aldehyde dehydrogenase ALDH₂ locus. *American.Journal of Human Genetics*, 35: 1107-1116

Yoshida, A. (1991). Genotypic polymorphisms of alcohol metabolizing enzymes and their significance for alcohol-related problems. In N. Palmer (Ed.), *Alcoholism: A Molecular Perspective* (pp. 127-138). New York: Plenum Press.

Biological Markers of Alcohol Consumption

Mikko Salaspuro
Research Unit of Alcohol Diseases, University of Helsinki, Finland

Alcohol consumption and associated incidence of alcohol related health-disorders increased considerably in most of the western countries from the 1950s to 1980 (Salaspuro, 1991). A significant decrease in alcohol consumption has thereafter occurred in many European countries, but nevertheless hospital inpatients still comprise a large number of alcoholics and heavy consumers. Especially in acute general medical admissions to hospitals, in emergency services and in trauma care alcohol abuse and/or excessive long term heavy alcohol consumption is frequently an essential contributory factor (Jarman and Kellett, 1979; Jariwalla et al., 1979; Skinner et al., 1984; Antti-Poika and Karaharju, 1986; Antti-Poika et al., 1988; Persson & Magnusson, 1987; Rodriques, 1988). On the other hand the failure of both general practitioners and emergency room physicians to recognize a large portion of excessively drinking patients is well documented (Barrison et al., 1980; Solomon et al., 1980; Anderson, 1985; Rydon et al., 1992) and their responsibility to pursue early identification has been stressed (Reyna et al., 1985; Sherin et al., 1982; Anderson, 1985). This contrasts with the assumption that treatment of alcohol problems is likely to produce better results at an early stage of alcohol abuse (Kristenson et al., 1983; Chick et al., 1985; Antti-Poika et al., 1988; Elvy et al., 1988; Wallace et al., 1988; Persson and Magnusson, 1989; Levine, 1990).

Questionnaires

A number of investigators have attempted to devise a simple and reliable screening questionnaire for the detection of excessive alcohol consumption and alcoholism. The most commonly used is the Michigan Alcoholism Screening Test (MAST) (Selzer, 1971). However, the MAST indentifies correctly only 50% of heavy drinkers (Saunders and Kershaw, 1980). The original version of the MAST consists of 25 questions but some abbreviated versions like the Brief-MAST (Pokorny et al., 1972), the Short Michigan Alcoholism Screening Test (SMAST, Selzer et al., 1975), the Malmö-MAST (Kristenson and Trell, 1982) and the Self-Administered Alcoholism Screening Test (SAAST, Stimmel et al., 1982) have also been proven to be useful. However, their reliability in the detection of alcohol-related problems in general practice has also been questioned (Rydon et al., 1992). Other questionnares include the Cage Questionnaire (Mayfield et al., 1974), the Mortimer-Filkins Test (Ennis and Vingilis, 1981), the computer assisted Reich (Reich et al., 1975) and MAST interview (Anderson, 1987), Münich Alcoholism Test (Feuerlein et al., 1977) and AUDIT M (WHO core screening instrument; Anderson,1990). The sensitivity of AUDIT M in the detection of hazardous alcohol consumption (>40g of pure alcohol daily for men and >20g for women) has been claimed to be 80% and specificity 89% (Anderson, 1990). Among young university students screening questionaires such as the modified Malmö-MAST can be recommended for the screening of heavy drinking and alcohol related problems (Nyström et al., 1993b).

It is generally accepted that the questionnaires rather well identify severe alcoholism with its dismal social consequences (Brown, 1979; Bernart et al., 1982; Saunders et al., 1980). Furthermore they have been successfully used in general practice and in mass screening of apparently healthy populations (Wallace et al., 1985 ; Kristenson et al., 1980; Kristenson & Trell, 1982). However, on an individual basis the reliability of personal interviews can be questioned (Orrego et al., 1985; Keso & Salaspuro, 1990a), and accordingly the search for a more objective biological laboratory marker of alcoholism and heavy drinking has been active.

Biological markers

Several laboratory abnormalities are associated with excessive alcohol consumption (Salaspuro, 1986, 1987, 1989; Lumeng, 1986; Watson et al., 1986; Chan, 1990; Salaspuro & Roine, 1993). It is well established that both in the detection of alcoholism as well as in the diagnosis of alcohol related organ damage the sensitivities and specificities of the laboratory markers vary considerably. In addition to ethanol and alcohol-induced tissue injury they may be influenced by many non-alcohol related diseases, enzyme-inducing drugs, nutritional factors, metabolic disorders, age, smoking and so forth (Salaspuro, 1986, 1987, 1989; Lumeng, 1986; Watson et al., 1986; Chan, 1990). None of the present or future laboratory tests can satisfy all the needs required of an ideal marker. It is, for example, clear that both markers reacting to alcohol abuse lasting for a few days (in the detection of relapses) as well as less sensitive markers reacting only to long lasting heavy drinking (screening of general population) are needed. The ideal test should be sensitive, specific, simple and inexpensive. We have to admit that so far none of the tests available fulfills all the criteria of an ideal marker (Salaspuro, 1986, 1987, 1989; Lumeng, 1986; Watson et al., 1986; Chan, 1990; Salaspuro and Roine, 1993). Especially in population studies, the sensitivities of even the newest markers have been shown to be poor (sensitivities < 26% with a specificity of 90% or higher; Nilssen et al., 1992).

Biological markers reflecting the physiological and/or pathological changes occurring in the body after alcohol use or abuse are also called *state markers*. They are aimed to detect, at an early stage, levels of alcohol consumption that are likely to be harmful in the long run. This allows intervention and treatment before severe pathological changes or negative social consequences associated with alcohol abuse have appeared. State markers have an important role in the follow-up of abstinence and may be the earliest indicators of relapses occurring during treatment (Morgan et al., 1981a; Shaw et al., 1979; Irwin et al., 1988). Consequently, their use in the studies on treatment evaluation can be considered to be essential (Keso & Salaspuro, 1989, 1990a,b,c). They may also function as a reinforcing feed-back mechanism during treatment of alcoholics, who thus have a possibility to follow the positive effects of abstinence on these tests.

Major conventional biological markers

1. Ethanol. A simple and specific evidence for recent alcohol use is the detection of alcohol in blood, breath, urine, sweat or saliva. As an example: regular determination of urinary alcohol concentration has been successfully used to assess the reliability of the self-reports on alcohol consumption by patients (Staun-Olsen & Thomsen 1979, Orrego et al., 1985, Caballeria et al., 1988). The test has also been suggested as routine for emergency admissions (Senior & Sloan, 1981).

This kind of testing, however, does not allow the distinction between acute and chronic alcohol use, unless it can be related to increased tolerance towards alcohol. Thus, according to the diagnostic criteria laid down by the National Council on Alcoholism (National Council on Alcoholism, 1972) the following are first level signs of alcoholism: 1. a blood ethanol concentration above 1 g/l in a routine examination, 2. 1.5 g/l in a patient showing no signs of clinical intoxication, or 3.0 g/l at any time.

Alcoholics have, due to metabolic tolerance, a faster rate of ethanol metabolism than non-alcoholics. It has therefore been suggested that this abnormality could be used in the detection of alcohol abuse by simple determination of ethanol elimination-rates after a small alcohol dose utilizing a breath alcohol analyzing device (Olsen et al., 1989). This method, however, requires repeated testing over a longer time period and is thus not well suited for routine use.

Gamma-glutamyl transferase (GGT). Gamma-glutamyl transferase is a well characterized membrane bound enzyme that is generally used in the diagnosis of hepato-biliary disorders (Teschke, 1985; Salaspuro, 1987). At present, it is the most commonly used single laboratory test for the detection of alcohol abuse.

Chronic heavy alcohol consumption has been shown to lead to an increased serum GGT activity in a variable percentage of patients (29-90%) in a number of studies performed during the last two decades (Rollason et al., 1972; Rosalki & Rau, 1972, Myrhed and Bergström, 1976, Kryszewski et al., 1977, Horner et al., 1979, Whitfield, 1981; Chick et al., 1981; Eckardt et al., 1981; Garvin et al., 1981; Gluud et al., 1981; Bernadt et al., 1982; Kristenson & Trell, 1982; Stamm et al., 1984b; Monteiro & Masur, 1985; Moussavian et al., 1985; Ishii et al., 1986; Halmesmäki et al., 1992). In contrast, acute alcohol consumption does not increase serum GGT activity (Clark et al., 1982; Devgun et al., 1985). Neither is it influenced by drinking of 60g of ethanol daily for three weeks (Salmela et al., 1993). However, increased serum activities of GGT are found in man after chronic alcohol consumption before the development of alcohol-related liver injury (Rollason et al., 1972).

In a random sample of middle-aged Swedish males, 16% had elevated serum GGT; in 75% of these the main reason was excessive alcohol consumption and in 2% it was a nonalcoholic liver disease (Kristenson et al., 1980). In another study on apparently healthy men, however, only 50% of elevated GGT values were due to alcohol (Penn et al., 1981). In hospital materials the prevalence of non-alcoholic origins of increased GGT is also high (Whitehead et al., 1981), and the diagnostic value of GGT in the detection of alcohol problems has therefore been questioned (Penn & Worthington, 1983).

The sensitivity of GGT in the detection of heavy drinking among young adult alcoholics is rather poor (15.6% or 37.5% with corresponding specificites of 95.1% or 90.2%, depending on the cut-off limit; Chan et al., 1987). The mean values of GGT, MCV and HDL-cholesterol may be higher in heavily drinking young university students than in occasional drinkers, but because of their poor sensitivity and specificity these measures cannot be recommended for screening purposes in this type of population (Nyström et al., 1993a).

Information about the correlation of GGT to alcohol consumption is controversial as some investigators have found a significant but low correlation between these two parameters (Papoz et al., 1981, Bell & Steensland, 1987) whereas others have not (Gluud et al., 1981; Poikolainen et al., 1985). On the other hand serum GGT correlates rather well (r = 0.55 - 0.66) with reported alcohol consumption in treated alcoholics with a rather low alcohol consumption (Orrego et al., 1985; Keso & Salaspuro, 1989).

The half-life of increased serum GGT is about 26 days (Orrego et al., 1985) and, consequently, in patients with very high initial GGT values, elevated levels can be found even after an abstinence period longer than one month. During abstinence of only a week GGT decreases in almost all alcoholics (Weill et al., 1988). Accordingly a decrease in GGT during total abstinence lasting not more than 7 days —even among those with values within the normal limits—is indicative of heavy alcohol consumption with a sensitivity of 90% (Weill et al., 1988).

In long-lasting alcoholism the activities of serum GGT tend to normalize (Wadstein and Skude, 1979; Morgan et al., 1981a), and this has been related to the length of the drinking episode, which is shortest in most severe alcoholics (Wadstein & Skude, 1979). The probability that the patient has more than six drinks per day increases from 20% to 50% when GGT exceeds 60 IU/l (Chick et al., 1981). In drinking debauches lasting less than 2 weeks, GGT stays within the normal limits (Wadstein& Skude, 1979). In debauches lasting 2-6 weeks GGT exceeded the upper limit of normal, and debauches of more than 6 weeks increased serum GGT values considerably (Wadstein and Skude, 1979).

The worst drawback concerning the use of GGT as a marker of alcohol abuse is its poor specificity. Elevated serum levels of GGT are most often confined to diseases of the pancreas and hepatobiliary system (Whitfield et al. 1972; Lum & Gambino 1972). The GGT level increases in all type of liver diseases and highest levels are seen in obstructive jaundice (Whitfield et al. 1972; Lum and Gambino 1972). The level of GGT correlates slightly with the degree of liver cell necrosis (Wu et al. 1976). Highly overlapping elevations of both serum and hepatic GGT are seen in alcoholic fatty liver, alcoholic hepatitis, alcohol-induced liver fibrosis, and alcoholic cirrhosis (Rollason et al. 1972; Seymour and Peters 1978; Nishimura et al. 1980; Wu et al. 1976; Ryback et al. 1982).

In addition to hepatobiliary diseases, elevated serum GGT is found in many other diseases.In relation to alcohol abuse the most important injury is perhaps pancreatitis. Others include:heart infarct, heart failure, coronary disease, nephrotic syndrome, diabetes mellitus (up to 57% with those with vascular complications), hepatic metastasis and severe trauma (Penn & Worthington 1983; Wadstein & Skude 1979; Agostini et al. 1965; Hedworth-Whitty et al. 1967; Konttinen et al. 1970).

In outpatient alcoholics the highest GGT values are found in patients with either liver cirrhosis or chronic persistent hepatitis (Gluud et al. 1981). Next come patients with chronic pancreatitis, diabetes mellitus, chronic renal disease and those with Yersinia-arthritis (Gluud et al. 1981). The third group is composed of "healthy" alcoholics and their mean GGT is in general lowest and often under the upper limit of normal (Gluud et al. 1981).

Drugs inducing the hepatic microsomal system may increase serum GGT levels. The most important drugs of this group are antiepileptics, anticoagulants (warfarin), and barbiturates (Rosalki et al. 1971; Whitfield, et al. 1973). In patients using these drugs a slightly elevated serum GGT value has no diagnostic importance, but it can be used in the follow-up study of the treatment of the alcohol problem provided that the medication is not changed and that it is taken regularly.

In men overweight by more than 30%, hyperlipidemia type IV, and excess use of carbohydrates have been related to increased serum GGT (Mörland et al. 1977; Mezey 1978). In an extensive population study serum GGT levels became gradually higher in men from 8 to 60 years of age, and decreased again after that. It was concluded that in older overweight men a slightly increased GGT value does not necessarily indicate an excessive alcohol consumption (Schiele et al. 1977). In women, GGT values start to increase after the age of sixteen. Between 40 and 50 years of age, GGT values of men are 75% higher than those of women (Schiele et al. 1977). In men but not in women there is a positive correlation between the weight and serum GGT levels (Sciele et al. 1977). Daily variation in the serum GGT level is minimal and the activity is not influenced by fasting (Rosalki et al. 1971). Consequently, a single determination is reliable.

Mean corpuscular volume (MCV). The association between macrocytosis (increased MCV) and alcoholism was found as early as the 1930s (Bianco & Jollife 1938). The mechanism behind alcohol-induced macrocytosis is unknown, but has been related to the direct toxicity of ethanol on erythroblasts. As a marker of excessive alcohol consumption it has been used since 1974 (Wu et al. 1974; Unger and Johnson 1974). In various materials increased MCV values are found in 26 - 94% of alcoholic patients (Wu et al. 1974; Unger & Johnson 1974; Chalmers et al. 1980, 1981; Morse and Hurt 1979; Morgan et al. 1981b; Chick et al. 1981; Korri et al. 1985; Tönnesen et al. 1986; Thiele and Thiele 1987).

Increased MCV value has been shown to correlate positively with the total amount of alcohol consumed and the length of the drinking period (Tönnesen et al. 1986). The probability that a patient uses over six drinks per day increases from 20% to 60%, when MCV increases from 90fl to 100fl (Chick et al. 1981). As a biological marker of heavy drinking, increased MCV is more specific than GGT. Other causes of increased MCV include vitamin B12 and folate deficiency (Carney and Sheffield 1978, 1980; Chalmers et al. 1980, 1981; Morgan et al. 1981b), liver disease, reticulocytosis, antiepileptics, age, smoking and menopause. Especially among women, in about a third of the cases the cause for macrocytosis may remain unexplained (Seppä et al. 1991). There is also some evidence that macrocytosis is more frequent in women than in men (Chalmers et al. 1980; Morgan et al. 1981b).

Due to the long survival of red cells, MCV normalizes slowly (within months) during abstinence (Renwick & Asker 1982). In some studies MCV has been shown to correlate better with the admitted alcohol consumption than GGT (Chick et al. 1981; Whitfield 1981). Most importantly MCV is inexpensive and can be easily determined in every clinical laboratory, which increases its availability. In addition to increased MCV, other haematologic parameters such as high red cell distribution width may be abnormal in alcoholics

(Seppä et al. 1992). Further studies are, however, still needed to establish their real clinical value.

Conventional biological markers with limited value

High density lipoprotein (HDL) cholesterol. High-density lipoprotein cholesterol (HDL-C) increases as a consequence of excessive alcohol consumption (Castelli et al. 1977). The mechanism behind the phenomenon increasing both HDL2- and HDL3 cholesterol concentrations is not known (Taskinen et al. 1982). Chronic administration of liver microsomal-system inducing drugs and vigorous physical exercise are other but rare factors capable of increasing HDL-C. Consequently HDL-C has been suggested to be a rather specific laboratory marker of alcoholism (Danielsson et al. 1978; Barboriak et al. 1980; Sanchez-Craig & Annis 1981; Hartung et al. 1983). On the other hand alcohol-induced liver injury may decrease HDL cholesterol level (Devenyi et al. 1981) and thereby hamper the reliability of the test.

Seventy-five grams of ethanol daily for 5 weeks has been shown to increase HDL-C (Belfrage et al. 1977). HDL-C returns to preconsumption levels in one to two weeks (Danielsson et al. 1978; Devenyi et al. 1981; Taskinen et al. 1982; Välimäki et al. 1986). The value of HDL cholesterol as a biological marker of alcohol consumption is increased by the fact that it functions also within the limits of normal values in patients without a significant liver injury. With respect to the general use of HDL-C as a biological marker of excessive alcohol consumption it can be concluded that HDL-C is better suited for the follow-up of abstinence in an individual patient than for the general screening of harmful drinking.

Apolipoproteins A-I and A-II. The concentrations of apolipoproteins (apo)A-I and A-II increase after heavy drinking and especially the increased apo A-II level has been suggested as a biochemical indicator of alcohol abuse (Puchois et al. 1984). Daily consumption of 60 g of pure ethanol for 3 weeks leads to elevated apo A-II levels (Välimäki et al. 1988) which, however, return rapidly to normal during abstinence. This renders the test unsuitable as a general screening instrument for excessive drinking.

Ferritin. A high serum ferritin concentration is a frequent finding in patients with hemochromatosis, hemosiderosis, various liver diseases, and inflammatory disorders. In addition serum ferritin may increase after chronic alcohol consumption (Jacobsson et al. 1978, Lundin et al. 1981; Kristenson et al. 1981; Välimäki et al. 1983; Chick et al. 1987). Up to 67% of heavy drinkers with elevated GGT levels, but without any signs of liver disease or manifest blood, gastrointestinal, or inflammatory disorder have been reported to have increased serum ferritin (Kristensson et al. 1981). Both the secreted and intracellular fractions of ferritin are increased in chronic alcoholics and they remain elevated after 11 days of abstinence (Moirand et al. 1991). The use of the test is hampered by its rather poor specificity. Therefore, it is doubtful whether serum ferritin concentration would offer any real advantages as compared, e.g., to GGT.

Alpha-amino-n-butyric acid to leucine ratio. Plasma alpha-amino-n-butyric acid (AANB) increases both in experimental animals and in man following chronic alcohol consumption (Shaw et al. 1976). However, protein malnutrition (Shaw & Lieber 1978) depresses the plasma AANB level, which evidently hampers the use of AANB as a biological marker of alcoholism, especially in chronic alcoholics. Therefore it is better to express AANB as a ratio relative to leucine (L), which is also depressed by protein restriction (Shaw et al. 1976). The specificity of the test is hampered by increased AANB : leucine ratios in nonalcoholic liver diseases (Morgan et al. 1977; Dienstag et al. 1978). Accordingly in later studies the AANB to leucine ratio has appeared to be of limited value as a biological marker of alcoholism (Jones et al. 1981; Herrington et al. 1981; Chick et al. 1982). The discrepancy is most probably due to the rapid normalization of AANB after cessation of alcohol consumption. Nevertheless the test may have some value in the follow-up of alcoholics in rehabilitation programs (Shaw et al. 1979). The determination of the AANB/L ratio is dependent on special laboratory facilities and, consequently the test is not ideal for routine use.

New and future biological markers

Markers of chronic alcohol consumption.

- *Carbohydrate deficient transferrin (CDT)*
An abnormal transferrin variant containing significantly lower concentrations of sialic acid, neutral galactose and N-acetylglucosamine has been observed in alcoholics (Stibler et al. 1986). This abnormality, first reported in 1978 (Stibler et al. 1978, 1979, 1980), has consequently been used successfully to detect problem drinking by several groups (Takase et al. 1985, Stibler et al. 1986, Stibler and Hultcrantz 1987; Schellenberg and Weill 1987, Storey et al. 1987, Behrens et al. 1988a,b, Kapur et al. 1989) and has been shown to be a highly specific

marker even in a racially mixed population (Behrens et al. 1988a). In these studies the sensitivity of the test to detect alcoholism has ranged from 76-91% and the specificity has been almost 100% with primary biliary cirrhosis being the only major disease group producing false positive values in approximately 30% of the cases (Stibler & Hultcrantz 1988; Stibler 1991; Bell et al. 1992). As the half-life of elevated levels is also suitable for a marker (around 2 weeks) and the test has been shown to react to a daily alcohol consumption exceeding 60 g of pure alcohol (Salmela et al. 1993), it has been considered as the most promising new test to detect alcohol abuse.

However, in the screening of heavy drinkers from the normal population, general practice or among drunken drivers (Gjerde et al. 1987, 1988; Poupon et al. 1989), as well as among young problem drinkers (Chan et al. 1989) and university students (Nyström et al. 1992), the sensitivity of the test to detect alcohol abuse has been far less satisfactory. Furthermore unavailability of a simple method to determine CDT concentration has so far limited its general use. Recent release of a commercially available kit (Pharmacia AB, Sweden) will hopefully solve this problem although the relatively high price and the somewhat poorer sensitivity of the test kit as compared to the original method may still limit the use of the test. Another method for CDT determination using isoelectric focusing and Western blotting has recently been suggested for routine use in clinical laboratories (Xin et al. 1991).

• *Blood and urinary β-hexosaminidase (β-Hex)*
β-hexosaminidase (β-Hex; n-acetyl–β-D-glucosaminidase) is a glycosidase, the activity of which is frequently increased in the sera of alcoholics admitted to detoxification treatment (Hultberg et al. 1980; Isaksson et al. 1985). The sensitivity of serum ß-Hex in the detection of heavy drinking has been reported to be better than that of GGT (86% for β-Hex, 47% for GGT; Kärkkäinen et al. 1990b). However, elevated serum levels of beta-hexosaminidase tend to decrease within days after the cessation of drinking (Kärkkäinen 1990, Fikärkkäinen et al. 1990a Wehr et al. 1991), which may hamper the use of the test in the early detection of heavy drinking. Furthermore among young university students β-Hex reflects heavy drinking poorly (Nyström et al. 1991). Most recently isoenzyme B of serum β-hexosaminidase has been reported to be a more sensitive and specific laboratory marker of alcoholism than GGT or total β-HEX (Hultberg et al. 1991).

The alcohol-induced increase in urinary β-HEX may, however, improve the diagnostic efficacy of the test (Kärkkäinen 1990). Moderate drinking of 60g of 100% ethanol daily for ten days is reflected in elevated serum but not in urinary β-HEX levels (Kärkkäinen et al. 1990). The specificity of increased serum and urinary β-HEX is comparable to that of GGT, i.e. abnormal values are also found in many other conditions including liver, renal and some other diseases. Furthermore strenous physical activity, aspirin intake and heat stress may all result in elevated urinary β-HEX levels (Roine et al. 1991). The analysis of β-Hex both in blood and urine is simple and inexpensive, which makes the test widely available in general practice.

- *Mitochondrial aspartate aminotransferase*

The activities of both hepatic and serum aspartate aminotransferase reflect two isoenzymes: cytosolic and mitochondrial. In the liver the mitochondrial isoenzyme is dominant, but in serum it represents only 4-12% of the total activity (Rej 1980). The amount of the mitochondrial isoenzyme (mASAT) increases in serum of alcoholics and especially the ratio of mitochondrial to total aspartate aminotransferase (mASAT/tASAT) has been shown to be a particularly sensitive marker of alcoholism (Nalpas et al. 1984, 1986). An acute drinking bout or non-alcoholic liver diseases do not affect this ratio. Neither do abstinent patients with alcoholic liver diseases exhibit increased mASAT concentrations.

These promising results are so far based mainly on the results of one group and other investigators have not been able to reproduce them either in a large unselected population (Schiele et al. 1989) or among young adult alcoholics (Chan et al. 1989). Further studies are clearly needed before the test can be recommended for widespread use. The lack of a simple and reliable analytical method has, however, to date made extensive testing difficult.

- *Urinary dolichol*

Dolichols are long-chain polyprenols essential for glycoprotein synthesis. Alcoholics have been found to have increased urinary dolichol concentrations and the test has therefore been suggested as a marker for alcohol abuse (Pullarkat et al. 1985, Roine et al. 1987ab), especially as urine samples are easy to obtain. The specificity of the test is, however, limited because some other common conditions are also associated with increased urinary dolichol excretion (Roine et al. 1989b). The use of the test is also hampered by the fairly rapid normalization of urinary dolichol concentrations after cessation of drinking (Roine 1988). Furthermore strenous physical activity, aspirin and heat stress increase urinary dolichols (Roine et al. 1991). Accordingly later studies have revealed the test to be a poor marker of alcoholism and therefore it cannot be recommended for general use (Stetter et al. 1991).

• *Acetaldehyde-hemoglobin adducts*
Acetaldehyde is the first metabolite in the hepatic oxidation of ethanol. It is rapidly further oxidized to acetate in the liver and is therefore normally not released in significant amounts to peripheral blood circulation except in alcoholics with accelerated ethanol oxidation or in those with decreased hepatic elimination of acetaldehyde (Lindros et al. 1980; Nuutinen et al. 1983). Measurable levels of acetaldehyde (0.2 to 68 μM) are found in the hepatic vein (Nuutien et al. 1984), but that naturally cannot per se be used as a marker for alcohol abuse. However, as a chemically very reactive substance acetaldehyde easily forms adducts with other substances. The number of adducts formed is proportional to the concentration and number of exposures to acetaldehyde (Stevens et al. 1981) and therefore it has been suggested that serum levels of acetaldehyde adducts could be used in the screening for alcohol abuse.

The adducts formed with hemoglobin or other constituents of red cells have been extensively studied (Stevens et al. 1981, Hoberman & Chiodo 1982, Peterson et al. 1988, Lucas et al. 1988; Hernández-Muñoz et al. 1989, Niemelä et al. 1990a) and may in the future emerge as useful markers, as more sensitive methods capable of detecting even small amounts of acetaldehyde adducts have recently been introduced (Peterson & Polizzi 1987, Peterson et al. 1988, Sillanaukee & Koivula 1990). With the most sensitive methods acetaldehyde-modified hemoglobins appear to have at least the same sensitivity to detect heavy drinking as the most widely accepted conventional tests GGT and MCV (Sillanaukee & Koivula 1990, Sillanaukee et al. 1991ab; Sillanaukee et al. 1992). However, the specificity of the test is hampered by the fact that these hemoglobin modifications are also found in diabetics and in social drinkers after a single acute dose (2g/kg) of alcohol (Sillanaukee & Koivula 1990; Sillanaukee et al. 1992).

• *Antibodies against acetaldehyde adducts*
The adducts formed with acetaldehyde may function as antigens and can consequently serve as target proteins leading to the formation of antibodies against acetaldehyde adducts (Israel et al. 1986; Hoerner et al. 1986, Niemelä et al. 1987, 1991a; Lin et al. 1990; Worrall et al. 1990). The fact that these antibodies are also found in individuals

with non-alcoholic liver diseases (Hoerner et al. 1988; Worrall et al. 1990) and in human volunteers following acute ethanol ingestion (Niemelä et al. 1990a), however, limits their use as a marker for alcohol abuse.

- *2,3-Butanediol, Salsolinol*

2,3-butanediol is an unusual metabolite of ethanol found in alcoholics. After ingestion of distilled spirits, 79% of alcoholic patients had a serum 2,3-butanediol concentration exceeding 5 µmol/l whereas only 5% of control subjects showed the same abnormality (Rutstein et al. 1983). Most recent evidence indicates that 2,3-butanediol may be derived at least in part from the ingestion of technical alcohol containing 2-butanol (Jones 1991). Extensive studies about the role of 2,3-butanediol in the detection of alcohol abuse are at the moment still lacking.

Increased urinary levels of a cyclic dopamine metabolite, salsolinol, are frequently found in alcoholics (Collins et al. 1979; Sjöquist et al. 1981b; Adachi et al. 1986). Also increased plasma levels of salsolinol sulphate have been reported in alcoholics (Faraj et al. 1989). Most recent evidence, however, indicates that urinary salsolinol excretion does not sufficiently distinguish between alcoholics and nonalcoholics (Feest et al. 1992).

- *Erythrocyte aldehyde dehydrogenase*

Erythrocyte aldehyde dehydrogenase activity (ALDH) has been reported by several groups (Agarwal et al. 1983, Takase et al. 1985, Towell et al. 1986) to be decreased in alcoholics. In one of these studies 78% of alcoholics showed low ALDH activity whereas only 30 % of controls had this abnormality. When combined with MCV, ALDH detected alcoholics with a sensitivity of 75% (Agarwal et al. 1983).

Although these studies are promising, further information about the sensitivity and specificity of the test is still needed before it can be recommended for routine use.

Markers of recent alcohol consumption.

- *Ethanol*

Small but increased levels of urinary ethanol (0.02 - 10 mM) can still be demonstrated by gas chromatography-mass spectrometry in abstaining active alcoholics at the 7th day after hospital admission (Tang 1987). The use of this test either in daily clinical routine or in the evaluation of treatment results has not yet been assessed.

• *Acetate*

Acetate is the second metabolite of ethanol oxidation. As it does not undergo hepatic oxidation during ethanol metabolism it is released to peripheral circulation at the same rate as alcohol is oxidized (Nuutinen at al. 1985). Accordingly it is an indicator of the rate of hepatic ethanol oxidation which, as a consequence of metabolic tolerance, is accelerated in alcoholics (Nuutinen et al. 1985). Serum acetate concentration can therefore serve as a marker of alcohol abuse with relatively good sensitivity and specificity (Korri et al. 1985). A limiting factor, however, is the fact that significant serum acetate concentrations are found only in the presence of alcohol in blood. Acetate is therefore best suited for screening of alcohol abuse in intoxicated emergency room patients or among drunken drivers (Roine et al. 1988b). Furthermore drugs known to enhance the the rate of ethanol elimination, such as glucocorticoids, may produce false positive results (Korri 1990).

• *Methanol*

Methanol is a congener in many alcoholic beverages and some methanol is also formed endogenously. Like ethanol, methanol is oxidized in the liver by alcohol dehydrogenase (ADH). The affinity of ADH for ethanol is, however, much higher than for methanol. Consequently the constant presence of alcohol in the body may inhibit elimination of methanol which therefore tends to accumulate in the blood. Based on this, methanol has been suggested as a marker for alcohol abuse (Bonte et al. 1985, Roine et al. 1989a). After disappearance of ethanol from blood, methanol is rapidly oxidized, and the test is therefore only suited for situations where ethanol is present. In this respect methanol, as a laboratory marker for alcohol abuse, is similar to acetate.

• *Urinary alcohol-specific product*

Stable acetaldehyde-protein adducts can be excreted in urine after protein degradation. The determination of these alcohol specific products has emerged as a new marker of alcohol abuse, especially as their disappearance appears to be slow. In one study the increased amount of alcohol specific products in urine correctly identified 79% of alcoholics abstinent for 24 hours and also 70% of alcoholics after an abstinence period of 7 days (Tang et al. 1986).

• *5-OH-tryptophol*

5-Hydroxytryptophol (5-HTOL) occurs in urine, and is normally a minor metabolite of serotonin. After ingestion of alcohol the catabolism of 5-HT is altered resulting in increased urinary levels of 5-HTOL. 5-HTOL can still be detected in urine several hours after ethanol itself is no longer detectable (Helander et al. 1992). Because urinary 5-HTOL may be strongly influenced by some dietary factors e.g., bananas, it is normally expressed as a ratio of 5-HTOL to 5-HIAAA. The test has been suggested for the detection of recent drinking, but further studies are still indicated in order to establish the true clinical value of this new marker.

Marker Combination

Several investigators have tried to combine two or more different laboratory tests to achieve better sensitivity and specificity in the screening for alcohol abuse. As an example: a combination of seven different laboratory tests reflecting hematologic abnormality, liver injury, cholestasis, effect of ethanol on lipids and tolerance to ethanol (MCV, ALAT, GGT, alkaline phosphatase, bilirubin, HDL-cholesterol and blood alcohol concentration) detected alcohol abuse with a sensitivity of 82% in males and 71% in females, whereas the value of the best single test (GGT) was increased in only 49% of these patients (Cushman et al. 1984). Similarly, combining an indicator of liver injury (GGT) with a hematologic marker (MCV) increased the sensitivity to detect alcohol abuse from 78% and 72% for the two tests alone, to 92%. However, the specificity of this combination was low (40%) (Stamm et al. 1984ab). The combination of acetate and GGT has been reported to correctly detect 71% of heavy drinkers while the percentage for GGT alone was only 35% (Korri et al. 1985). Thus the combination of several markers may increase the sensitivity to detect alcohol abuse, but may do this at the cost of decreased specificity.

The sensitivity of the different tests can also be improved by the application of discriminant function analysis to combinations of biological markers. Employing this method MCV, log10 of GGT and log 10 of alkaline phosphatase correctly detected over 80% of patients with excessive alcohol consumption in a hospital sample of 512 patients (Chalmers et al. 1981). A quadratic multiple discriminant function analysis using 24 different laboratory tests classified 100% of medical ward alcoholics as alcoholic and 100% of medical controls as nonalcoholic (Ryback et al. 1982). Among young adult alcoholics a stepwise linear discriminant analysis using urea nitrogen, potassium and MCV has been shown to correctly classify 89% of alcoholics and 92% of non-alcoholics (Chan et al. 1987). With different test combinations these results have been confirmed by Eckardt et al.

(1981), Bernadt et al. (1984), Hillers et al. (1986), Shaper et al. (1985) & Sillanaukee (1992). Consequently, discriminant function analysis of blood test results appears to be a potentially useful tool in the detection of alcohol abuse.

Tests for Differential Diagnosis

ASAT/ALAT ratio

The ratio of aspartate aminotransferase to alanine aminotransferase (ASAT/ALAT) has been postulated to be a far more reliable indicator of alcohol induced liver damage than either of the enzymes alone. As patients with alcoholic liver diseases—at least partly due to pyridoxal 5'-phosphate depletion—have a low serum ALAT activity in relation to ASAT activity, a ratio of ASAT/ALAT over 1.5 has been said to be indicative and a ratio over 2 highly suggestive of alcohol related liver damage (Cohen and Kaplan 1979, Correia et al. 1981, Spech & Liehr 1983). Our own clinical experience with this ratio regarding the detection of early alcohol abuse without liver involvement, has however, not been very encouraging.

GGT/alkaline phosphatase ratio

Combining the values of GGT and alkaline phosphatase activities to form a GGT/alkaline phosphatase-ratio has been reported to discriminate well between individuals with nonalcoholic and alcoholic liver disease. A ratio of more than 1.4 was found to detect alcoholic liver disease with a specificity of 78% (Lai & Lok 1982). This could, however, not be confirmed in another study (Spech & Liehr 1983).

Glutamate dehydrogenase (GDH)

Glutamate dehydrogenase is an intramitochondrial enzyme found in the centrolobular area of hepatic acinus from which alcohol-induced liver injury usually originates. Theoretically it could therefore serve as an ideal marker for alcohol induced organ pathology, and indeed it has been introduced as a reliable marker for alcoholic liver injury (Van Waes & Lieber 1977, Worner & Lieber 1980). However, recent alcohol consumption may increase serum and hepatic GDH activities independently of the underlying liver histology (Mills et al. 1981). On the other hand, serum GDH activity falls rapidly toward normal after cessation of heavy drinking (Worner & Lieber 1980). These facts render the test less suitable as a diagnostic aid for alcoholic liver injury. In addition, the original findings concerning the usefulness of GDH as a marker for alcoholic liver injury have been disputed in two other studies (Mills et al. 1981; Jenkins et al. 1982).

Immunoglobulin A

Serum concentration of immunoglobulin A is frequently increased in alcoholics and it has been reported that the ratio of immunoglobulin A to immunoglobulin G (IgA/IgG-ratio) may be useful in differentiating alcoholic from non-alcohol liver disease (Iturriaga et al. 1977; Spech & Liehr 1983).

Procollagen type III-peptide (PIIIP), other markers of fibrosis and acetaldehyde adduct antibodies

An important task for a clinician when treating alcoholic patients with hepatic damage is to distinguish between the three stages of alcoholic liver disease (fatty liver, alcoholic hepatitis, alcohol cirrhosis). This has conventionally been done by liver biopsy which, however, as an invasive method cannot be repeated as frequently as may be desired. Blood tests to aid the differential diagnosis of hepatic involvement are, therefore, clearly needed. The determination of amino-terminal procollagen type III peptide seems to emerge as the most promising of such blood tests presently available (Rohde et al. 1979; Schuppan et al. 1986). This test has been reported to be helpful in monitoring fibrogenesis in alcoholic liver injury (Nakano et al. 1983, Niemelä et al. 1983, Savolainen et al. 1984) and can also distinguish between alcoholic fatty liver and alcoholic hepatitis with high efficacy.

Most recently it has been proposed that both fibrogenesis and basement membrane formation (propeptide of type III collagen, type IV collagen and laminin) are associated with the severity of liver disease, the degree of alcoholic hepatitis as well as with alcohol intake, which are all important determinants of prognosis in alcoholic liver disease (Niemelä et al. 1990b). Furthermore antibodies to acetaldehyde modified epitopes in the central area of the hepatic acinus can be used to differentiate alcoholic from nonalcoholic liver injury (Niemelä et al. 1991b).

Use of Markers in Clinical Practice

In the hospital emergency

A significant number of patients seeking help from hospital emergency rooms are heavy drinkers or alcoholics (Jarman & Kellett 1979;
Jariwalla et al. 1979; Skinner et al. 1984; Antti-Poika & Karaharju
1986; Antti-Poika et al. 1988; Persson & Magnusson 1987; Rodriques
& Cami 1988). On the other hand they most often stay as "hidden"
alcoholics or heavy drinkers (Barrison et al. 1980; Solomon et al. 1980;
Anderson 1985; Rydon et al. 1992). Therefore, it is important that
effort is made to discover their underlying alcohol problems and to
refer them to adequate treatment (Reyna et al. 1985; Sherin et al. 1982;
Anderson 1985, 1990). In this respect the most simple test to use in a
hospital emergency room is the determination of blood alcohol concentration (BAC) by a portable breathanalyzer or semiquantitatively
from saliva by a dipstick (Peachey & Kapur 1986). As discussed
earlier in this review, BAC when related to the clinical status of
intoxication in an individual patient can give valuable clues regarding possible alcohol abuse. In addition to standard laboratory parameters other relatively simple tests, which can be used in
intoxicated patients, include serum acetate and methanol concentrations.

In early detection and secondary prevention

Gamma-glutamyl transferase is probably the test that has most successfully been used in the early detection of heavy drinking. One
example of this is a large Swedish study in which middle-aged men
were screened for alcohol abuse using GGT. Those with increased
GGT activity were divided into an intervention and non-interven-
tion group and followed for several years. The results of this study
showed clearly that even minimal intervention is efficient in significantly reducing alcohol related sickness and mortality (Kristenson et
al. 1983). Similar positive results have been reported from other
intervention studies (Chick et al. 1985, Antti-Poika et al. 1988, Elvy et
al. 1988; Wallace et al. 1988, Persson & Magnusson 1989; Levine
1990).

At the moment the second most useful test for large scale screening of heavy drinking is MCV. Like GGT, MCV is routinely available
in most laboratories and the determination of MCV is inexpensive.

The studies concerning CDT as a marker for alcohol abuse have been promising and, consequently, this test may in the near future emerge as a useful instrument for the early detection and secondary prevention of alcohol related problems. The relatively high price of the test and the lower sensitivity of the commercially available kit may, however, limit its use in screening of large unselected populations.

In in-patient treatment

In a hospital setting, a physician is more often concerned about possible alcohol related organ pathology than with the detection of alcohol abuse per se. Consequently the tests needed are those indicating liver injury (aspartate- and alanine aminotransferases, GGT, alkaline phosphatase, bilirubin, immunoglobulin A, hepatitis antigens etc.), pancreatic involvement (amylase, lipase, trypsin) or possible vitamin deficiencies (thiamine, pyridoxal phosphate) that might underlie neurologic disturbances. However, as suggested by many recent studies, in-patient and emergency units of general hospitals are places in which the early detection and intervention of alcohol abuse should be highly encouraged (Solomon et al. 1980, Barrison et al. 1980, Holt et al. 1980, Chick et al. 1985, Babor et al. 1986, Persson & Magnusson 1987, Antti-Poika et al. 1988, Elvy et al. 1988, Rodriques & Cami 1988, Persson & Magnusson 1989; Anderson 1990).

In the follow-up and in the evaluation of treatment results

In the follow-up of abstinence in alcoholics, it is most important to reliably detect relapses in drinking as early as possible. In this respect, the detection of ethanol in blood or urine is a simple and reliable method. As it also gives evidence of alcohol use without any latency, testing for the presence of alcohol in blood, urine or breath should be an essential part of the follow-up visits after detoxification Orrego et al. 1985; Caballeria et al. 1988).

The other conventional state markers also have an important role in the follow-up of abstinence and may be the earliest indicators of relapses occurring during treatment (Shaw et al. 1979, Monteiro and Masur 1986, Fantozzi et al. 1987, Irwin et al. 1988, Keso & Salaspuro 1989, 1990abc). In addition to their use as reinforcing feed-back factors in the treatment of alcoholics, their use in the studies on treatment evaluation significantly improves the reliability of the study (Keso & Salaspuro 1989, 1990abc).

The determination of HDL-cholesterol (although not valuable in screening for alcohol abuse), may also be utilized in the follow-up of abstinence in an individual patient. Other simple tests which would react to alcohol abuse of short duration—for example 1-2 days—are, however, still clearly needed.

References

Adachi, J., Mizoi, Y., & Fukunaga, T. (1986). Individual difference in urinary excretion of salsolinol in alcoholic patients. *Alcohol and Alcoholism*, 3: 371-376.

Agarwal, D.P., Tobar-Rojas, L., Harada, S., & Goedde, H.W. (1983). Comparative study of erythrocyte aldehyde dehydrogenase in alcoholics and control subjects. *Pharmacology, Biochemistry and Behavior*, 18: [Suppl. 1]: 89-95.

Agostini, A., Ideo, G., & Stabilini, R. (1965). Serum gamma-glutamyltranspeptidase activity in myocardial infarction. *British Heart Journal*, 27: 688-690.

Anderson, J.L. (1987). Computerized MAST for college health service. *Journal of American College Health*, 36: 83-88.

Anderson, P. (1985). Managing alcohol problems in general practice. *British Medical Journal*, 290: 1873-1875.

Anderson, P. (1990). Management of drinking problems. *WHO Regional Publications, European Series*, No. 32, 1 - 168.

Antti-Poika, I., & Karaharju, E. (1986). Alcohol and accidents —A prospective study in a casualty department. *Annales Chirurgiae et Gynaecologiae*, 75: 304-307.

Antti-Poika, I., Karaharju, E., Roine, R., & Salaspuro M. (1988). Intervention of heavy drinking—a prospective and controlled study of 438 consecutive injured male patients, *Alcohol and Alcoholism*, 23: 115-121.

Babor, T.F., Ritson, E.B., & Hodgson, R.J. (1986). Alcohol-related problems in the primary health care setting: a review of early intervention strategies, *British Journal of Addiction*, 81: 23-46.

Barboriak, J.J., Jacobson, G.R., Cushman, P., Herrington, R.E., Lipo, R.F., Daley, M.E. & Anderson, A.J. (1980). Chronic alcohol abuse and high density lipoprotein cholesterol. *Alcoholism, Clinical and Experimental Research* 4: 346-349.

Barrison, I.G., Viola, L., & Murray-Lyon, I.M. (1980). Do housemen take an adequate drinking history? *British Medical Journal*, 281: 1040.

Behrens, U.J., Worner, T.M., Braly, L.F., Schaffner, F., & Lieber, C.S. (1988a). Carbohydrate-deficient transferrin, a marker for chronic alcohol consumption in different ethnic populations. *Alcoholism, Clinical and Experimental Research*, 12: 427-432.

Behrens, U.J., Worner, T.M., & Lieber, C.S. (1988b). Changes in carbo-hydrate-deficient transferrin levels after alcohol withdrawal. *Alcoholism, Clinical and Experimetal Research*, 12: 539-544.

Belfrage, P., Berg, B., Hägerstrand, I., Nilsson-Ehle, P., Törnqvist, H., & Wiebe, T. (1977). Alterations of lipid metabolism in healthy volunteers during long-term ethanol intake. *European Journal of Clinical Investigation*, 7: 127-131.

Bell, H. & Steensland, H. (1987). Serum activity of gammaglutamyl-transpeptidase (GGT) in relation to estimated alcohol consumption and questionnaires in alcohol dependence syndrome. *British Journal of Addiction*, 82: 1021-1026.

Bell, H., Tallaksen, C., Sjäheim, T., Weberg, R., Raknerad, I.V., Örjasäter, H., Try, K.,and Haug, E. (1991). Serum carbohydrate-deficient transferrin as a marker of alcohol consumption in patients with chronic liver diseases. *Alcoholism, Clinical and Experimental Research*, 17: 246-252

Bernadt, M.W., Mumford, J., & Murray, R.M. (1984). A discriminant-function analysis of screening tests for excessive drinking and alcoholism. *Journal of Studies on Alcohol*, 45: 81-86.

Bernadt, M.W., Mumford, J., Taylor, C., Smith, B., & Murray, R.M. (1982). Comparison of questionnaire and laboratory tests in the detection of excessive drinking and alcoholism. *Lancet, i:* 325-328.

Bianco, A., & Jolliffe, N. (1938). The anemia of alcohol addicts. Observations as to the role of liver disease, achlorhydria nutritional factors and alcohol on its production. *American Journal of Medical Sciences*, 196: 414-420.

Bonte, W., Kühnholz, B., & Ditt, J. (1985). Blood methanol levels and alcoholism. In M. Valverius (Ed.), *Punishment and/or treatment for driving while under the influence of alcohol and other drugs. International Committee on Alcohol, Drugs and Traffic Safety, ICADDS* (pp. 255-259). Stockholm.

Brown, R.A. (1979). Use of Michigan Alcoholism Screening Test with hospitalized alcoholics, psychiatric patients, drinking drivers, and social drinkers in New Zealand. *American Journal of Drug and Alcohol Abuse*, 6: 375-381.

Caballeria, J., Torres, M., Camps, J., Parés, A., Reixach, M., & Rodés. (1988). Urine ethanol assessment: a helpful method for controlling abstinence in alcoholic liver disease. *Alcohol and Alcoholism*, 23: 403-407.

Carney, M.W., & Sheffield, B. (1978). Serum Folate and B12 & haematological status of in-patient alcoholics. *British Journal of Addiction*, 73: 3-7.

Carney, M.W., & Sheffield, B. (1980). The hemogram and the diagnosis of alcoholism. *Journal of Studies on Alcohol*, 41: 744-748.

Castelli, W.P., Doyle, J.T., Gordon, T., Hames, C.G., Hjortland, M.C., Hulley, S.B., Kagan, A., & Zukel, W.J. (1977). Alcohol and blood lipids. The cooperative lipoprotein phenotyping study. *Lancet, ii*: 153-155.

Chalmers, D.M., Chanarin, I., MacDermott, S., & Levi, A.S. (1980). Sex-related differences in the haematological effects of excessive alcohol consumption. *Journal of Clinical Pathology*, 33: 3-7.

Chalmers, D.M., Rinsler, M.G., MacDermott, S., Spicer, C.C., & Levi, A.J. (1981). Biochemical and haematological indicators of excessive alcohol consumption. *Gut*, 22: 992-996.

Chan, A.W.K. (1990). Biochemical markers for alcoholism. In M. Windle, & J.S. Searles (Eds.), *Children of alcoholics: Critical perspectives* (pp. 39-71). The Guilford Press, New York, NY.

Chan, A.W.K., Leong, F.W., Schanley, D.L., Welte, J.W., Wieczorek, W., Rej, R., Whitney, RB (1989). Transferrin and mitochondrial aspartate aminotransferase in young adult alcoholics. *Drug and Alcohol Dependence*, 23: 13-18.

Chan, A.W.K., Welte, F.W., & Whitney, R.B. (1987). Identification of alcoholism in young adults by blood chemistries. *Alcohol*, 4: 175-179.

Chick, J., Kreitman, N., & Plant, M. (1981). Mean cell volume and gamma-glutamyl- transpeptidase as markers of drinking in working men. *Lancet, i*: 1249-1251.

Chick, J., Lloyd, G., & Crombie, E. (1985). Counselling problem drinkers in medical wards: a controlled study. *British Medical Journal*, 290: 965-967.

Chick, J., Longstaff, M., Kreitman. M.P., Thatcher, D., & Waite, J. (1982). Plasma alfa-amino-n-butyric acid leucine ratio and alcohol consumption in working men and in alcoholics. *Journal of Studies on Alcohol*, 43: 583-587.

Chick, J., Pikkarainen, J., & Plant, M. (1987). Serum ferritin as a marker of alcohol consumption in working men. *Alcohol and Alcoholism*, 22: 75-77, 1987.

Clark, P.M.S., Kricka, L.J., & Zaman, S. (1982). Drivers, binge drinking, and gamma- glutamyl transpeptidase. *British Medical Journal,* 285: 1656.

Cohen, J.A., & Kaplan, M.M. (1979). The SGOT/SGPT ratio —an indicator of alcoholic liver disease. *Digestive Diseases and Sciences,* 24: 835-838.

Collins, M.A., Nijm, W.P., Borge, G.F., Teas, G., & Goldfarb, C. (1979). Dopamine-related tetrahydroisoquinolines: Significant urinary excretion by alcoholics after alcohol consumption. *Science,* 167: 1184-1186.

Correia, J.P., Alves, P.S., & Camilo, E.A. (1981): SGOT-SGPT ratios. *Digestive Diseases and Sciences,* 26: 284.

Cushman, P., Jacobson, G., Barboriak, J.J., & Anderson, A.J. (1984). Biochemical markers for alcoholism: sensitivity problems. *Alcoholism, Clinical and Experimental Research,* 8:253-257.

Danielsson, B., Ekman, R., Fex, G., Johansson, B.G., Kristenson, H., Nilsson-Ehle, P., & Wadstein, J. (1978). Changes in plasma high density lipoproteins in chronic male alcoholics during and after abuse. *Scandinavian Journal of Clinical and Laboratory Investigation,* 38: 113-119.

Devenyi, P., Robinson, G.M., Kapur, B.M., Roncari, D.A.K. (1981). High-density lipoprotein cholesterol in male alcoholics with and without severe liver disease. *American Journal of Medicine,* 71: 589-594.

Devgun, M.S., Dunbar, J.A., Hagart, J., Martin, B.T., & Ogston, S.A. (1985). Effects of acute and varying amounts of alcohol consumption on alkaline phosphatase, aspartate transaminase, and gamma-glutamyltransferase. *Alcoholism, Clinicial and Experimental Research,* 9: 235-237.

Dienstag, J.L., Carter, E.A., Wands, J.R., Isselbacher, K.J., & Fisher, J.E. (1978). Plasma alfa-amino-n-butyric acid to leucine ratio. Nonspecificity as a marker of for alcoholism. *Gastroenterology,* 75: 561-565.

Eckardt, M.J., Ryback, R.S., Rawlings, R.R., & Graubard, B.I. (1981). Biochemical diagnosis of alcoholism. A test for the discriminating capabilities of gamma-glutamyl transpeptidase and mean corpuscular volume. *Journal of the American Medical Association,* 246:2707-2710.

Elvy, G.A., Wells, J.E., & Baird, K.A. (1988). Attempted referral as intervention for problem drinking in the general hospital. *British Journal of Addiction,* 83: 83-89.

Ennis, P., & Vingilis, E. (1981). The validity of a revised version of the Mortimer-Filkins Test with impaired drivers in Oshawa, Ontario. *Journal of Studies on Alcohol*, 42: 685-688.

Fantozzi, R., Caramelli, L., Ledda, F., Moroni, F., Masini, E., Blandina, P., Botti, P., Peruzzi, S., Zorn, A.M., & Mannaioni, P.F. (1987). Biological markers and therapeutic outcome in alcoholic disease: a twelve-year survey. *Klinische Wochenschrift*, 65: 27-33.

Faraj, B.A., Camp, V.M., Davis, D.C., Lenton, J.D., & Kutner, M. (1989). Elevation of plasma salsolinol sulfate in chronic alcoholics as compared to nonalcoholics. *Alcoholism, Clinical and Experiemntal Research*, 13: 155-163.

Feest, U., Kemper, A., Nickel, B., Rabe, H., & Koalick, F. (1992). Comparison of salsolinol excretion in alcoholics and nonalcoholic controls. *Alcohol*, 9: 49-52.

Feuerlein, W., Ringer, C., Kufner, H., & Antons, K. (1977). Diagnose des Alkoholismus der Münchener Alkoholismustest (MALT). *München Medisinische Wochenschrift*, 119: 1275-1282.

Garvin, R.B., Foy, D.W., & Alford, G.S. (1981). A critical examination of gamma-glutamyl transpeptidase as a biochemical marker for alcohol abuse. *Addiction Behaviors*, 6: 377-383.

Gjerde, H., Johnsen, J., Bjorneboe, A., Bjorneboe, G.-E. & Morland, J. (1988): A comparison of serum carbohydrate-deficient transferrin with other biological markers of excessive drinking. *Scandinavian Journal of Clinical and Laboratory Investigation*, 48:1-6.

Gjerde, H., & Mörland, J. (1987). Concentrations of carbohydrate-deficient transferrin in dialysed plasma from drunken drivers. *Alcohol and Alcoholism*, 22: 271-276.

Gluud, C., Andersen, I., Dietrichson, O., Gluud, B., Jacobsen, A., & Juhl, E. (1981) Gamma-glutamyltransferase, aspartate aminotransferase and alkaline phosphatase as markers of alcohol consumption in out-patient alcoholics. *European Journal of Clinical Investigation*, 11: 171-176.

Halmesmäki, E., Roine, R., & Salaspuro, M. (1992). Gammaglutamylstransferase, aspartate and alanine aminotransferases and their ratio, mean cell volume and urinary dolichol in pregnant alcohol abusers. *British Journal of Obstetrics and Gynaecology*, 99: 287-291.

Hartung, G.H., Foreyt, J.P., Mitchell, R.E., Mitchell, J.G.M., Reeves, R.S., & Gotto, A.M. (1983). Effect of alcohol intake on high-density cholesterol levels in runners and in inactive men. *Journal of the American Medical Association*, 249: 747-750.

Hedworth-Whitty, R.B., Whitfield, J.B & Richardson, R.W. (1967). Serum gamma-glutamyl-transpeptidase activity in myocardial ischaemia. *British Heart Journal,* 29: 432-438.

Helander, A., Beck, O., Jacobsson, G., Wikström, T., & Borg, S. (1992). Characterization of elevated urinary 5-hydroxytryptophol as a marker of recent alcohol consumption. *Alcoholism, Clinical and Experimental Research,* 16: 607.

Hernández-Muñoz, R., Baraona, E., Blacksberg, I., & Lieber, C.S. (1989). Characterization of the increased binding of acetaldehyde to red blood cells in alcoholics. *Alcoholism, Clinical and Experimental Research,* 13: 654-659.

Herrington, R.E., Jacobsen, G.R., Daley, M.E., Lipo, R.F., Biller, H.B., & Weissgerber, C. (1981). Use of the plasma alpha-amino-n-butyric acid: leucine ratio to identify alcoholics. An unsuccessful test. *Journal of Studies on Alcohol,* 42: 492-499.

Hillers, V.N., Alldredge, J.R., & Massey, L.K. (1986). Determination of habitual alcohol intake from a panel of blood chemistries. *Alcohol and Alcoholism,* 21: 199-205.

Hoberman, H.D., & Chiodo, S.M. (1982). Elevation of the hemoglobin A1 fraction in alcoholism. *Alcoholism, Clinical and Experimental Research,* 6: 260-266.

Hoerner, M., Behrens, U.J., Worner, T., & Lieber, C.S. (1986). Humoral immune response to acetaldehyde adducts in alcoholic patients. *Research Communication in Chemical Pathology and Pharmcalogy,* 54: 3-12.

Hoerner, M., Behrens, U.J., Worner, T.M., Blacksberg, I., Braly, L.F., Schaffner, F., & Lieber, C.S. (1988). The role of alcoholism and liver disease in the appearance of serum antibodies against acetaldehyde adducts. *Hepatology,* 8: 569-574.

Holt, S., Stewart, I.C., Dixon, J.M.J., Elton, R.A., Taylor, T.V., & Little, K. (1980). Alcohol and the emergency service patient. *British Medical Journal,* 281: 638-640.

Horner, F., Kellen, J.A., Kingstone, E., Maharaj, N, & Malkin, A. (1979). Dynamic changes of serum gamma-glutamyl transferase in chronic alcoholism. *Enzyme,* 24: 217-223.

Hultberg, B., Isaksson, A., Berglund, M., & Moberg, A.-L. (1991). Serum ß-hexosaminidase isoenzyme: A sentitive marker for alcohol abuse. *Alcoholism, Clinical and Experimental Research,* 15: 549-552.

Hultberg, B., Isaksson, A., & Tiderström, G. (1980). ß-hexosaminidase, leucine-aminopeptidase, cystidyl aminopeptidase, hepatic enzymes and bilirubin in serum of chronic alcoholics with acute ethanol intoxication. *Clinica Chimica Acta*, 105: 317-323.

Irwin, M., Baird, S., Smith, T.L., & Schuckit, M. (1988). Use of laboratory tests to monitor heavy drinking by alcoholic men discharged from a treatment program. *American Journal of Psychiatry*, 145: 595-599.

Isaksson, A., Blanche, C., Hultberg, B., & Joelsson, B. (1985). Influence of ethanol on the human serum level of ß-hexosaminidase. *Enzyme*, 33: 162-166.

Ishii, H., Ebihara, Y., Okuno, F., Munakata, Y., Takagi, T., Arai, M., Shigeta, S. & Tsuchiya M (1986). Gamma-glutamyl transpeptidase activity in liver of alcoholics and its histochemical localization. *Alcoholism, Clinical and Experimental Research*, 10: 81-85.

Israel, Y., Hurwitz, E., Niemelä, O., & Armon, R. (1986) Monoclonal and polyclonal anti-bodies against acetaldehyde-containing epitopes in acetaldehyde-protein adducts. *Proceedings of the National Academy of Sciences of the United States of America*, 83: 7923-7927.

Iturriaga, H., Pereda, T., Estevez, A., & Ugarte, G. (1977). Serum immunoglobulin changes in alcoholic patients. *Annales of Clinical Research*, 9: 39-43.

Jacobsson, A., Norden, A., Qvist, J., & Wadstein, J. (1978). Serum ferritin — a new marker for alcoholism? *Acta Societatis Medicorum Suecanae*, 87: 3314-3316.

Jariwalla, A.G., Adams, P.H., & Hore, B.D. (1979). Alcohol and acute general medicine admissions to hospital. *Health Trends*, 11: 95-97.

Jarman, C.M.B., & Kellett, J.M. (1979: Alcoholism in general hospital. *British Medical Journal*, 2: 469-472.

Jenkins, W.J., Rosalki, S.B., Foo, Y., Scheuer, P.J., Nemesanszky, E., & Scherlock, S. (1982). Serum glutamate dehydrogenase is a not a reliable marker of liver cell necrosis in alcoholics. *Journal of Clinical Pathology*, 35: 207-210.

Jones, A.W. (1991). 2,3-butanediol in blood from drinking technical alcohol containing 2-butanone. *Lancet* 338: 1090.

Jones, J.D., Morse, R.M., & Hurt, R.D. (1931). Plasma alpha-amino-n-butyric acid/leucine ratio in alcoholics. *Alcoholism, Clinical and Experimental Research*, 5: 363-365.

Kapur, A., Wild, G., Milford-Ward, A., & Triger, D.R. (1989). Carbohydrate deficient transferrin: a marker for alcohol abuse. *British Medical Journal*, 299: 427-431.

Kärkkäinen, P. (1990). Serum and urinary β-hexosaminidase as markers of heavy drinking. *Alcohol and Alcoholism*, 25: 365-369, 1990.

Kärkkäinen, P., Jokelainen, K., Roine, R., Suokas, A., & Salaspuro, M. (1990a). The effects of moderate drinking and abstinence on serum and urinary β-hexosaminidase levels. *Drug and Alcohol Dependence*, 25: 35-38.

Kärkkäinen, P., Poikolainen, K., & Salaspuro, M. (1990b). Serum ß-hexosaminidase as a marker of heavy drinking. *Alcoholism, Clinical and Experimental Research, 14*: 187-190.

Keso, L., & Salaspuro, M. (1989). Laboratory markers as compared to drinking measures before and after inpatient treatment for alcoholism. *Alcoholism, Clinical and Experimental Research,* 13: 449-452.

Keso, L., & Salaspuro, M. (1990a). Comparative value of self-report and blood tests in assessing outcome amongst alcoholics. *British Journal of Addiction*, 85: 209-215.

Keso, L., & Salaspuro, M. (1990b). Inpatient treatment of employed alcoholics: a randomized clinical trial on Hazelden-type and traditional treatment. *Alcoholism, Clinical and Experimental Research,* 14: 584-589.

Keso, L., & Salaspuro, M. (1990c). Laboratory tests in the follow-up of treated alcoholics: How often should testing be repeated? *Alcohol and Alcoholism*, 25: 359-363.

Konttinen, A., Härtel, G., & Louhija, A. (1970). Multiple serum enzyme analyzes in chronic alcoholics. *Acta Medica Scandinavica*, 188: 257-264.

Korri, U.-M. (1990). The effect of glucocorticoids, beta-2-adrenoreceptor agonists, theophylline and propranol on the rate of ethanol elimination and blood acetate concentration in humans. *Alcohol and Alcoholism*, 25: 519-522.

Korri, U.-M., Nuutinen, H., & Salaspuro, M. (1985). Increased blood acetate: a new laboratory marker of alcoholism and heavy drinking. *Alcoholism, Clinical and Experimental Research*, 9: 468-471.

Kristenson, H., Fex, G., & Trell, E. (1981). Serum ferritin, gamma-glutamyltranspeptidase and alcohol consumption in middle-aged men. *Drug and Alcohol Dependence*, 8: 43-50.

Kristenson, H. & Trell, E. (1982). Indicators of alcohol consumption: Comparisons between a questionnaire (Mm-MAST), interviews and serum gamma-glutamyl transferase (GGT) in a health survey of middle-aged males. *British Journal of Addiction*, 77:297-304.

Kristenson, H., Trell, E., Fex, G., & Hood, B. (1980). Serum gamma-glutamyltransferase: statistical Distribution in a middle-aged male population and evaluation of alcohol habits in individuals with elevated levels. *Preventive Medicine*, 9: 108-119.

Kristenson, H., Öhlin, H., Hultén-Nosslin, M.-B., Trell, E., & Hood, B. (1983). Identification and intervention of heavy drinking in middle-aged men: Results and follow-up of 24-60 months of long-term study with randomized controls. *Alcoholism, Clinical and Experimental Research,* 7: 203-209.

Kryszewski, A., Bardzik, I., Kilkowska, K., Vogel-Pienkowska, M., & Schminda, R. (1977). Gamma-glutamyltranspeptidase activity in serum and liver in chronic alcoholism. Possible usefulness as a test of abstinence. *Acta Medica Polona,* 18: 199-211.

Lai, C.L., Ng, R.P., & Lok, A.S.F. (1982). The diagnostic value of the ratio of serum gamma-glutamyl transpeptidase to alkaline phosphatase in alcoholic liver disease. *Scandinavian Journal of Gastroenterology,* 17: 41-47.

Levine, J. (1990). The relative value of consultation, questionnaires and laboratory investigation in the identification of excessive alcohol consumption. *Alcohol and Alcoholism,* 25: 539-553.

Lin, R.C., Lumeng, L., Shahidi, S., Kelly, T., & Pound, D.C. (1990). Protein-acetaldehyde adducts in serum of alcoholic patients. *Alcoholism, Clinical and Experimental Research,* 14: 438-443.

Lindros, K.O., Stowell, A., Pikkarainen, P.O., & Salaspuro, M. (1980). Elevated blood acetaldehyde in alcoholics with accelerated ethanol elimination. *Pharmacology, Biochemistry and Behavior,* 13: Suppl. 1, 119-124.

Lucas, D., Menez, J.F., Bodenez, P., Baccino, E., Bardou, L.G., & Floch, H.H. (1988). Acetaldehyde adducts with haemoglobin: determination of acetaldehyde released from haemoglobin by acid hydrolysis. *Alcohol and Alcoholism,* 23: 23-31.

Lum, G., & Gambino, S.R. (1972). Serum gamma-glutamyltranspeptidase activity as an indicator of disease of liver, pancreas or bone. *Clinical Chemistry,* 18: 358-362.

Lumeng, L. (1986). New diagnostic markers of alcohol abuse. *Hepatology,* 6: 742-745.

Lundin, L., Hallgren, R., Birgegard, G., & Wide, L. (1981). Serum ferritin in alcoholics and the relation to liver damage, iron state and erythropoetic activity. *Acta Medica Scandinavica,* 209: 327-331.

Mayfield, D., McLeod, G., & Hall, P. (1974). The CAGE questionnaire: Validation of a new alcoholism screening instrument. *American Journal of Psychiatry,* 131: 1121-1123.

Mezey, E. (1978). Alcohol consumption and gamma-glutamyltransferase activity. *Gastroenterology,* 74: 632-633.

Mills, P.R., Spooner, R.J., Russell, R.I., Boyle, P., & MacSween, R.N.M. (1981). Serum glutamate dehydrogenase as a marker of hepatocyte necrosis in alcoholic liver disease. *British Medical Journal, 283*: 754-755.

Moirand, R., Lescoat, G., Delamaire, D., Lauvin, L., Campion, J.P., Deugnier, Y., & Brissot, P. (1991). Increase in glycosylated and nonglycosylated serum ferritin in chronic alcoholism and their evolution during alcohol withdrawal. *Alcoholism, Clinical and Experimental Research, 15*: 963-969.

Monteiro, M.G., & Masur, J. (1985). Diagnostic of alcoholism: How useful is the combination of gammaglutamyl transferase with different biochemical markers? *Drug and Alcohol Dependence, 16*: 31-37.

Morgan, M.Y., Colman, J.C., & Sherlock, S. (1981a). The use of a combination of peripheral markers for diagnosing alcoholism and monitoring for continued abuse. *Alcohol Alcohol, 16*: 167-177.

Morgan, M.Y., Camilo, M.E., Luck, W., Sherlock, S., & Hoffbrand, A.V. (1981b). Macrocytosis in alcohol-related liver disease: its value for screening. *Clinical and Laboratory Haematology, 3*: 35-44.

Morgan, M.Y., Milsom, J.P., & Sherlock, S. (1977). Ratio of plasma alpha-amino-n-butyric acid to leucine ratio: diagnostic value. *Science, 197*: 1183-1185.

Morse, R.M., & Hurt, R.D. (1979). Screening for alcoholism. *Journal of the American Medical Association, 242*: 2688-2690.

Moussavian, S.N., Becker, R.C., Piepmeyer, J.L., Mezey, E., & Bozian, R.C. (1985). Serum gamma-glutamyl transpeptidase and chronic alcoholism. Influence of alcohol ingestion and liver disease. *Digestive Diseases and Sciences, 30*: 211-214.

Myrhed, M., & Bergström, K. (1976). Liver enzymes in alcohol-discordant twins. *Acta Medica Scandinavica, 200*: 87-91.

Mörland, J., Huseby, N.E., Sjöblom, M., & Strömme, J.H. (1977). Does chronic alcohol consumption really induce hepatic microsomal gamma-glutamyltransferase activity? *Biochemical and Biophysical Research Communications, 77*: 1060-1066.

Nakano, H., Kawasaki, T., Miyamura, M., Fukuda, Y., & Imura, H. (1983). Serum levels of N-terminal type III procollagen peptide in normal subjects and comparison to hepatic fibrosis. *Acta Hepatologica Japonica, 24*: 1230-1234.

Nalpas, B., Vassault, A., Charpin, S., Lacour, B., & Berthelot, P. (1986). Serum mitochondrial aspartate aminotransferase as a marker of chronic alcoholism: diagnostic value and interpretation in a liver unit. *Hepatology, 6*: 608-614.

Nalpas, B., Vassault, A., Le Guillou, A., Lesgourgues, B., Ferry, N., Lacour, B., & Berthelot, P. (1986). Serum activity of mitochondrial aspartate aminotransferase: a sensitive marker of alcoholism with or without alcoholic hepatitis. *Hepatology*, 4: 893-896.

National Council on Alcoholism, The Criteria Committee. (1972). Criteria for the diagnosis of alcoholism. *Annals of Internal Medicine*, 77: 249-258.

Niemelä, O., Halmesmäki, E., & Ylikorkala, O. (1991a). Hemoglobin-acetaldehyde adducts are elevated in women carrying alcohol-damaged fetuses. *Alcoholism, Clinical and Experimental Research*, 15: 1007-1010.

Niemelä, O., Israel, Y., Mizoi, Y., Fukunaga, T., & Eriksson, C.J.P. (1990a). Hemoglobin - acetaldehyde adducts in human volunteers following acute ethanol ingestion. *Alcoholism, Clinical and Experimental Research*, 14: 838-841.

Niemelä, O., Juvonen, T., & Parkkila, S. (1991b). Immunohistochemical demonstration of acetaldehyde-modified epitopes in human liver after alcohol consumption. *Journal of Clinical Investigation*, 87: 1367-1374.

Niemelä, O., Klajner, F., Orrego, H., Vidins, E., Blendis, L., & Israel, Y. (1987). Antibodies against acetaldehyde-modified protein epitopes in human alcoholics. *Hepatology*, 7: 1210-1214.

Niemelä, O., Risteli, J., Blake, J.E., Risteli, L., Compton, K.V., & Orrego, H. (1990b). Markers of fibrogenesis and basement membrane formation in alcoholic liver disease. *Gastroenterology*, 98: 1612-1619.

Niemelä, O., Risteli, L., Sotaniemi, E.A., & Risteli, J. (1983). Aminoterminal propeptide of type III procollagen in serum in alcoholic liver disease. *Gastroenterology*, 85: 254-259.

Nilssen, O., Huseby, N.E., Höyer, G., Brenn, T., Schirmer H., & Förde, O.H. (1992). New alcohol markers —how useful they are in population studies: The Svalbard study 1988-89:*Alcoholism, Clinical and Experimental Research*, 16: 82-86.

Nishimura, M., Hasumura, Y., & Takeuchi, J. (1980). Effect of an intravenous infusion of ethanol on serum enzymes and lipids in patients with alcoholic liver disease. *Gastroenterology*, 78: 691-695.

Nuutinen, H., Lindros, K., Hekali, P., & Salaspuro, M. (1985). Elevated blood acetate as indicator of fast ethanol elimination in chronic alcoholics. *Alcohol*, 2: 623-626.

Nuutinen, H., Lindros, K., & Salaspuro, M. (1983). Determinants of blood acetaldehyde level during ethanol oxidation in chronic alcoholics. *Alcoholism, Clinical and Experimental Research*, 7: 163-168.

Nuutinen, H.U., Salaspuro, M., Valle, M., & Lindros, K.O. (1984). Blood acetaldehyde concentration gradient between hepatic and antecubital venous blood in ethanol intoxicated alcoholics and controls. *European Journal of Clinical Investigation*, 14: 306-311.

Nyström, M., Peräsalo, J., Pikkarainen, J., & Salaspuro, M. (1993a). Conventional laboratory tests as indicators of heavy drinking in young university students. Scandinavian Journal of Primary Care, 11: 44-49.

Nyström, M., Peräsalo, J., & Salaspuro, M. (1991). Serum ß-hexosaminidase in young university students. *Alcoholism, Clinical and Experimental Research*, 15: 877-880.

Nyström, M., Peräsalo, J., & Salaspuro, M. (1992). Carbohydrate-deficient transferrin (CDT) in serum as a possible indicator of heavy drinking in young university students. *Alcoholism, Clinical and Experimental Research*, 16: 93-97.

Nyström, M., Perasalo, J., & Salaspuro, M (1993b). Screening for heavy drinking and alcohol related problems in young university students; the Cage, the Mm-MAST and the Trauma score questionnaires. *Journal of Studies on Alcohol*, in press.

Olsen, H., Sakshaug, J., Duckert, F., Stromme, J.H., & Morland, J. (1989). Ethanol elimination-rates determined by breath analysis as a marker of recent excessive ethanol consumption. *Scandinavian Journal of Clinical Laboratory Investigation*, 49: 359-365.

Orrego, H., Blake, J.E., & Israel, Y. (1985). Relationship between gamma-glutamyl transpeptidase and mean urinary alcohol levels in alcoholics while drinking and after alcohol withdrawal. *Alcoholism, Clinical and Experimental Research*, 9: 10-13.

Papoz, L., Warnet, J.-M., Péguignot, G., Eschwege, E., Claude, J.R., Schwartz, D. (1981). Alcohol consumption in a healthy population. Relationship to gamma-glutamyl transferase activity and mean corpuscular volume. *Journal of the American Medical Association*, 245:1748-1751.

Peachey, E., & Kapur, B.M. (1986). Monitoring drinking behavior with the alcohol dipstick during treatment. *Alcoholism, Clinical and Experimental Research*, 10: 663-666.

Penn, R., Worthington, L.J., Clarke, C.A., & Whitfield, A.G.W. (1981). Gamma-glutamyl- transpeptidase and alcohol intake. *Lancet, i*: 894.

Penn, R., & Worthington, D.J. (1983). Is serum gammaglutamyltransferase a misleading test? *British Medical Journal*, 286: 531-535.

Persson, J. & Magnusson, P.-H. (1987). Prevalence of excessive or problem drinkers among patients attending somatic outpatient clinics: a study of alcohol related medical care. *British Medical Journal*, 295: 467-472.

Persson, J., & Magnusson, P.-H. (1989). Early intervention in patients with excessive consumption of alcohol: A controlled study. *Alcohol*, 6: 403-408.

Peterson, C.M., Jovanovic-Peterson, L., & Schmid-Formby, F. (1988). Rapid association of acetaldehyde with hemoglobin in human volunteers after low dose ethanol. *Alcohol*, 5: 371-374.

Peterson, C.M., & Polizzi, C.M. (1987). Improved method for acetaldehyde in plasma and hemoglobin-associated acetaldehyde: Results in teetotalers and alcoholics reporting for treatment. *Alcohol*, 4: 477-480.

Poikolainen, K., Kärkkäinen, P., & Pikkarainen, J. (1985). Correlations between biological markers and alcohol intake as measured by a diary and questionnaire in men. *Journal of Studies on Alcohol*, 46: 383-387.

Pokorny, A.D., Miller, B.A., & Kaplan, H.B. (1972). The Brief MAST: A shortened version of the Michigan Alcoholism Screening Test. *American Journal of Psychiatry*, 129: 342-345.

Poupon, R.E., Schellenberg, F., Nalpas, B., & Weill, J. (1989). Assessment of the transferrin index in screening heavy drinkers from general practice. *Alcoholism, Clinical and Experimental Research*, 4: 549-553.

Puchois, P., Fontan, M., Gentilini, J.-L., Gelez, P., & Fruchart J.-C. (1984). Serum apolipoprotein A-II, a biochemical indicator of alcohol abuse. *Clinica Chimica Acta*, 185: 185-189.

Pullarkat, R.K., & Raguthu, S. (1985). Elevated urinary dolichol levels in chronic alcoholics. *Alcoholism, Clinical and Experimental Research*, 9: 28-30.

Rej, R. (1980). An immunochemical procedure for determination of mitochondrial aspartate aminotransferase in human serum. *Clinical Chemistry*, 26: 1694-1700.

Reich, T., Robins, L.N., Woodruff, R.A., Taibleson, M., Rich, C., & Cunningham, L. (1975). Computer assisted derivation of a screening interview for alcoholism. *Archives of General Psychiatry*, 32: 847-852.

Renwick, J.H., and Asker, R.L. (1982). The time course of response of erythrocyte volume to ethanol and to its withdrawal. *Clinical and Laboratory Haematology*, 4: 325-326.

Reyna, T.M., Hollis, H.W., & Hulsebus, R.C. (1985). Alcohol-related trauma. The Surgeon's responsibility. *Annals of Surgery*, 201: 194-197.

Rodriguez, M.E. & Lami (1988). Alcoholism among inpatients in a general hospital in Barcelona, Spain. *International Journal of Addiction,* 23: 29-46.

Rohde, H., Vargas, L., Hahn, E.G., Kalbfleisch, H., Bruguera, M., & Timpl, R. (1979). Radioimmuno-assay for type III procollagen peptide and its application to human liver disease. *European Journal of Clinical Investigation,* 9: 451-459.

Roine, R. (1988). Effects of moderate drinking and alcohol abstinence on urinary dolichol levels. *Alcohol,* 5: 229-231.

Roine, R.P., Eriksson, C.J.P., Ylikahri, R., Penttilä, A., & Salaspuro, M. (1989a). Methanol as a marker of alcohol abuse. *Alcoholism, Clinical and Experimental Research,* 13: 172-175.

Roine, R., Heinonen, T., Salmela, K., Heikkonen, E., Suokas, A., Luurila, O.J., Koskinen, P., Palo, J., & Salaspuro, M. (1991). Strenous physical activity, aspirin and heat stress increase urinary dolichols: evidence for lysosomal origin of urinary dolichols. *Clinica Chimica Acta,* 204: 13-22.

Roine, R.P., Humaloja, K., Hämäläinen, J., Nykänen, I., Ylikahri, R., & Salaspuro, M. (1989b). Significant increases in urinary dolichol levels in bacterial infections, malignancies and pregnancy but not in other clinical conditions. *Annals of Medicine,* 21:13-16.

Roine, R.P., Korri, U.M., Ylikahri, R., Penttilä, A., Pikkarainen, J., & Salaspuro, M. (1988b). Increased serum acetate as a marker of problem drinking among drunken drivers. *Alcohol,* 23:123-126.

Roine, R.P., Turpeinen, U., Ylikahri, R., & Salaspuro, M. (1987a). Urinary dolichol—a new marker of alcoholism. *Alcoholism, Clinical and Experimental Research,* 11: 525-527.

Roine, R.P., Ylikahri, R., Koskinen, P., Suokas, A., Hämäläinen, J. & Salaspuro, M. (1987b). Effect of heavy weekend drinking on urinary dolichol levels. *Alcohol,* 4:509-511.

Rollason, J.G., Pincherle, G., & Robinson, D. (1972). Serum gamma glutamyl-transpeptidase in relation to alcohol consumption. *Clinica Chimica Acta,* 39: 75-80.

Rosalki, S.B., & Rau, D. (1972). Serum gamma-glutamyl transpeptidase activity in alcoholism. *Clinica Chimica Acta,* 39: 41-47.

Rosalki, S.B., Tarlow, D., & Rau, D. (1971). Plasma gamma-glutamyl-transpeptidase elevation in patients receiving enzyme-inducing drugs. *Lancet, ii:* 376-377.

Rutstein, D.D., Veech, R.L., Nickerson, R.J., Felver, M.E., Vernon, A.A., Needham, L.L., Kishore, P., Thacker, S.B. (1983). 2,3-butanediol: an unusual metabolite in the serum of severely alcoholic men during acute intoxication. *Lancet, ii:* 534-537.

Ryback, R.S., Eckhardt, M.J., Felsher, B., & Rawlings, R.R. (1982). Biochemical and hematologic correlates of alcoholism and liver disease. *Journal of the American Medical Association*, 248: 2261-2265.

Rydon, P., Redman, S., Sanson-Fisher, R.W., & Reid, A.L.A. (1992). Detection of alcohol-related problems in general practice. *Journal of Studies on Alcohol*, 53: 197-202.

Salaspuro, M. (1986). Conventional and coming laboratory markers of alcoholism and heavy drinking. *Alcoholism, Clinical and Experimental Research*, 10: 5S-12S.

Salaspuro, M. (1987). Use of enzymes for the diagnosis of alcohol-related organ damage. *Enzyme, 37*: 87-107.

Salaspuro, M. (1989). Characteristics of laboratory markers in alcohol related organ damage. *Scandinavian Journal of Gastroenterology*, 24: 769-780.

Salaspuro, M. (1991). Epidemiological aspects of alcohol and alcoholic liver disease, ethanol metabolism, and pathogenesis of alcoholic liver injury. In N. McIntyre, J.-P. Benhamou, J. Bircher, M. Rizzetto, & J.O. Rodes (Eds.), *Oxford textbook of Clinical Hepatology* (pp. 791-810). *Oxford University Press*.

Salaspuro, M. & Roine, R. (1993). *Alcohol*. In D.A. Noe (ed.), Laboratory Medicine: The selection and interpretation of clinical laboratory studies, (pp. 554-564). Williams & Wilkins

Salmela, K., Laitinen, K., Nyström, M., & Salaspuro, M. (1993). Carbohydrate-deficient transferrin during three week's moderate alcohol consumption. *Alcoholism, Clinical and Experimental Research*, 18: 228-230.

Sanchez-Graig, M., & Annis, H.M. (1981). Gamma-glutamyltranspeptidase and high density lipoprotein cholesterol in male problem drinkers: Advantages of a composite index for predicting alcohol consumption. *Alcoholism, Clinical and Experimental Research*, 5: 540-544.

Saunders, W.M., & Kershaw, P.W. (1980). Screening tests and self-identification in the detection of alcoholism—findings from a community study. *British Journal of Addiction*, 75: 37-41.

Savolainen, E.R., Goldberg, B., Leo, M.A., Velez, M., & Lieber, C.S. (1984). Diagnostic value of serum procollagen peptide measurements in alcoholic liver disease. *Alcoholism, Clinical and Experimental Reserach*, 8: 384-389.

Schellenberg, F., & Weill, J. (1987). Serum desialotransferrin in the detection of alcohol abuse. Definition of a Tf index. *Drug and Alcohol Dependence*, 19: 181-191.

Schiele, F., Artur, Y., Varasteh, A., Wellman, M., & Siest, G. (1989). Serum mitochondrial aspartate aminotransferase activity: Not a useful marker of excessive alcohol consumption in an unselected population. *Clinical Chemistry,* 35: 926-930.

Schiele, F., Guilman, A.M., Detienne, H., & Siest, G. (1977). Gamma-glutamyltransferase activity in plasma: statistical distributions, individual variations, and reference intervals. *Clinical Chemistry,* 23: 1023-1028.

Schuppan, D., Dumont, J.M., Kim, K.Y., Hennings, G., & Hahn, E.G. (1986). Serum concentration of the aminoterminal procollagen type III peptide in the rat reflects early formation of connective tissue in experimental liver cirrhosis. *Journal of Hepatology,* 3: 27-37.

Selzer, M.L. (1971). The Michigan Alcoholism Screening Test: The quest for a new diagnostic instrument. *American Journal of Psychiatry,* 127: 1653-1658.

Selzer, M.L., Vinokur, A., & Van Rooijen, L. (1975). A Self-Administered Short Michigan Alcoholism Screening Test (SMAST). *Journal of Studies on Alcohol,* 36: 117-126.

Senior, J.R., & Sloan, B.P. (1981). Emergency measurement of stat, timed, serum ethanol levels for medical management. *Alcoholism, Clinical and Experimental Research,* 5: 6-11.

Seppä, K. Laippala, P. & Saurni, M. (1991). Macrocytosis as consequence of alcohol abuse among patients in general practice. *Alcoholism, Clinical and Experimental Research,* 15: 871-876.

Seppä, K., Sillanaukee, P., & Koivula, T. (1992). Abnormalities of hematological parameters in heavy drinkers and alcoholics. *Alcoholism, Clinical and Experimental Research,* 16:117-121.

Seymour, C.A., & Peters, T.J. (1978). Changes in hepatic enzymes and organelles in alcoholic liver disease. *Clinical Science and Molecular Medicine,* 55: 383-389.

Shaper, A.G., Pocock, S.J., Ashby, D., Walker, M., & Whitehead T.P. (1985). Biochemical and haematological response to alcohol intake. *Annals of Clinical Biochemistry,* 22: 50-61.

Shaw, S., & Lieber, C.S. (1978). Plasma amino acid abnormalities in the alcoholic. Respective role of alcohol, nutrition, and liver injury. *Gastroenterology,* 74: 677-682.

Shaw, S., Stimmel, B., & Lieber, C.S. (1976). Plasma alpha-amino-n-butyric acid to leucine ratio: An empirical biochemical marker of alcoholism. *Science,* 194: 1057-1058.

Shaw, S., Worner, T., Borysow, M.F., Schmitz, R.E., & Lieber, C.S. (1979). Detection of alcoholism relapse: Comparative diagnostic value of MCV, GGT, and AANB. *Alcoholism, Clinical and Experimental Research*, 3: 297-301.

Sherin, K.M., Piotrowski, Z.H., Panek, S.M., & Doot, M.C. (1982). Screening for alcoholism in a community hospital. *Journal of Family Practice*, 15: 1091-1095.

Sillanaukee, P. (1992). The diagnostic value of a discriminant score in the detection of alcohol abuse. *Archives of Pathology and Laboratory Medicine*, 116: 924-929.

Sillanaukee, P., & Koivula, T. (1990). Detection of a new acetaldehyde-induced hemoglobin fraction HbA_{1ach} by cation exchange liquid chromatography. *Alcoholism, Clinical and Experimental Research*, 14: 842-846.

Sillanaukee, P., Seppä, K., & Koivula, T. (1991a). Effect of acetaldehyde on hemoglobin: HbA_{1ach} as a potential marker of heavy drinking. *Alcohol and Alcoholism*, 8: 377-381.

Sillanaukee, P., Seppä, K., & Koivula, T. (1991b). Association of a haemoglobin- acetaldehyde adduct with questionnaire results on heavy drinkers. *Alcohol and Alcoholism*, 26: 519-525.

Sillanaukee, P., Seppä, K., Koivula, T., Israel, Y., & Niemelä, O. (1992). Acetaldehyde-modified hemoglobin as a marker of alcohol consumption: Comparison of two new methods. *Journal of Laboratory and Clinical Medicine*, 120: 42-47.

Sjöquist, B., Borg, S., & Kvande, H. (1981a). Catecholamine derived compounds in urine and cerebrospinal fluid from alcoholics during and after long-standing intoxication. *Substance and Alcohol Actions Misuse*, 2: 63-72.

Sjöquist, B., Borg, S., & Kvande, H. (1981b). Salsolinol and methylated salsolinol in urine and cerebrospinal fluid from healthy volunteers. *Substance and Alcohol Actions Misuse* 2:73-77.

Skinner, H.A. (1979). A multivariate evaluation of the MAST. *Journal of Studies on Alcohol*, 40: 831-844.

Skinner, H.A., Holt, S., Schuller, R., Roy, J., & Israel, Y. (1984). Identification of alcohol abuse using laboratory tests and a history of trauma. *Annals of Internal Medicine*, 101: 847-851.

Solomon, J., Vanga, N., Morgan, J.P., & Joseph, P. (1980). Emergency-room physicians' recognition of alcohol misuse. *Journal of Studies on Alcohol*, 41: 583-586.

Spech, H.J., & Liehr, H. (1983). Was leisten SGOT/SGPT-, GGT/AP- und IgG/IgA -Quotienten differential diagnostisch bei fortgeschrittenen Leberkrankheiten? *Zeitschrift für Gastroenterologie*, 21: 89-96.

Stamm, D., Hansert, E., & Feuerlein, W. (1984a). Excessive consumption of alcohol in men as a biological influence factor in clinical laboratory investigations. *Journal of Clinical Chemistry and Clinical Biochemistry,* 22: 65-77.

Stamm, D., Hansert, E., & Feuerlein, W. (1984b). Detection and exclusion of alcoholism in men on the basis of clinical laboratory findings. *Journal of Clinical Chemistry and Clinical Biochemistry,* 22: 79-96.

Staun-Olsen, P., & Thomsen, A.C. (1979). Serum ethanol estimations in the control of alcohol abstinence in patients with liver disease. *Scandinavian Journal of Gastroenterology,* 14:785-789.

Stetter, F., Gaertner, H.J., Wiatr, G., Mann, K., & Breyer-Pfaff, U. (1991). Urinary dolichol—A doubtful marker of alcoholism. *Alcoholism, Clinical and Experimental Research,* 15: 938-941

Stevens, V.J., Fantl, W.J., Newman, C.B., Sims, R.V., Cerami, A., & Peterson, C.M. (1981). Acetaldehyde adducts with hemoglobin. *Journal of Clinical Investigation,* 67: 361-369.

Stibler, H. (1991). Carbohydrate-deficient transferrin in serum: a new marker of potentially harmful alcohol consumption reviewed. *Clinical Chemistry,* 37: 2029-2037.

Stibler, H., Allgulander, C., Borg, S., & Kjellin, K.G. (1978). Abnormal microheterogeneity of transferrin in serum and cerebrospinal fluid in alcoholism. *Acta Medica Scandinavica,* 204:49-56.

Stibler, H., Borg, S., & Allgulander, C. (1979). Clinical significance of abnormal heterogeneity of transferrin in relation to alcohol consumption. *Acta Medica Scandinavica,* 206: 275-281.

Stibler, H., Borg, S., & Allgulander, C. (1980). Abnormal microheterogeneity of transferrin—a new marker of alcoholism. *Substance and Alcohol Actions Misuse,* 1: 247-252.

Stibler, H., Borg, S., & Joustra, M. (1986). Micro anion exchange chromatography of carbohydrate-deficient transferrin in serum in relation to alcohol consumption (Swedish patent 8400587-5). *Alcoholism, Clinical and Experimental Research,* 10: 535-544.

Stibler, H., & Hultcrantz, R. (1987). Carbohydrate deficient transferrin (CDT) in serum in patients with liver diseases. *Alcoholism, Clinical and Experimental Research,* 11: 468-473.

Stimmel, B., Sturiano, V., Cohen, M., Korts, D., Hanbury, R., & Jackson, G. (1982). The ability of a Self-Administered Alcohol Screening Test (mSAAST) to detect future excessive alcohol consumption in persons on methadone maintenance. *Alcoholism, Clinical and Experimental Research,* 6: 362-368.

Storey, E.L., Anderson, G.J., Mack, U., Powell, L.W., & Halliday, J.W. (1987). Desialylated transferrin as a serological marker of chronic excessive alcohol ingestion. *Lancet, i*:1292-1294.

Takase, S., Takada, A., Tsutsumi, M., & Matsuda, Y. (1985). Biochemical markers of chronic alcoholism. *Alcohol*, 2: 405-410.

Tang, B.K. (1987). Detection of ethanol in urine of abstaining alcoholics. *Canadian Journal of Physiology and Pharmacology*, 65: 1225-1227.

Tang, B.K., Devenyi, P., Teller, D., & Israel, Y. (1986). Detection of an alcohol spesific product in urine of alcoholics. *Biochemical and Biophysical Research Communications*, 140: 924-927.

Taskinen, M.-R., Välimäki, M., Nikkilä, E.A., Kuusi, T., Enholm, C., & Ylikahri, R. (1982). High density lipoprotein subfractions and postheparin plasma lipase in alcoholic men before and after withdrawal. *Metabolism*, 31: 1168-1174.

Teschke, R. (1985). Gamma-glutamyltransferase and other markers for alcoholism. In H. Seitz & Y. Kommerell (Eds.), *Alcohol-related diseases in gastroenterology* (pp. 48-64). Berlin Springer Verlag.

Thiele, G., & Thiele, J. (1987). Die Bedeutung der Makrozytose als indikator für einen chronischen alkoholabusus. *Zeitschrift für die Gesamte Innere Medizin und ihre Grenzgebiete*, 42: 53-56.

Tonnesen, H., Hejberg, L., Frobenius, S. & Andersen, J.R. (1986). Erythrocyte mean cell volume—correlation to drinking pattern in heavy alcoholics. *Acta Medica Scandinavica*, 219: 515-518.

Towell, J.F. 3d., Barboriak, J.J., Townsend, W.F., Kalbfleisch, J.H. & Wang, R.I. (1986). Erythrocyte aldehyde dehydrogenase: assay of a potential biochemical marker of alcohol abuse. *Clinical Chemistry*, 32: 734-738.

Unger, K.W. & Johnson, D.Jr. (1974). Red cell mean corpuscular volume: a potential indicator of alcohol usage in working population. *American Journal of Medical Sciences*, 267: 281-289.

Välimäki, M., Härkönen, M,. & Ylikahri, R. (1983). Serum ferritin and iron levels in chronic male alcoholics before and after ethanol withdrawal. *Alcohol Alcohol*, 18: 255-260.

Välimäki, M., Nikkilä, E.A., Taskinen, M.-R., & Ylikahri, R. (1986). Rapid decrease in high density lipoprotein subfractions and postheparin plasma lipase activities after cessation of chronic alcohol intake. *Atherosclerosis*, 59: 147-153.

Välimäki, M., Taskinen, M.-R., Ylikahri, R., Roine, R., Kuusi, T., & Nikkilä, E.A. (1988). Comparison of the effects of two different doses of alcohol on serum lipoproteins, HDL-subfractions and apolipoproteins A-I and A-II. A controlled study. *European Journal of Clinical Investigation*, 18: 472-480.

Van Waes, L., & Lieber, C.S. (1977). Glutamate dehydrogenase: a reliable marker of liver cell necrosis in the alcoholic. *British Medical Journal*, 2: 1508-1510.

Wadstein, J., & Skude, G. (1979). Serum ethanol, hepatic enzymes and length of debauch in chronic alcoholics. *Acta Medica Scandinavica*, 205: 317-318.

Wallace, P., Cutler, S., & Haines, A. (1988). Randomised controlled trial of general practitioner intervention in patients with excessive alcohol consumption. *British Medical Journal*, 297: 663-668.

Watson, R.R., Mohs, M.E., Eskelson, C., Sampliner, R.E., & Hartmann, B. (1986). Identification of alcohol abuse and alcoholism with biological parameters. *Alcoholism, Clinical and Experimental Research*, 10: 364-385.

Wehr, H., Czartoryska, B., Górska, D., & Matsumoto, H. (1991). Serum ß hexosaminidase and α-mannosidase activities as markers of alcohol abuse. *Alcoholism, Clinical and Experimental Research*, 15: 13-15.

Weill, J., Schellenberg, F., Le Goff, A.-M., Benard, J.-Y. (1988). The decrease of low serum gamma glutamyl transferase during short-term abstinence. *Alcohol*, 5:1-3.

Whitehead, T.P., Pandov, H., & Clark, D.M. (1981). Gammaglutamyl-transpeptidase and alcohol problems. *Lancet, i*: 663.

Whitfield, J.B. (1981). Alcohol-related biochemical changes in heavy drinkers. *Australian and New Zealand Journal of Medicine*, 11: 132-139.

Whitfield, J.B., Moss, D.W., Neale, G., Orme, M., & Breckeridge, A. (1973). Changes in plasma-gammaglutamyltranspeptidase activity associated with alterations in drug metabolism in man. *British Medical Journal*, 274: 316-318.

Whitfield, J.B., Pounder, R.E., Neale, G., & Moss, D.W. (1972). Serum gamma-glutamyl-transpeptidase activity in liver disease. *Gut, 13*: 702-708.

Worner, T.M., & Lieber, C.S. (1980). Plasma glutamate dehydrogenase: a marker of alcoholic liver injury. *Pharmacological and Biochemical Behavior*, 13: [Suppl. 1]: 107-110.

Worrall, S., DeJersey, J., Shanley, B.C., & Wilce, P.A. (1990). Antibodies against acetaldehyde-modified epitopes: Presence in alcoholic, non-alcoholic liver disease and control subjects. *Alcohol Alcohol*, 25: 509-517.

Wu, A., Chanarin, I., & Levi, A.J. (1974). Macrocytosis of chronic alcoholism. *Lancet i*: 829-830.

Wu, A., Slavin, G., & Levi, A.J. (1976). Elevated serum gamma-glu-tamyltransferase (transpeptidase) and histological liver damage in alcoholism. *American Journal of Gastroenterology*, 65: 318-323.

Xin, Y., Lasker, J.M., Rosman, A.S., & Lieber, C.S. Isoelectric focus-ing/western blotting: A novel and practical method for quantita-tion of carbohydrate-deficient transferrin in alcoholics. *Alcoholism, Clinical and Experimental Research*, 15: 814-821.

Gender Related Issues In Alcohol Problems Research—a Special Need Group?

Ilana B. Glass-Crome
St. Bartholomew's Hospital Medical College
London, UK

After a period of relative neglect during the 1930s to 1960s, the "disease model" era (Jellinek 1960), the last two decades have witnessed the emergence of a risk group: alcohol problems and women (Thom, in press; Blume 1986, 1990) has portrayed the "female drinker." She describes how from Biblical times the image of the drinking woman has embraced notions of being victimised. She was perceived as immoral, aggressive, promiscuous, and her behaviour as inappropriate and irresponsible when compared to drinking men. Attitudes to the sexes became polarised, double standards were pervasive and women with alcohol problems became marginalised. Not surprisingly, this vicious circle breeds shame, guilt and low self esteem. It engenders stigma and prejudice, desperation and denial and so makes for difficulty in seeking help and detection (Moore et al 1989; Konovsky & Wilsnack 1982).

This review will demonstrate, contrary to the stereotyped picture described above, that there is a growing realisation of the heterogeneity in women's drinking patterns, and that the study of sex differences is a valuable method of analysing the biological, social and psychological determinants and consequences of drinking behaviour.

Epidemiology

Data on prevalence is available from a wide range of sources. National surveys of drinking practices, overall consumption, hospital admission rates, general practice attendance, community surveys and criminal justice system statistics are a few components of the data patchwork (Plant 1990). This wealth of different methodologies might still not capture representative samples. Gaps in information result from lack of detection. To some extent this is related to the stigma of admitting to being a drinking female. Those afflicted might never reach hospital, even though they might experience alcohol related problems and might, as mortality statistics reveal, even die much earlier from alcohol related illnesses than a control group. The focus of the sample may not be reflective of problems associated with women's drinking compared to men, i.e., workplace accidents, drunk and disorderly offences, and drunken driving convictions.

Despite these inadequacies, consumption data from international surveys indicate that clear differences do exist between men and women (Wilsnack et al 1984). Women are predominantly lighter drinkers in that they drink less often, in smaller amounts, and have a different beverage choice when compared to men. Overall, women have fewer alcohol related problems. Spontaneous remission occurs more often, fewer dependence symptoms develop and women take more psychoactive drugs than men (Fillmore 1987a).

Hilton (1988) reviewed a number of surveys in the United States since 1971 and showed that there had been little change over that time period. Seventy-five percent of men and 60% of women were drinkers, and between 14-20% of men and 3-6% of women fell into the heavy drinking category. Women predominantly abstained or were light drinkers. In the National Household Survey by the United States Census Bureau (1989), 34.5% of male and 14.1% of females had drunk once a week or more in the previous year. This pattern of a 2:1 ratio in general population surveys is a consistent one (Clayton et al 1986).

In the United Kingdom, data from the Office of Population Censuses and Surveys (1990) estimated that 4% of women were drinking more than 35 units of alcohol per week in comparison to 14% of men. Crawford (1986) showed that 5% of men and 2% of women were drinking over the safe limit recommended by the Royal College of Psychiatrists. These figures must be interpreted against the background of accumulating evidence of greater vulnerability by women to the effects of alcohol.

Data relating to use of services also emphasises the disparity of presentation. Recent studies which indicate that between 15% and 27% of female admissions to the wards of a general hospital have alcohol related problems suggests that the prevalence may be similar to male admissions to general hospital beds (Watson et al 1991; Lockhart et al 1986). King (1986) uncovered a far greater discrepancy in general practice. He detected 3.7% of female and 27.6% of male attenders at a general practice were drinking above 35 units of alcohol per week, whereas 1.3% females and 13.6% males were drinking over safe limits of 51 units per week.

Ghodsian and Power's 1987 study which surveyed young people demonstrated that, at age 23, 12% of males were drinking over 50 units of alcohol per week and 2% of females were drinking over 35 units of alcohol per week. A survey of elderly people with alcohol problems identified 9% of men and 4% of women "at risk", i.e., drinking above 21 and 14 units per week respectively (Bristow and Clare 1992). Fillmore (1987a) studied cohort effects and revealed that, although drinking decreased with age, men always drank more than women.

In specialist settings alcohol problems may precipitate the manifestation of particular problems: Halliday et al (1986) found that 11% of obstetric cases but 19% of gynaecological cases presenting to an obstetric and gynaecology clinic were heavy drinkers.

Toner et al (1991) estimated that 30% of women and 42.2% of men who were psychiatric inpatients were using alcohol and Dobkin et al (1991) diagnosed alcoholism in 73.5% men and 26.5% of women in a psychiatric hospital.

Thus while alcohol problems are found in a sizeable group of female patients attending a range of hospital departments and general practice, there remains a disparity between the numbers of men and women who present and the extent of their drinking problem.

With such diverse sources of information and a variety of diagnostic categories, there has been concern about the possibilities of exaggerating or minimising the problem.

One group of researchers (Jenkins 1986; Wilsnack et al 1984; OPCS 1990; Roman 1988) refutes the convergence hypothesis (Fillmore 1987b) that practices in women are beginning to mimic that of the male population. A controversy has emerged regarding the stability of drinking patterns in women. For instance, Williams and Debakey (1992) find no evidence of stability in drinking practices in males and females as abstention rates declined and heavy drinking increased between 1983 and 1988.

Furthermore, there is increasing evidence that the differences in drinking practices are associated in a complex relationship of a wide variety of factors, which may be gender related in the sociocultural matrix. These factors are marital status, employment, educational attainment, religion, ethnicity (including cultural sub-groups), age, socioeconomic level, parental drinking patterns, family size, social contacts, genetic and biological background, and concurrent smoking, all of which may influence drinking habits and presentation of problems (Roman 1988).

In summary, therefore, the evidence points to women drinking less by abstaining more or drinking less frequently. This appears to be consistent across national and international boundaries, even though definitions of drinking categories may differ. It is important to bear in mind that women seem to need less alcohol to experience a similar level of damage as men. There is also further evidence—or lack of it—which raises the issues of differential presentation, use of services and stability of pattern. This suggests that questionnaires have not been developed which would reveal ways in which women differ from men in their drinking practices.

"Women Have to Drink Less" . . . the Adverse Consequences of Heavy Drinking

Mortality and morbidity provide some indication of the adverse consequences of heavy drinking. A number of studies have shown that female alcoholics have between 4.5 - 5.2 times the expected death rate of the general population and life span is decreased by fifteen years in these women (Smith & Cloninger 1981; Smith et al 1983; Lindberg & Agren 1988). In 1988 in the United States 5% of deaths overall were due to alcohol, and death from alcohol related causes were more common in women.

Women are more likely to become intoxicated on a given dose of alcohol when compared to men. This has been explained by more rapid absorption, and by the fact that women have less body water so that alcohol reaches a higher concentration in the tissues and in the blood. Additional evidence points to body weight being the important variable in determining the peak blood alcohol concentration (Mello 1986; Mezey 1990). Lieber and his colleagues (Frezza et al 1990; Lieber 1991) have demonstrated differential gastric metabolism in females compared to males. The increased bioavailability of ethanol resulting from decreased gastric oxidation of ethanol in women may contibute to the enhanced vulnerability of women to acute and chronic complication of alcoholism.

Hilton (1987) reported that women develop more problems if they drink equal amounts of alcohol as men, as did Wilsnack et al (1987). Ashley et al (1977) confirmed that even though lifetime prevalence of alcoholism is the same, problems develop more quickly in women.

Hilton (1988) showed that women who drank were more isolated and drank on a greater number of occasions. At similar levels to men, women became more intoxicated, experienced more conflict and problems in their marital relationships but were less likely to lose control of their drinking.

When coping styles and personality traits were addressed, alcoholic men were more assertive than alcoholic women, who scored more highly on passivity, aggression, depression and conflict (Conte et al 1991; Olenick & Chalmers 1991). While moderate doses of alcohol produce aggression in women (Gustafson 1991), alcoholic women compared to normal women were less confident, less socially desirable, more depressed, more passive, more anxious and more submissive (Birnbaum et al 1983; Orford and Keddie 1985; Roman, 1988).

The findings in a group of studies corroborate a different constellation of presentations of alcohol related problems and psychiatric disorders (Allan 1991). In general female alcoholics have more psychiatric symptoms than male alcoholics (Ojchagen et al 1991). In the Epidemiologic Catchment Area Study (Miller & Rees 1991) nearly half those diagnosed as having alcoholism had a secondary diagnosis, with alcoholic women having higher rates of depression and psychiatric disorder. Mendelson et al (1986) reported that women with alcohol related problems were more frequently diagnosed as having neurotic and psychiatric disorders than men.

Hesselbrock et al (1985a, 1985b) found that 80% of women with alcohol problems were likely to have one or more additional diagnoses, especially major depression and phobic disorder, and these preceded the alcohol abuse. Similarly, Helzer and Pryzbeck (1988) reported that while 44% of alcoholic men had a second diagnosis, 65% of female alcoholics had a dual diagnosis. Depression more commonly preceded the alcohol problems in women, and this suggests the alcohol might mediate negative emotional states in women. Women exceeded men in all diagnoses except anti-social personality disorder. Ross et al (1988) demonstrated equal numbers of alcoholic patients with affective disorders, but anxiety and eating disorders were more prevalent in women. While the latter seems to be of particular relevance in female patients (Beary et al 1986; Pelever and Fairburn 1990; Bulik 1991), Weiss et al (1992) have described methodological problems in dual-diagnosis research in substance misusers.

There is some suggestion that women might be more vulnerable to the effects of alcohol (Harper et al 1990). Acker (1986) and Jacobson (1986) demonstrated that women were more likely to develop alcoholic brain damage: drinking histories were shorter, peak alcohol consumption was lower, psychological test performance was worse and scan abnormalities were greater than in men (Harper et al 1990).

Likewise, a number of studies have drawn attention to the rapid development of alcoholic liver disease in women: the course of the illness is shorter, the daily mean alcohol consumption is less (40 gm alcohol per day) and the prognosis is poorer when compared to men (Barrison et al 1985; Johnson & Williams 1985; Norton et al 1987). Yet women are less likely to have been identified as having alcoholic liver disease and to have received appropriate treatment for it, and women with alcoholic liver disease received more psychiatric treatment for non-alcohol related problems, (Saunders et al 1981; Saunders et al 1985). These findings could be interpreted as indicating that at the time of presentation and diagnosis women are faring poorly as compared to men.

The association of moderate alcohol intake with the development of breast cancer has been repeatedly reported (Willett et al 1987; Schatzkin et al 1987). The relationship between moderate amounts of alcohol (up to 17 1/2 units per week) and cardiovascular risk factors has not been resolved, and though some research suggests that there is a protective effect this conclusion must be cautiously interpreted (Razay et al 1992).

Alcohol metabolism is affected by female sex hormones (Sutker et al 1983a). One study has suggested that since aldehyde dehydrogenase is modulated by female sex steroids, women who are on the pill or pregnant may be at greater risk from the toxic effects of ethanol consumption (Jeavons & Zeiner 1984), while another has shown a decreased rate of ethanol metabolism across the menstrual cycle in female social drinkers on oral contraceptives (Jones and Jones 1984).

Alcohol affects the hypothalamic-pituitary axis (Sutker et al 1983b). The relationship between blood alcohol levels and the menstrual cycle is complex. Blood alcohol levels are influenced by progesterone which increases after ovulation and decreases with the onset of the menses (Lex 1991). Tate and Charette (1991) examined alcohol intake and physical and affective distress in normally menstruating women and found no association.

Thus, women apparently differ from men in many aspects of presentation of psychiatric, physical and metabolic consequences and complications of alcohol abuse. Whether this relates predominantly to a particular sensitivity to the effects of alcohol or to social factors in the treatment process or a combination needs refinement.

Fetal Alcohol Syndrome (FAS): An Example of the Evolving Interest in Women's Problems and Alcohol

Since women's alcohol problems were not taken seriously during the early part of the century it is perhaps not surprising that most authorities were dismissive of potential damage to the fetus. That alcohol had an impact on fetal health was described in Trotter (1804) and even earlier. Gradually as interest in women's issues was developing, Lecomte (1950), Lemoine et al (1968) and Ulleland (1972) published descriptions of a cluster of anomalies linked by maternal alcohol abuse, and increased risk of stillbirth, low birth weight and small for dates babies were related to alcohol consumption.

Just as women's health issues were being publicised a turning point was established by Jones et al in 1973 (Jones & Smith 1973; Jones et al 1973) when the syndrome was named "fetal alcohol syndrome". Since then workers in many countries have reported the syndrome, and alcohol is established as the major preventable cause of birth and neonatal morbidity (Chasnoff 1991).

More recently fetal alcohol syndrome and fetal alcohol effect (FAE) have been delineated. The main features of fetal alcohol syndrome are growth retardation, mental handicap and abnormal features of the head and face. Cardiac and neurological abnormalities, behavioural difficulties, genitourinary problems, cleft palate, finger print and palmar crease abnormalities are termed fetal alcohol effect or alcohol related birth defect.

Epidemiological research in the western world indicates a prevalence of fetal alcohol syndrome of 1-3/1000 live births and fetal alcohol effect of 4-6/1000 live births (Ihlen et al 1990). There is marked variation in different parts of the world for reasons which are not clear. It is noteworthy that this does fall far short of the numbers of women drinking abusively as only 30% of women who drink 70 gm of absolute alcohol/day have babies with fetal alcohol syndrome, though drinking histories can be very unreliable and under-reporting needs to be taken into account (Halmesmaki et al

1987; Morrow-Tlucak et al 1989). The special sensitivity of some women to the adverse effects of alcohol during pregnancy reflects the more general concern about the routes and mechanisms of susceptibility to alcohol.

Cost benefit analysis has recently become another facet of alcohol problems research. Abel and Sokol (1991) have estimated that 1200 children with FAS are born in the USA each year and this costs at least $73.6 million/year to treat.

Knupfer (1991) has incisively explored whether dose response effects could give any indication of a "safe limit" in pregnant women. She exposed the inadequate research methodology in the studies which had been carried out: there was variation and hence confusion in the use of terminology for quantity and patterns of consumption. Such shortcomings resonate through the literature of alcohol problems. Furthermore, Knupfer emphasised that multiple confounding variables, e.g., smoking, other drug use, and lifestyle may interact with drinking to affect pregnancy.

The jury is still out on this vital issue (Poikolainen 1991). Blume (1991) reiterates that since there is no convincing proof that social drinking is harmless, it is better to err on the side of caution.

A detailed understanding of this complex issue has implications not only for FAS but for alcohol problems research as a whole: the relationship of the timing, quantity and pattern of drinking to the development of harmful effects; the problem of confounding variables, e.g., under-reporting, other drug use and abuse, general lifestyle; difficulties in identification and assessment of serious consequences; the impact of the spouse or significant other in altering the course of the illness; accessibility, intervention and prevention (Heller et al 1988; Waterson et al 1990; Masis & May 1991).

Genetics and Neuroscience: "Sins of Fathers" —Sons of Alcoholic Fathers

The vast majority of studies in which the genetic component of alcoholism has been investigated have drawn on male probands.

The earlier twin studies (Kaij 1960; Hrubec & Omenn 1981) all focused on male children of alcoholic fathers. The study of Gurling et al (Gurling 1989) included a group of female alcoholics, and this was the only study which failed to demonstrate any difference between mono- and dizygotic twins. Pickens et al (1991) studied male and female twins: while male twins exhibited a difference in concordance between monozygotic and dizygotic twins, this was not the case in females.

Adoption studies, too, have mostly used adopted away sons of alcoholic fathers since female samples were small. There have been serious criticisms of diagnostic categories, design and follow up of these studies. Goodwin's group (1973) showed that there was a three fold difference in the likelihood of developing alcoholism in the adopted away sons of alcoholic parents. Goodwin et al (1977) did study a small group of adopted away females but the sample size precluded any meaningful conclusions. However, there appeared to be an equal incidence of alcohol problems whether the biological parents were alcoholic or not.

Bohman (1978) confirmed the three-fold increase in alcohol abuse in adopted away sons of alcoholic parents and demonstrated the highest rates of alcoholism in adopted away daughters of alcoholic mothers, although once more, the sample was small. This confirms the findings of Midanik (1983) who reported that more women than men admitted to a family history of drinking problems. Reich's (1988) study of first degree relatives of male and female alcoholics showed similar numbers of alcoholic relatives.

Cadoret et al (1978, 1985, 1987) also examined a male and female sample. These studies underlined the importance of biological factors in predicting the development of alcoholism. Increased alcohol abuse was found among male and female adoptees who had first degree biological relatives with problem drinking. However, drinking in the adoptive home was also found to influence alcohol abuse in male adoptees, indicating some environmental influence.

On the basis of Bohman's study, Cloninger et al (1981) have identified Type 1 (milieu-limited) and Type 2 (male-limited) alcoholism, and recently it has been suggested that this typology can be applied to female drinkers. Cloninger et al (1986) suggest that genetic factors in women with a family history of alcoholism is expressed differently, i.e., the female counterpart of "male-limited" alcoholism is expressed as somatization as opposed to impulsivity, belligerence and criminality. Glenn and Nixon (1991) recently modified Cloninger's classification to use age of onset rather than symptomatology as a discriminating factor and found that female alcoholics presented in both Type 1 and Type 11 categories. Early onset was linked with a Type II profile.

Longitudinal studies have pursued the sons of fathers, and generally examined the effects of growing up in a home where father's drinking was a part of the environment. Vaillant (1983) followed up male subjects for 30 years. His conclusion was that psychosocial factors were of lesser importance in comparison to genetic factors in the development of later alcoholism. McCord (1988) also reviewed outcome in sons of alcoholic fathers; Rydelius (1981) carried out a twenty year study on children of alcoholic fathers; and Werner (1986) linked resilience of children of alcoholic fathers to qualities in the child's mother. There is no reason why studies on the sons and daughters of alcoholic parents cannot be tackled simultaneously.

Implementation of the latest techniques in molecular biology in the study of psychiatric disorders will allow an opportunity not to limit study of the genetic component of the transmission of alcoholism to men only. These new approaches, as described in this volume, could also ensure that similar diagnostic techniques can be applied across studies. There are serious difficulties when attempting to compare findings across different countries and cultures.

A constellation of studies have focused on electrophysiological responses in males at risk of developing alcoholism—sons of alcoholic fathers or family history positive young men (Cohen et al 1991; Pfefferbaum et al 1991). No similar studies appear to have been published on sons of alcoholic mothers or daughters of alcoholic parents. The electrophysiological studies have been complemented by a range of studies which investigate the subjective responses (mood, intoxication), body sway (Mills & Bisgrove 1983), and hormonal changes (cortisol, prolactin) to alcohol ingestion in controlled conditions (Schuckit 1984; Schuckit 1985; Schuckit & Gold 1988; Schuckit et al 1991; Moss et al 1989). The objective has been to identify ways in which sons of alcoholics differ from sons of non-alcoholics. Generally, sons of alcoholics have been shown to be less sensitive or responsive to a challenge dose of alcohol, to differ in the development of tolerance to alcohol (Newlin & Thomson 1991), and to show a different cognitive (Hewett et al 1991) and personality profile (Whipple & Noble 1991) when compared to the sons of non-alcoholics.

This body of work deserves replication in a female population: it is extraordinary that this has not been done.

Treatment: The Myth of the Poorer Prognosis

As described on the section on epidemiology, women may present to treatment agencies with alcohol problems seemingly less frequently than men. Reasons for this under-representation may be related to many features of the treatment process in addition to reasons outlined in the section on epidemiology, such as inadequate identification, referral to appropriate agencies and availability of suitable facilities.

Many factors in the treatment process may militate against women making gains. There are factors such as transport and accessibility which relate to the family responsibilities of caring for children or elderly members of the family, and economic factors. Further, there are attitudes of providers of care which may be expressed as lack of sensitivity, of detection, and/or of onward referral to appropriate agencies providing suitable treatment facilities. In addition there may be the sociocultural factors of stigma and prejudice. In order to fairly evaluate outcome measures any treatment research must take into account the lack of resources with which women go into treatment.

Classic studies were presumably conducted on male alcoholics rather than females because of the different rates of presentation to services (Edwards et al 1977; Vaillant 1983). Vannicelli and Nash (1984) reviewed alcoholism treatment studies and found that 23 of 259 studies described female alcoholics only, while 37% described mixed or female only samples. Only 30% of the studies distinguished between the sexes on presentation of the data and 7.8% of the 64,000 patients were female. This is discordant with national drinking surveys.

Thom (1986, 1987) has described how women have different perceptions about the role alcohol problems play in their lives. Since women were less likely to feel that alcohol was the main problem in their lives, they are reluctant to ask for help especially if it involves being labelled an alcoholic or psychiatric patient. In keeping with other reports, women also complain of depression and anxiety with greater frequency than men. In later studies, Thom et al. (1992a, b) report that although men have higher prior expectations from an alcohol clinic, at the end of the first consultation women were more likely to rate helpfulness higher. These findings have implications for availability and accessibility to treatment services.

Vanicelli (1987) and Annis and Liban (1980) reviewed outcome in the studies that included female alcoholics: outcome was similar to or better than men. Thus, their conclusion was that women do *not* have poorer prognosis. Jarvis (1992) presents a meta-analysis of 26 treatment studies. She found that women had better treatment outcome than men during the first twelve months whereas men were better after one year. Thus, women may flourish with shorter term, self-help manuals and behavioural therapies, while men appear to find longer-term group therapies effective (Sanchez-Craig et al 1991). This discrepancy may be due to the treatment system being male oriented: men may feel more comfortable in the group situation; women may feel lacking in confidence in mixed sex groups. Women may be traumatised by sexual abuse, have different psychiatric problems such as anxiety and depression, may be unsupported by their spouse or others and may have to drop out of treatment due to lack of support: such antecedents and consequences may set women apart from men in the treatment setting (Turnbull & Gomberg 1991). Women may therefore need different kinds of longer-term help.

Data on "what works" for men cannot be extrapolated to women (Beckman & Amaro 1987). Treatment needs of women require identification (Glass-Crome 1992) so that services can be matched to the specific problems which confront alcoholic women (Allan & Cooke 1986). Help with social support, single sex groups, outreach facilities, or female therapists are some of the resources which might serve women well. Dahlgren and Willander (1989) report an initiative where women did appreciably better in programmes designed for them specifically. Copeland and Hall (1992) report that some women drop out of treatment less if the service is oriented to women.

There is insufficient information on which to conclude that women "do worse" in treatment. What is evident is that stability and support is associated with a better outcome. Thus, if social attitudes change, entry to appropriate services may be facilitated and the provision of help may be oriented to the difficult social reality of the female drinker (Duckert 1988). Further, if support is sustained and strengthened it may be possible to mitigate the opposition for treatment from spouses, friends, family and the workplace. Only then will researchers in the treatment field be in a position to test outcome in both alcoholic males and females.

While most countries accept the special requirements of women, very few are able to provide such facilities (Institute of Medicine 1990). In the United Kingdom although counselling services may frequently have female counsellors, there are few specialist services for women and very few which can accommodate children (Alcohol Concern 1992).

Policy—A Case for Positive Discrimination?

The Public Health Task Force on Women's Health Issues (Ray & Braude 1984) focused on the issue that sex differences have not been routinely studied. At a recent conference on the policy implications of substance misuse, one delegate calculated that only 15% of all the participants and speakers at the conference were women (Babor 1992). Admittedly, this is a crude measure of the priority which women's issues have held in the scientific and policy making community. But it is substantiated by the glaring imbalance—as outlined above—in the manner in which the nature and extent of these problems are addressed.

The majority of women are drinking, and many will experience problems as a result. Some authorities argue that women will develop more serious physical and psychological problems than men for a given quantity of alcohol. The consequences of these problems may be devastating for the woman herself, her family and her community.

Yet, while this review has provided evidence that women with alcohol (and drug) problems are sufficiently burdensome to the health and social well-being of every country, only a fraction of the research effort has been oriented towards women.

There is a fundamental need for an integrated research effort which is directed at redressing the balance of activity which has hitherto focused on men. This involves allocating and designating specific funds for women's needs.

Studies on prevalence of alcoholism in women in the community and the treatment services available for women of all ages and socioeconomic and ethnic groups have important implications for the development of services. Longitudinal studies using male and female subjects and parents would establish any differential consequences of genetic factors and environmental antecedents.

Study of gender differences in a multidisciplinary research strategy which encompasses sociology, history, anthropology, pharmacology, neurophysiology, neuropsychology, psychology, and neuroendocrinology would prove enormously valuable.

Clinical issues such as the potential protective effect of alcohol in cardiovascular disease, the rapid progression of liver and brain damage, the mechanism of fetal alcohol syndrome, the association with cancers and endocrine abnormalities, the relationship to the course of psychiatric illnesses and other addictive substance misuse are some of the many areas to be researched in both sexes.

Prevention and treatment related issues remain the most urgent, since women have received such bad press on the basis of so few studies. The desirability of special treatment programmes must be evaluated: does increased accessibility decrease drop-out rate, are female polysubstance abusers or those with dual diagnosis properly diagnosed, what is the prognosis for adolescent and elderly alcohol abusers, and how successful is treatment matching in terms of outcome, what questionnaires and outcome measures are best suited to thoroughly assess improvement in women, and what measures can enhance prevention at the community level?

The differing, changing and interacting social contexts for both men and women have to be explored. This is one case where the compartmentalisation of disciplines will obstruct the advance of knowledge.

For while this review has sought to place the problem of the female alcoholic in the social context, it has simultaneously through this exploration revealed those areas which are conspicuous by their absence.

Sadly these are the biological dimensions. Hopefully this analysis will serve as a catalyst for promoting a policy on alcohol and women. One is led to believe that only positive discrimination will place this area on the research agenda in any worthwhile and meaningful fashion.

Acknowledgements

I would like to thank Betsy Thom for helpful comments on this paper. Margaret Prendergast and Annabelle Short provided excellent secretarial assistance.

References

Abel, E.L. & Sokol, R.J. (1991). A revised conversative estimate of the incidence of FAS and its economic impact. *Alcoholism: Clinical and Experimental Research*, 15: 514-524.

Acker, C. (1986). Neuropsychological deficits in alcoholics: the relative contributions of gender and drinking history. *British Journal of Addiction*. 81: 395-403.

Alcohol Concern. (1992) A woman's guide to alcohol.Alcohol Concern: London.

Allan, C.A. & Cooke D. (1986). Women, life events and drinking problems. *British Journal of Psychiatry*, 148: 462.

Allan, C.A. (1991) Psychological symptoms, psychiatric disorder and alcohol dependence amongst men and women attending a community-based voluntary agency and an alcohol treatment unit, 86: 419-427.

Annis, H.M. & Liban, C. B. (1980). Alcoholism in women: treatment modalities and outcomes. In: Kalant, O.J. (Ed). *Alcohol and drug problems in women: research advances in alcohol and drug problems.* New York: Plenum. Volume 5, pg 384-422. .

Ashley, M. J., Olin, J. S., Le Riche, W. H., Kornaczewski, A., Schmidt, W. & Rankin, J. G. (1977). Morbidity in alcoholics: Evidence of accelerated development of physical disease in women. *Archives of Internal Medicine.* 137: 883-887.

Babor, T. (1992). Towards a science policy analysis on research on substance problems. In: Edwards, G. & Strang, J. (Ed). *Drugs, alcohol and tobacco—making the science and policy connections.* Oxford University Press Oxford.

Barrison, I. G., Waterson, E. J. & Murray-Lyon, I. M. (1985).Adverse effects of alcoholism in pregnancy. 80: 11-22.

Beary, M.D., Lacey, J.H. ,and Merry, J. (1986) Alcoholism and eating disorders in women of fertile age. *British Journal of Addiction.* 81: 389-393.

Beckman, L.J. & Amaro, H. (1987) Patterns of women's use of alcohol treatment agencies. In: Wilsnack and Beckman (Eds) *Alcohol problems in women.*New York: Guildford Press.

Birnbaum, I.M., Taylor, T.H., & Parker, E.S. (1983) Alcohol and sober mood state in female social drinkers. *Alcoholism: Clinical and Experimental Research.* 7: 362-367.

Blume, S.B. (1991) The problems of quantifying alcohol consumption. *British Journal of Addiction.* 86: 1059-1060.

Blume, S.B. (1990) Chemical dependency in women: important issues. *American Journal of Drug and Alcohol Abuse.* 16: 297-302.

Blume, S.B. (1986). Women and alcohol: a review. *Journal of the American Medical Association.* 256: 1467-1470.

Bohman, M. (1978). Some genetic aspects of alcoholism and criminality. *Archives of General Psychiatry.* 35: 269-276

Bohman, M., Sigvardsson, S. & Cloninger, C.R. (1981). Maternal inheritance of alcohol abuse cross-fostering analysis of adopted women. *Archives of General Psychiatry.* 38: 965-969.

Bristow, M.F. & Clare, A.W. (1992). Prevalence and characteristics of at-risk drinkers among elderly acute medical in-patients. *British Journal of Addiction.* 87: 291-294.

Bulik, C.M. (1991). Family history of bulimic women with and without comorbid alcohol abuse or dependence. *American Journal of Psychiatry.* 148: 1267-1268 .

Cadoret, R.J. (1978). Inheritance of alcoholism in adoptees. *British Journal of Psychiatry.* 132: 252-258.

Cadoret, R.J. Gath, A., O'Gorman, T.W., Troughton, E. & Heywood, E. (1985). Alcoholism and anti-social personality. *Archives of General Psychiatry.* 42: 161-167.

Cadoret , R. J., Troughton, E. & O'Gorman, T.W. (1987). Genetic and environmental factors in alcohol abuse and anti-social personality. *Journal of Studies on Alcohol.* 48: 1-8.

Chasnoff, I.J. (1991). Drugs, alcohol, pregnancy and the neonate—pay now or later. *Journal of the American Medical Association.* 266: 1567-1568.

Clayton, RL., Voss, H.L., Robbins, C. & Skinner, W.F. (1986). Gender differences in drug use: An epidemiological perspective. In B.A. Ray and M.C. Braude (Eds). *Women and drugs: a new era for research.* pp 80-99. NIDA Research Monograph No. 65. Rockville: MD NIDA.

Cloninger, C.R., Sigvardsson, S., Reich, T. & Bohman, M. (1986). Inheritance of risk to develop alcoholism. In M.C. Braude and H.M. Chao (Eds). *Genetic and biological markers in drug abuse and alcoholism* NIDA Research Monograph No 66: 86-96. Washington DC US Government Printing Office.

Cloninger, C.R., Bohman, M. & Sigvardsson, S. (1981). Inheritance of alcohol abuse: Cross fostering analysis of adopted men. *Archives of General Psychiatry.* 38: 861-868.

Cohen, H.L., Porjesz, B. & Begleiter, H. (1991). EEG characteristics in males at risk for alcoholism. *Alcoholism: Clinical and Experimental Research.* 15: 858-861.

Conte, H.R., Plutchik, A., Picard, S., Galanter, M. & Jacoby, J. (1991). Sex differences in personality traits and coping styles of hospitalised alcoholics. *Journal of Studies on Alcohol.* 52: 26-32.

Cook, C.C.H. & Gurling, H., M.D. (1990). The genetic aspects of alcoholism and substance abuse. In: *The Nature of Drug Dependence,* Edwards, G. and Lader, M. (Eds), Oxford: Oxford University Press.

Copeland, J. & Hall, W. (1992). A comparison of predictors of treatment drop-out of women seeking drug and alcohol treatment in a specialist women's and two traditional mixed-sex treatment services. *British Journal of Addiction.* 87: 883-890.

Crawford, A. (1986). Adults at risk: a comparison of heavy drinkers in three areas of Britain. *Drug and Alcohol Dependence.* 18: 301-309.

Dahlgren, L. & Willander, A. (1989). Are special treatment facilities for female alcoholics needed? A controlled 2-year follow-up study from a specialised female unit (EWA) versus a mixed male/female treatment facility. *Alcoholism: Clinical and Experimental Research.* 13: 499-504.

Dobkin, P., Dongier, M., Cooper, D. & Hill, J.M. (1991). Screening for alcoholism in a psychiatric hospital. *Canandian Journal of Psychiatry.* 36: 39-45.

Duckert, F. (1988). Recruitment into alcohol treatment: a comparison between male and female problem drinkers recruited to treatment in two different ways. *British Journal of Addiction.* 83: 285-293.

Edwards, G., Orford, J., Egert, S., Guthrie, S., Hawther, A., Hensman, C., Mitcheson, M., Oppenheimer, E. & Taylor, C. (1977). Alcoholism: a controlled trial of treatment and advice. *Journal of Studies on Alcohol.* 38: 1004-1031.

Fillmore, K.M. (1987a). Women's drinking across the life course as compared to men's. *British Journal of Addiction.* 82: 801-81.

Fillmore, K.M. (1987b). When angels fall: Women's drinking as cultural preoccupation and as reality. In: Wilsnack, S.C. and Beckman, L.J. (Eds). *Alcohol problems in women.* New York: Guilford Press.

Frezza, M., DiPadova, C., Pozzato, G., Terpin, M., Baraona, E. & Lieber, C.S. (1990). High blood alcohol levels. The rate of decreased alcohol dehydrogenase activity and first pass metabolism. *New England Journal of Medicine.* 322: 95-99.

Ghodsian, M. & Power, C. (1987). Alcohol consumption between the ages of 16 and 23 in Britain: a longitudinal study. *British Journal of Addiction.* 82: 175-180.

Glass-Crome, I.B. (1992). Training: a vital ingredient for alcohol treatment services. *Current Opinion in Psychiatry.* 5: 436-440

Glenn, S.W. & Nixon, S. J. (1991) Applications of Cloninger's subtypes in a female alcoholic sample. *Alcoholism: Clinical and Experimental Research.* 15: 851-857.

Goodwin, D.W., Schulsinger, F., Knop, H., Medwick, S. & Guze, S.B. (1977). Alcoholism and depression in adopted out daughters of alcoholics. *Archives of General Psychiatry.* 31: 751-755.

Goodwin, D.W., Schulsinger, F., Miller, N., Hermansen,L., Winokur, G. & Guze, S.B. (1987). Drinking problems in adopted and non adopted sons of alcoholics. Archives of General Psychiatry. 31: 164-169.

Goodwin, D., Schulsinger, F., Hermansen, L., Guze, S.B. & Winokur, G. (1973). Alcohol problems in adoptees raised apart from alcoholic biological parents. *Archives of General Psychiatry.* 28: 238-243.

Gurling, H.M.D. (1989). The genetic predisposition to alcoholism adn the effects of alcoholism on brain structure and function. M.D. Thesis University of London.

Gustafson, R. (1991). Aggressive and non-aggressive behavior as a function of alcohol intoxication and frustration in women. *Alcholism Clinical and Experimental Research*, 15: 886-892.

Halliday, A., Booher, B., Cleary, P., Aronson, M. & Delbanco, T. (1986). Alcohol abuse in women seeking gynaecologic care. *Obstetrics and Gynaecology*. 68: 322-326.

Halmesmaki, E., Raivio, K.O. & Ylikorkala, O. (1987). Patterns of alcohol consumption during pregnancy. *Obstetrics and Gynaecology*. 69: 594-597.

Harper, C.G., Smith, N.A. & Kril, J.J. (1990). The effects of alcohol on the female brain—a neuropathological study. *Alcohol and Alcoholism* 25: 445-448.

Heller, J., Anderson, H.R., Bland, J.M., Brooke, O.G., Peacock, J.L., & Stewart, C.M. (1988). Alcohol in pregnancy: patterns and association with socio-economic psychological and behavioural factors. *British Journal of Addiction*, 83: 541-551.

Helzer, J. & Pryzbek, T. (1988). The co-occurrence of alcoholism with other psychiatric disorders in the general population and its impact on treatment. *Journal of Studies on Alcohol*, 49: 219-224.

Hesselbrock, M.N., Meyer, R.E., & Keener, J. J .(1989a). Psychopathology in hospitalised alcoholics. *Archives of General Psychiatry*, 42: 1050-1055.

Hesselbrock, M.N., Weideman, M.A., & Reed, H.B. (1985b). Effect of age, sex, drinking history and antisocial personality on neuropsychology of alcoholics. *Journal of Studies on Alcohol*, 46: 313-320.

Hewett, L.J., Nixon, S.J., Glenn, S.W., & Parsons, O.A. (1991). Verbal fluency deficits in female alcoholics. *Psychology* , 47: 716-719.

Hilton, M.E. (1988). Trends in US drinking patterns: further evidence from the past 20 years. *British Journal of Addiction*, 83: 269-278.

Hilton, M.E. (1987). Drinking patterns and drinking problems in (1984). Results from the general population survey. *Alcoholism: Clinical and Experimental Research*, 11: 167-175.

Hrubec, Z.& Omenn, G . (1981) Evidence of genetic predisposition to alcoholic cirrhosis and psychosis: Twin concordances for alcoholism and its biological end points by zygosity among male veterans. *Alcoholism: Clinical and Experimental Research* , 5: 207-215.

Ihlen, B.M., Amundsen, A., Sande, H.A.,& Daae, L (1990). Changes in the use of intoxicants after onset of pregnancy. *British Journal of Addiction* 85: 1627-1633.

Institute of Medicine (1990) *Broadening the base of treatment for alcohol problems*. National Academy Press Washington DC.

Jacobson, R. (1986). Female alcoholics: a controlled CT brain scan and clinical study. *British Journal of Addiction*, 81: 661-669.

Jarvis, T.J. (1992) Implications of gender for alcohol treatment research: a quantitative and qualitative review. *British Journal of Addiction*, 87: 1249-1262

Jeavons, C.M. & Zeiner, A.R. (1984). Effects of elevated female sex steroids on ethanol and acetaldehyde metabolism in humans. *Alcoholism: Clinical and Experimental Research*, 8: 352-358.

Jellinek, E.M. (1960). *The Disease Concept of Alcoholism*. Hillhouse Press New Haven.

Jenkins R (1986). Sex differences in alcohol consumption and its associated morbidity in young civil servants. *British Journal of Addiction*, 81: 525-535.

Johnson, R.D. & Williams, R. (1985). Genetic and environmental factors in the individual susceptibility to the development of alcoholic liver disease. *Alcohol and Alcoholism*, 20: 137-160.

Jones K.L., Smith, D.W., Ulleland, C.N., & Streissguth, A.P. (1973). Patterns of malformation in offspring of alcoholic mothers. *Lancet*, 1: 1267-1271.

Jones, K.L. & Smith, D.W. (1973). Recognition of the foetal alcohol syndrome in early infancy. *Lancet*, 2: 999-1001.

Jones, M.K. & Jones, B.M. (1984). Ethanol metabolism in women taking oral contraceptives. *Alcoholism: Clinical and Experimental Research*, 8: 24-28.

Kaij, L. (1960). *Alcoholism in twins: studies of the etiology and sequels of abuse of alcohol*. Alquist and Wiksell Stockholm.

King, M. (1986). At risk drinking among general practice attenders: prevalence, characteristics and alcohol related problems. *British Journal of Psychiatry*, 148: 533-540.

Knupfer, G. (1991). Abstaining for fetal health: the fiction that even light drinking is dangerous. *British Journal of Addiction*, 86: 1063-1074.

Konovsky, M. & Wilsnack, S.C. (1982). Social drinking and self-esteem in married couples. *Journal of Studies on Alcohol*, 43, 319-333.

Lecomte, M. (1950). Elements d'heredopathologie. *Scalper*, 103: 1133-1145.

Lemoine, P., Harronseau, H., Borteyru, J.P. & Menuet, J.C. (1968)Les enfants de parents alcooliques: Anomalies observées à propos des 127 cas. *Quest Medicale*, 25: 476-482

Lex, B.W. (1991). Some gender differences in alcohol and polysubstance users. *Health Psychology*, 10: 121-132.

Lex, B.W., Lukas, S.E., Greenwal,d N.E. & Mendelson, J.H. (1988). Alcohol induced change in body sway in women at risk for alcoholism. A pilot study. *Journal of Studies on Alcohol*, 49: 346-356.

Lieber C S (1991). Pathways of ethanol metabolism and related pathology. In: T N Palmer (Ed). *Alcoholism: A Molecular Perspective. Plenum Press New York.*

Lindberg, S. & Agren, G. (1988). Mortality among male and female hospitalised alcoholics in Stockholm 1962-1983. *British Journal of Addiction*, 83: 1193-1200.

Lockhart, S.P., Carter, Y.H., Straffen, A.M., Pang, K.K., McLaughlin, J., and Baron, J.H. (1986) Detecting alcohol consumption as a cause of emergency general medical admissions. *Journal of the Royal Society of Medicine*. 79: 132-136.

McCord, J. (1988). Identifying developmental paradigms leading to alcoholism. *Journal of Studies in Alcohol*, 49: 357-362.

McKenna, T. & Pickens, R. (1981) Alcoholic children of alcoholics. *Journal of Studies on Alcohol*, 42: 1021-1029.

Masis, K.B. & May, P.A. (1991). A comprehensive local program for the prevention of fetal alcohol syndrome. *Public Health Report*, 106: 484-489.

Mello, N.K. (1986). Drug use patterns and premenstrual dysphoria. In: Ray, B.A. and Braude, M.C. (Eds). *Women and drugs: a new era for research*. NIDA Research Monograph 65. NIDA Washington DC.

Mendelson, J.H., Babor, T.F., Mello, N.K. & Pratt, H. (1986) Alcoholism and prevalence of medical and psychiatric disorders. *Journal of Studies on Alcohol*, 47: 361-366.

Mezey, E. (1990). Alcoholism metabolism in men and women—Reply. *Alcoholism (NY)*, 14: 785-786.

Midanik, L. (1983) Familial alcoholism and problem drinking in a national drinking practices survey. *Addictive Behaviour*, 8:133-141.

Miller, N.S. & Rees, R.K. (1991). Drug and alcohol dependence and psychiatric populations: the need for diagnosis, intervention and training. *Comprehensive Psychiatry*, 32: 268-272.

Mills, K.C. & Bisgrove, E.Z. (1983). Body sway and divided attention performance under the influence of alcohol: dose-response differences between males and females. *Alcoholism: Clinical and Experimental Research*, 7: 393-397.

Moore, R.D., Bone, L.R., Geller, G., Mamon, J.A., Stokes, E.J. & Levine, D.M. (1989). Prevalence detection and treatment of alcoholism in hospitalised patients. *Journal of the American Medical Association*, 261: 403-408.

Moss, H.B., Yao, J.K. & Maddock, J.M. (1989). Responses by sons of alcoholic fathers to alcoholic and placebo drinks: perceived mood, intoxication and plasma prolactin. *Alcoholism: Clinical and Experimental Research*, 13: 252-257.

Morrow-Tlucah, et al. (1989). National Institute on Drug Abuse (1989). National Household Survey on Drug Abuse: Population estimates (1988). US Government Printing Office: Washington DC.

Newlin, D.B. & Thomson, J.B. (1991). Chronic tolerance and sensitization to alcohol in sons of alcoholics. *Alcoholism: Clinical and Experimental Research*, 13: 399-405.

Norton, R., Batey, R., Dwyer, T. & MacMahon, S. (1987). Alcohol consumption and the risk of alcohol related cirrhosis in women. *British Medical Journal*, 295: 80-82.

Office of Population Censuses and Surveys (1990). HMSO: London.

Ojehagen, A., Berglund, M., Appel, C.P., Nilsson, B. & Skjaerris, A. (1991). Psychiatric symptoms in alcoholics attending out-patient treatment. *Alcoholism: Clinical and Experimental Research*, 15: 640-646.

Olenick, N.L. & Chalmers, D.K. (1991). Gender specific drinking styles in alcoholics and non-alcoholics. *Journal of Studies on Alcohol*, 52: 325-330.

Orford, J. & Keddie, A. (1985). Gender differences in the functions and effects of moderate and excessive drinking. *British Journal of Clinical Psychology*, 24: 265-279.

Peacock, J.L., Bland, J.M., Anderson, H.R. (1991). Effects on birthweight of alcohol and caffeine consumption in smoking women. *Journal of Epidemiology and Community Health*, 45: 159-163.

Pelever, R. & Fairburn, C. (1990). Eating disorders in women who abuse alcohol. *British Journal of Addiction*, 85: 1633-1638.

Pfefferbaum, A., Ford, J.M., White, P.M. & Mathalon, D. (1991). Event-related potentials in alcoholic men P3 amplitude reflects family history but not alcoholic consumption. *Alcoholism: Clinical and Experimental Research*, 15: 839-850.

Pickens, R.W., Svikis, D.S., Megue, M., Lykken, D.T., Heston, L., & Clayton, P.J. (1991). Heterogeneity in the inheritance of alcoholism—a study of male and female twins. *Archives of General Psychiatry*, 48: 19-28.

Plant, M.L. (1990). Women and alcohol : a review of international literature on the use of alcohol. World Health Organisation, Geneva.

Poikolainen, K. (1991). Abstain from poisoning your unborn child. *British Journal of Addiction*, 86: 1060-1061.

Ray, B.A. & Braude, M.C. (Eds). 1986 Women and drugs: a new era for research. NIDA Research Monograph 65. National Institute of Drug Abuse, Washington DC.

Razay, G., Heaton, K.W., Bolton, C.H. & Hughes, A.O. (1992). Alcohol consumption and its relation to cardiovascular risk factors in British women. *British Medical Journal*, 304: 80-83.

Reich, T., Cloninger, C.R, Van Eerdewegh P., Rice, J.P. & Mullaney, J. (1988). Secular trends in the familial transmission of alcoholism. *Alcoholism : Clinical and Experimental Research*, 12: 458-464.

Roman, P.M. (1988). Women and alcohol use: a review of the research literature. National Institute of Alcohol Abuse and Alcoholism, Washington.

Ross, H.E., Glaser, F.B., & Stiansnys. (1988). Sex differences in the prevalence of psychiatric disorders in patients with alcohol and drug problems. *British Journal of Addiction*, 83: 1179-1192.

Royal College of General Practitioners. (1986). Alcohol: a balanced view. Royal College of General Practitioners London.

Royal College of Psychiatrists. (1986). Alcohol—our favourite drug. Tavistock London.

Rydelius, P.A. (1981). Children of alcoholic fathers. *Acta Paediatrica Scandinavica Supplement*, 286: 1-89.

Sanchez-Craig, M., Spivak, K. & Davila, R. (1991). Superior outcome of females over males after brief treatment for the reduction of heavy drinking: replication and report of therapist effects. *British Journal of Addiction*, 86: 867-876.

Saunders, J.B., Wodak, A.D. & Williams, R. (1985). Past experience of advice and treatment for drinking problems of patients with alcoholic liver disease. *British Journal of Addiction*, 80: 51-56.

Saunders, J.B., Davis, M. & Williams, R. (1981). Do women develop alcoholic liver disease more readily than men? *British Medical Journal*, 282: 1140-1143.

Schatzkin, A., Jones, Y., Hoover, R.N., Taylor, P.R., Brinton, L.A., Ziegler, R.G., Harvey, E.B., Carter, C.L., Licitra, L.M., Dufour, M.C. & Larson, D.B. (1987). Alcohol consumption and breast cancer in the epidemiologic follow-up study of the first National Health and Nutritious Examination Survey. *New England Journal of Medicine, 316: 1169-1173.*

Schuckit, M.A., Duthie, L.A., Mahler, H.I.M., Irwin, M. & Montiero, M. (1991). Subjective feelings and changes in body sway following diazepam in sons of alcoholics and control subjects. *Journal of Studies on Alcohol*, 52: 601-608.

Schuckit, M.A. & Gold, E. (1988). A simultaneous evaluation of multiple markers of ethanol/placebo challenges in sons of alcoholics and controls. *Archives of General Psychiatry*, 45: 211-216.

Schuckit, M.A. (1985). Ethanol induced changes in body sway in men at high alcoholism risk. *Archives of General Psychiatry*, 42: 375-375.

Schuckit, M.A. (1984). Subjective responses to alcohol in sons of alcoholics and control subjects. *Archives of General Psychiatry*, 42: 879-884.

Smart, R.G. (1979). Female and male alcoholics in treatment: Characteristics at intake and recovery rates. *British Journal of Addiction*, 74: 275-281.

Smith, E.M. & Cloninger, C.R. (1981). Alcoholic females: mortality at 12 year follow up. *Focus on women*, 2: 1-13.

Smith, E.M., Cloninger, C.R. & Bradford, S. (1983) Predictors of mortality in alcoholic women: A prospective follow-up study. *Alcoholism Clinical and Experimental Research*, 7: 237-243.

Smith, L. (In press). A literature review: help seeking in alcohol dependent females. *Alcohol and Alcoholism*.

Sutker, P.B., Tabakoff, B., Goist, K.C. & Randall, C.L. (1983a). Acute alcohol intoxication, mood states and alcohol metabolism in women and men. *Pharmacology Biochemistry and Behaviour*, 18: 349-354.

Sutker, P.B., Libet, J.M., Allain, A.N. & Randell, C.L. (1983b). Alcohol use, negative mood states and menstrual cycle phases. *Alcoholism: Clinical and Experimental Research*, 7: 327-331.

Tate, D.L. & Charette, L.(1991). Personality, alcohol consumption and menstrual distress in young women. *Alcohol : Clinical and Experimental Research*, 15: 647-652.

Thom, B., Brown, C., Drummond, C., Edwards, G. & Mullan, M. (1992a). The use of services for alcohol problems: the general practitioner and specialist alcohol clinic. *British Journal of Addiction*, 87: 613-624.

Thom, B., Brown, C., Drummond, C., Edwards, G. & Mullan, M. (1992b). Engaging patients with alcohol problems in treatment : the first consultation. British Journal of Addiction 87 601-612.

Thom, B. (In press). *Woman and alcohol—the emergence of an at risk group*. In: Gender drink and drugs, Maryon McDonald (Ed). Berg: Oxford and New York.

Thom, B. (1987). Sex differences in help-seeking for alcohol problems: 2—Entry into treatment. *British Journal of Addiction*, 82: 989-997.

Thom, B. (1986). Sex differences in help-seeking for alcohol problems: 1—The barriers to help-seeking. *British Journal of Addiction*, 81: 777-788.

Thom, B. (In press). Women and alcohol—The emergence of an at risk group. In: *Gender drink and drugs*, Maryon McDonald (Ed)., Berg Oxford and New York.

Toner, B.B., Shugar, G., Campbell, B. & Gasbarro, D. (1991). Pattern of substance abuse in psychiatric in-patients. *Canadian Journal of Psychiatry*, 36: 381-383.

Trotter, T. (1804). An essay medical philosophical and chemical on drunkenness and its effects on the human body. Longman, Hurst, Rees and Urme London. Republished (1988). Routledge London.

Turnbull, J.E. & Gomberg, E.S.L. (1991). The structure of drinking related consequences in alcoholic women. *Alcoholism (NY)*. 15: 29-38.

Ulleland, C.N. (1972). The offspring of alcoholic mothers. *Annals of the New York Academy of Science* ,197: 167-169.

Vaillant, G.E. (1983). *The natural history of alcoholism*. Cambridge MA: Harvard University Press.

Vannicelli, M. & Nash, L.(1984). Effect of sex bias on women's studies on alcoholism. *Alcoholism: Clinical and Experimental Research*, 8: 334-336.

Vannicelli, M. (1987). Treatment outcome of alcoholic women: the state of the art in relation to sex bias and expectancy effects. In: Wilsnack S and Beckman (Eds). *Alcohol problems in women*, New York: Guilford, pp. 369-419.

Waterson, E.J., Evans, C. & Murray-Lyon, I.M. (1990). Is pregnancy a time of changing drinking and smoking patterns for fathers as well as mothers? *British Journal of Addiction*, 85: 389-396.

Watson, H.E., Kershaw, P.W. & Davies, J.B. (1991). Alcohol problems among women in a general hospital. *British Journal of Addiction*, 86: 889-894.

Weiss, R.D., Mirin, S.M. & Griffin, M.L. (1992). Methodological considerations in the diagnosis of coexisting psychiatric disorders in substance abusers. *British Journal of Addiction*, 87: 179-188.

Werner, E.E. (1986). Resilient offspring of alcoholics: a longitudinal study from birth to age 18. *Journal of Studies on Alcohol*, 47: 34-40.

Whipple, S.C. & Noble, P. (1991). Personality characteristics of alcoholic fathers and their sons. *Journal of Studies on Alcohol*, 52: 331-337.

Williams, G.D. & DeBakey, S.F. (1992). Changes in levels of alcohol consumption: United States 1983-1988. British Journal of Addiction 87: 643-648.

Williamson S.M., Williamson, D.F., Kendrick, J. S., Anda, R.F. & Byers, T. (1991). Trends in alcohol consumption by pregnant women. *Journal of the American Medical Association*, 265: 876-879.

Willett, W.C., Stampfer, M.J., Colditz, G.A., Rosner, B.A., Hennekens, C.H. and Speizer, F.E. (1987). Moderate alcohol consumption and the risk of breast cancer. *New England Journal of Medicine*, 316: 1174-1180.

Wilsnack, S.C. (1987). Drinking, sexuality and sexual dysfunction in women. In: Wilsnack, S.C. and Beckman, L.J. (Eds). *Alcohol problems in women*. New York: Guilford Press.

Wilsnack, S.C. & Beckman, L.J. (1987). *Alcohol problems in women*. New York: Guilford.

Wilsnack, R.W., Wilsnack, S.C. & Klassen, A.D. (1984). Women's drinking and drinking problems: patterns from 1981 national survey. *American Journal of Public Health*, 74: 1231-1238.

Neurobiology of Alcohol's Actions and the Addictive Process

J. E. Dildy-Mayfield and R. A. Harris
University of Colorado Health Sciences Center
Department of Pharmacology

Neuroscience has undergone explosive growth during the past ten years and neurobiological studies of alcohol action progressed dramatically during those years. Advances in the molecular biology of brain genes and proteins as well as patch clamp electrophysiology have revolutionized the study of brain function and these techniques have been vigorously applied to studies of alcohol action. In this brief review, we summarize some of the most exciting and promising recent studies of effects of acute and chronic alcohol exposure on mammalian brain function. Space does not allow us to be comprehensive or to cite all of the relevant literature. Rather, we have attempted to cite useful review articles and key recent publications.

Physical Properties of Membranes

Historically, membrane lipids have been implicated as potential sites of action of ethanol and other intoxicant-anesthetics. For about 100 years, it has been appreciated that the potency of anesthetic agents, including alcohols, can be accurately predicted by their solubility in biological lipids (Seeman, 1972). This is true not only for anesthetic potency but also for other behavioral and physiological actions including ataxia and hypothermia. This relationship provides compelling evidence that the site of action (at least the site for many actions) of ethanol is hydrophobic in nature. This led to the postulate that this site is the lipid bilayer and that ethanol acts by partitioning into these lipids, altering their physical properties and thereby changing membrane function, perhaps through perturbation of intrinsic membrane proteins.

A detailed discussion of data supporting this hypothesis is beyond the scope of this review but is presented by Hunt (1985) and more recently by Deitrich et al. (1989). In brief, studies with fluorescent probes, electron paramagnetic resonance probes, and nuclear magnetic resonance of endogenous lipid atoms all provide remarkably consistent evidence that ethanol disorders ("fluidizes") membrane lipids. More importantly, this disordering is reduced in membranes from animals selected for genetic insensitivity to ethanol and in animals made tolerant by chronic ethanol administration. The genetic studies provide the most compelling evidence that effects of ethanol on membrane physical properties are closely related to acute ethanol sensitivity *in vivo* (Hitzemann et al., 1991). During chronic ethanol ingestion there is evidence of membrane adaptation (mentioned above) that may be related to development of tolerance, but the role of membrane physical properties in physical dependence is less clear. Most investigators find that chronic ethanol exposure produces decreased membrane fluidity, but this change is small and is not related to genetic differences in development of physical dependence (Buck & Harris, 1991).

Presently, the critical issue is whether perturbation of membrane lipids by ethanol is causally related to behavioral actions of the drug or is merely an epiphenomenon of little real importance. An argument raised against a lipid site of action is that the changes in physical properties produced by reasonable concentrations (e.g., 10-100 mM) of ethanol are quite small and have not been shown to be responsible for any of the known neurochemical or neurophysiological actions of ethanol (discussed in subsequent sections of this review). An alternative explanation is that ethanol interacts with hydrophobic regions of membrane proteins within the lipid bilayer. In this model, action on the protein is proportional to the concentration of ethanol in the bilayer. Thus, genetic selection or chronic treatment could change partitioning of ethanol into the bilayer (as shown in several studies) and thereby change action at a protein site. Importantly, membrane disordering is also directly proportional to the concentration of ethanol in the bilayer; thus, membrane disordering will perfectly reflect the action of ethanol on proteins but there need not be any causal relationship between the two actions of ethanol. Detection of drug-induced changes in membrane function that result from changes in membrane physical properties has proven difficult and frustrating, and the role of membrane physical properties in acute and chronic actions of ethanol remains to be rigorously defined.

Neuronal Electrical Activity

For a detailed review of the effects of ethanol on neuronal electrical activity in various brain regions, see Deitrich et al. (1989). The effects of ethanol on firing rate and patterns of single cells have revealed both depressant and excitatory actions. Ethanol increased single-unit activity and/or the regularity of firing in cerebellar Purkinje cells in *in vivo* and *in vitro* systems (Franklin & Gruol, 1987). Low doses of ethanol have been reported to excite whereas higher doses inhibited Purkinje cell activity (Urrutia & Gruol, 1992). In brain slices, ethanol altered both the rate and pattern of activity (George and Chin, 1984). Genetic studies of the ethanol sensitivity of Purkinje cells showed that tissue from long-sleep (ethanol-sensitive, LS) mice was more sensitive to depression of cell firing by ethanol compared to short-sleep (ethanol-insensitive, SS) mice, and that tolerance to the depressant effects of ethanol could be demonstrated in these lines; other studies have also provided evidence for electrophysiological sensitivity to ethanol correlating with behavioral ethanol sensitivity (see Deitrich et al., 1989).

As reviewed by Deitrich et al. (1989), depending on the anesthetic used, ethanol decreased firing in the inferior olive, in addition to producing depressant actions in the locus coeruleus. Decreased unit activity was generally produced by ethanol in raphe nuclei, hippocampal, and medial septal neurons. However, in the ventral tegmental area and substantia nigra, ethanol increased spontaneous activity or rate of firing. The ventral tegmental area and nucleus accumbens are rich in dopamine-containing neurons, and studies support a role for these neurons in mediating the rewarding properties of drugs of abuse (see Koob, 1992). For example, ethanol increases extracellular dopamine levels in the nucleus accumbens, and dopamine receptor antagonists injected into the nucleus accumbens decrease ethanol self-administration, indicating a role for activation of the mesolimbic dopamine system in the reinforcing properties of ethanol.

In terms of ethanol's effects on synaptic transmission, decreased evoked population spike responses were recorded in various hippocampal regions, and disruption of synaptic transmission by ethanol has also been observed in the locus coeruleus, cerebellum, cerebral cortex, and spinal cord (see Deitrich et al., 1989). Moreover, ethanol typically interferes with synaptic plasticity mechanisms. For example, ethanol blocks hippocampal long-term potentiation (LTP) (Mulkeen et al., 1987; Sinclair and Lo, 1986). LTP refers to long lasting increases in synaptic transmission following brief periods of high-frequency stimulation, and has been studied as a cellular mechanism which may underlie learning and memory *in vivo*. Overall, ethanol has depressant actions on single-unit activity, synaptic transmission, and certain forms of synaptic plasticity.

Ion Channels

Excitatory amino acids

NMDA (N-methyl-D-aspartate) receptor-operated channels.
Glutamate is the most abundant excitatory transmitter in the CNS, and glutamate receptors of the NMDA subtype open channels allowing Ca^{2+} and Na^+ influx and K^+ efflux. NMDA receptors exist in a complex consisting of NMDA receptor-operated cation channels, sites positively modulated by glycine and polyamines, and sites negatively modulated by Zn^{2+}, Mg^{2+}, and PCP (phencyclidine)-like compounds. In preparations from embryonic or neonatal and adult tissue, ethanol inhibited NMDA single channel currents, NMDA-mediated cyclic guanosine monophosphate (cGMP) production and $^{45}Ca^{2+}$ influx, NMDA-induced increases in $[Ca^{2+}]_i$, and NMDA-stimulated neurotransmitter release (for review see Gonzales, 1990). Lima-Landman and Albuquerque (1989) demonstrated two effects for ethanol, where low concentrations (1.74-8.65 mM) facilitated activation of NMDA current without changing mean open time, whereas higher ethanol concentrations (86.5-174 mM) decreased frequency of opening and channel lifetime. Mean open times of single NMDA channels were also decreased by the n-alkanols butanol, pentanol, and octanol (McLarnon et al., 1991). Population EPSPs mediated by NMDA were inhibited by 25-37% in the presence of 25-100 mM ethanol in adult rat hippocampal slices (Lovinger et al., 1990). The most sensitive preparation appears to be isolated adult dorsal root ganglion neurons in which NMDA-activated current was inhibited by ethanol concentrations as low as 2.5 mM with an IC_{50} estimate of 10 mM ethanol (White et al., 1990b). Ethanol inhibition of NMDA-mediated responses has also been observed *in vivo* in that ethanol (2 g/kg) injected intraperitoneally protected against NMDA-induced convulsions in rats (Kul-

karni et al., 1990). Furthermore, ethanol *in vivo* inhibited NMDA-stimulated electrophysiological activity but only in a subset of neurons tested (Simson et al., 1991).

Chronic ethanol ingestion increased the number of glutamate binding sites in rat brain synaptosomes (Michaelis et al., 1978), and convulsions during chronic ethanol withdrawal were attenuated by a glutamate receptor antagonist (Freed & Michaelis, 1978). Recent studies have addressed the role of NMDA receptors specifically following chronic ethanol treatment. An upregulation of NMDA receptor complexes (Grant et al., 1990; Gulya et al., 1991) and increased NMDA-mediated $[Ca^{2+}]_i$ have been observed after chronic ethanol exposure (Iorio et al., 1992), but no functional change in NMDA-stimulated norepinephrine release from cortical slices was observed from chronically ethanol treated rats (Brown et al., 1991). Furthermore, no changes in ethanol's inhibition of NMDA-mediated responses have been reported after chronic ethanol (Brown et al., 1991; White et al., 1990a). There was also no evidence for development of *in vitro* tolerance to ethanol's inhibition of NMDA-mediated currents in *Xenopus* oocytes expressing rat hippocampal mRNA (Dildy-Mayfield and Harris, 1992). However, the NMDA antagonists, MK-801 [(+)-5-methyl-10,11-dihydro-5H-dibenzo[a,d]cyclohepten-5,10- imine maleate)] and ketamine, blocked development of rapid tolerance to ethanol-induced motor impairment in rats (Khanna et al., 1992). In addition, competitive and non-competitive NMDA antagonists decreased ethanol withdrawal seizures (Grant et al., 1990; Liljequist, 1991), and genetic evidence for a role of NMDA receptors was provided by the finding of a higher number of NMDA receptors in hippocampus of withdrawal seizure prone (WSP) mice than withdrawal seizure resistant (WSR) mice (Valverius et al., 1990).

Using a rat model of Fetal Alcohol Syndrome, prenatal ethanol exposure was shown to block the inhibitory action of NMDA on carbachol-induced phosphatidylinositol hydrolysis in hippocampal slices (Noble and Ritchie, 1989). Prenatal ethanol exposure resulted in an approximately 50% decrease in hippocampal glutamate binding in 45 day old rats (Farr et al., 1988). This has been linked with a long-lasting decrease in excitatory neurotransmission in the hippocampus of fetal alcohol exposed rats. In fact, prenatal ethanol exposure decreased the sensitivity of hippocampal slices from adult offspring to NMDA (Morrisett et al., 1989).

Current research interests involve the mechanism(s) by which ethanol inhibits NMDA-mediated functions in various neuronal preparations. Hoffman et al. (1989) reported that the percent ethanol inhibition of NMDA-stimulated cGMP accumulation in cerebellar granule cells decreased as the NMDA concentration increased. However, a noncompetitive mechanism of action for ethanol's inhibition of NMDA-stimulated increases in $[Ca^{2+}]_i$ and $[^3H]$norepinephrine release has been observed (Dildy-Mayfield & Leslie, 1991; Gonzales & Woodward, 1990). An interaction of ethanol with Mg^{2+} was reported in the hippocampal CA1 region of adult rats in that the ethanol inhibition of NMDA responses was enhanced in the presence of Mg^{2+} (Martin et al., 1991; Morrisett et al., 1991). Gonzales and Woodward (1990) did not find any interaction between ethanol and sites for Mg^{2+} or glycine in NMDA-stimulated $[^3H]$norepinephrine release from rat cortical slices. Although ethanol's inhibition of NMDA-mediated increases in $[Ca^{2+}]_i$ (Dildy-Mayfield & Leslie, 1991) and endogenous dopamine release (Woodward & Gonzales, 1990) was also not affected by the external Mg^{2+} concentration, increasing concentrations of glycine were able to reverse the ethanol inhibition in these studies. In cultured cerebellar granule cells, NMDA-mediated cGMP production was enhanced by 10 µM glycine, but in the presence of 50 and 100 mM ethanol, the ability of glycine to potentiate NMDA responses decreased (Hoffman et al., 1989). Rabe and Tabakoff (1990) suggested that glycine at high concentrations can reverse ethanol's inhibitory effects on NMDA-stimulated Ca^{2+} uptake into primary cultures of cerebellar neurons. However, as reported in cortical slices (Gonzales & Woodward, 1990), an interaction of ethanol with the glycine site was also not observed in cultured hippocampal neurons (Peoples & Weight, 1992).

Other conflicting evidence exists regarding the phencyclidine (PCP) site as a possible site of action for ethanol. Ethanol did not appear to affect the PCP site in cerebellar granule cells since an additive type of inhibition was observed with ethanol and 10 nM PCP (Hoffman et al., 1989). However, Dildy-Mayfield and Leslie (1991) suggested a possible interaction between ethanol inhibition of NMDA-stimulated increases in $[Ca^{2+}]_i$ and the PCP site in the presence of higher MK-801 concentrations. Behavioral studies showed that pigeons trained to discriminate between ethanol and saline injections by responding on an "ethanol" versus "saline" key, when injected with PCP or MK-801, responded on the "ethanol" key (Grant and Barrett, 1989).

In summary, ethanol has been clearly shown to acutely inhibit various NMDA-mediated responses in biochemical and electrophysiological studies, and a role for NMDA receptors in ethanol withdrawal seizures has also been reported. Despite the neurochemical evidence for an ethanol interaction with the glycine co-agonist site on the NMDA complex, a definitive site(s) of action for ethanol's inhibition of various NMDA-mediated events remains unresolved at present. Cloning of the NMDA receptor has revealed different subtypes and splice variants of the receptor, and this receptor diversity may account for the diversity of ethanol actions associated with NMDA receptor function.

Non-NMDA receptor-operated channels. Ethanol also inhibits responses mediated by other subtypes of excitatory amino acid (EAA) receptors. Originally, alcohols of increasing chain length were reported to inhibit kainate- and quisqualate-stimulated increases in $^{22}Na^+$ flux to a greater extent than NMDA, glutamate, or aspartate responses in striatal slices (Teichberg et al., 1984). Although the higher chain length alcohols were more selective for kainate and quisqualate as compared to NMDA, 100 mM ethanol produced approximately equal inhibition (20%) of non-NMDA and NMDA-induced responses.

Subsequent studies showed that ethanol inhibited responses activated by kainate and quisqualate, but the inhibition was much weaker than that observed with NMDA (Hoffman et al., 1989; Lovinger et al., 1989, 1990). However, recent data from our laboratory suggests that ethanol can produce similar inhibition of NMDA and non-NMDA-induced currents in *Xenopus* oocytes expressing rat hippocampal mRNA (Dildy-Mayfield & Harris, 1992a,b). We observed that the degree of ethanol inhibition increased as the concentration of kainate decreased, and in the presence of 50-100 mM ethanol, low kainate concentration responses were inhibited by 30-50% which was similar to the ethanol inhibition of NMDA currents. Current research in our laboratory involves ethanol's effect on kainate/AMPA clones (e.g., GluR1-6) expressed in oocytes and provides further support for significant ethanol inhibition at non-NMDA channels (see Dildy-Mayfield et al., 1991). In terms of the effects of chronic ethanol on kainate receptors, Freed and Michaelis (1978) reported that ethanol-dependent mice showed a supersensitivity to kainate-induced seizures compared to controls. We have recently provided evidence for development of ethanol tolerance at kainate receptor-operated channels in oocytes following 1-2 days of *in vitro* ethanol exposure (Dildy-Mayfield & Harris, 1992a).

GABA$_A$ receptor-operated channels

γ-Aminobutyric acid (GABA) is the major inhibitory neurotransmitter in mammalian brain; perhaps 70% of central neurons are inhibited by GABA, primarily through its actions on GABA$_A$ receptors. Binding of GABA to these receptors activates a chloride conductance that generally hyperpolarizes neurons. The GABA$_A$ receptor/chloride channel complex is composed of membrane spanning protein subunits that form both a chloride channel and binding sites for GABA as well as barbiturates, benzodiazepines and some convulsant drugs (e.g., picrotoxin). A number of different GABA$_A$ receptor subunits have been cloned and sequenced (Olsen and Tobin, 1990). This receptor represents a prime candidate for ethanol action because of compelling evidence that pharmacologically similar agents such as barbiturates, benzodiazepines and even volatile anesthetics exert many of their actions by enhancing GABAergic function.

Behavioral studies showed that GABA$_A$ agonists enhanced ethanol actions whereas GABA$_A$ antagonists produced the opposite actions, providing indirect evidence that ethanol might increase central GABAergic transmission. Indeed, a number of neurochemical studies showed that low concentrations (5-50 mM) of ethanol enhanced the GABA-activated uptake of ^{36}Cl$^-$ by brain membranes. Electrophysiological studies have also shown ethanol enhancement of GABA action in brain, but there are also electrophysiological and neurochemical studies that failed to detect any action of ethanol on GABA$_A$ function (see Deitrich et al., 1989). In particular, hippocampal GABA$_A$ receptors appear less likely to be affected by ethanol than cortical or cerebellar receptors. From these findings it is clear that ethanol does not affect all GABA receptors under all assay conditions and raise the question of what factors influence the ethanol sensitivity of the GABA$_A$ system.

One variable that has been explored in some detail is genetics. Ethanol enhancement of GABA action varies markedly among selected lines of rodents and individual mice of a heterogeneous stock. In general, these differences in ethanol action on GABA$_A$ receptor function are closely related to genetic differences in behavioral sensitivity to ethanol (Harris & Allan, 1989). These genetic correlations provide evidence that ethanol enhances GABA action *in vivo* and that this action of ethanol is one determinant of genetic differences in acute sensitivity to ethanol. These studies raise the question of what is the molecular basis for the diversity of ethanol sensitivity of

GABA$_A$ receptors and provide justification for detailed biochemical studies of this receptor system.

Molecular aspects of the GABA$_A$ receptor provide important clues to the action of ethanol on this complex. As mentioned above, the GABA$_A$ receptor is postulated to be a heteropentameric complex for which, based on the cloning and sequencing of at least 16 different receptor subunits, multiple receptor subtypes exist. The subunits are differentially located throughout the brain and the subunit composition of a receptor defines its pharmacology. For example, the presence of a γ_2 subunit in the receptor complex appears to confer benzodiazepine sensitivity to the receptor. Recently, two forms of the γ_2 receptor have been identified: the original form (now known as γ_{2S}) and an alternatively spliced variant ($_{\gamma 2L}$). We showed that the γ_{2L} form of the subunit is critical for ethanol potentiation of the GABA$_A$ receptor (Wafford et al., 1991). Antisense (hybrid arrest) deletions of γ_{2L} but not α_1, β_1, γ_1 or γ_3 subunits prevent ethanol potentiation of GABA$_A$ receptor responses in oocytes expressing whole brain mRNAs. Furthermore, expression in oocytes of $\alpha_1\beta_1\gamma_{2L}$ cRNAs, but not $\alpha_1\beta_1\gamma_{2S}$ cRNAs results in GABA$_A$ receptor responses that are potentiated by ethanol (Wafford et al., 1991). The specific subunit requirement for ethanol action and the differential brain distribution of the γ_{2L} subunit may explain why certain subpopulations of neurons are sensitive to ethanol.

In addition to the subunit composition of the receptor, the post-translational state of the receptor may also be important for observing ethanol effects. Protein phosphorylation is widely recognized as the primary mechanism for post-translational control of protein activity, and clear evidence has linked phosphorylation to regulation of receptor function. The mechanisms by which ethanol could influence the in situ phosphorylation of proteins, and the GABA$_A$ receptor in particular, are not known. There have been a number of reports that ethanol could influence protein phosphorylation. For instance, ethanol has been reported to increase cyclic adenosine monophosphate (cAMP) levels by enhancing G_s activation (see below). Moreover, ethanol may increase resting levels of intracellular Ca^{2+} via mobilization of intracellular Ca^{2+} stores. Conversely, during neuronal stimulation, ethanol may decrease intracellular Ca^{2+} by blockade of voltage sensitive Ca^{2+} channels or the NMDA receptor complex.

However, the strongest evidence that modulation of phosphorylation may underlie the effect of ethanol on GABA$_A$ receptor function has come from two separate studies. As discussed above, a new subunit (γ_{2L}) of the GABA$_A$ receptor was found to be necessary for the potentiating effects of ethanol (Wafford et al., 1991). This subunit differed from the other γ_2 subunit (γ_{2S}) by only a single stretch of eight amino acids. Moreover, these eight amino acids contain a consensus sequence site for phosphorylation by protein kinase C. In subsequent work it has recently been determined that substitution of an alanine for the serine in that consensus sequence eliminates the effect of ethanol on the GABA$_A$ receptor, (Wafford& Whiting, 1992).

In a separate group of studies Palmer and colleagues examined the effects of ethanol on GABA responses in cerebellar Purkinje cells (Lin et al., 1991). These authors found that ethanol would potentiate GABA inhibition of Purkinje cell firing only if it was coapplied with norepinephrine or isoproterenol. These data strongly suggest that activation of the β-adrenergic/adenylyl cyclase/protein kinase A system modifies the sensitivity of the Purkinje cell GABA$_A$ receptor to ethanol, most likely through phosphorylation of the receptor or some other modulatory constituent of the cell. Thus, inconsistencies in the literature regarding the ability of ethanol to enhance GABA action may be due to requirement for the γ_{2L} subunit of the GABA$_A$ receptor and the requirement for the proper phosphorylation state of the receptor for ethanol action.

Regarding the role of GABA$_A$ receptors in ethanol tolerance and dependence, acute injection of a high dose of ethanol (4 g/kg, i.p.) or chronic ingestion of lower concentrations results in a marked tolerance to effects of ethanol on GABA-activated ^{36}Cl$^-$ flux, without altering the actions of GABA agonists (see Buck and Harris, 1991). We also found that a single injection of ethanol enhances the inhibition of GABA action by benzodiazepine inverse agonists, indicating rapid functional changes in the GABA$_A$ receptor in response to ethanol. Furthermore, behavioral studies show that development of acute tolerance to ethanol ataxia can be blocked by injection of flumazenil, a benzodiazepine antagonist, providing additional evidence to link acute tolerance and the GABA$_A$ system (Buck and Harris, 1991).

There are four effects of chronic ethanol treatment on GABA$_A$ receptors that are of particular interest: 1. Decreased ability of ethanol to potentiate GABA action; 2. Decreased ability of a benzodiazepine agonist to potentiate GABA; 3. Increased ability of beta-carboline and benzodiazepine inverse agonists to inhibit GABA action; and 4. Changes in brain levels of mRNAs coding for specific GABA$_A$ receptor subunits. Because these neurochemical changes would tend to offset acute actions of ethanol and produce seizure sensitivity, anxiety, etc., they provide plausible mechanisms for development of tolerance and/or dependence. In addition, chronic ethanol treatment has been shown to reduce the action of $GABA_A$ agonists, reduce receptor binding of benzodiazepine agonists, and increase binding of benzodiazepine inverse agonists; however, these actions have not been detected in all studies (see Buck & Harris, 1991). Two effects of chronic ethanol ingestion, increased action of benzodiazepine inverse agonists and decreased levels of α_1 subunit mRNA, are greater in withdrawal seizure prone (WSP) than withdrawal seizure resistant (WSR) mice, providing a genetic correlation with development of ethanol withdrawal seizures. The effects of chronic ethanol ingestion on mRNA levels, namely decreases in levels of α_1 and α_2 with increases in γ_3 and no change in γ_{2S} or γ_{2L}, are particularly tantalizing because the α subunits contain benzodiazepine binding sites but γ_{2S} or γ_{2L} is required for benzodiazepine action and only γ_{2L} will allow ethanol action. Thus, chronic ethanol may produce a shift in the α and γ subunit composition of the $GABA_A$ receptor (i.e., less α_1 and α_2, more γ_3) possibly leading to the observed changes in action of benzodiazepine agonist and inverse agonists and ethanol. These subtle and complex changes suggest a practical application, namely that benzodiazepines with unique subunit specificity may be useful in treating alcohol withdrawal.

In summary, there is considerable evidence from behavioral, neurochemical, electrophysiological, and genetic studies that actions of ethanol on $GABA_A$ receptors are responsible for some aspects of ethanol intoxication, tolerance and dependence.

5-HT₃ -receptor-operated channels

In contrast to G-protein coupled serotonin (5-hydroxytryptamine) receptors such as the 5-HT₁, 5-HT₂, and 5-HT₄ receptors, the 5-HT₃ receptor subtype activates a ligand gated ion channel with permeability to Na^+ and K^+, producing a rapid, desensitizing depolarizing response. Although ethanol abuse has been linked with serotonergic systems (Sellers et al., 1992), its interaction with the specific 5-HT₃ receptor subtype has just recently been investigated. The first report showed that ethanol potentiated 5-HT currents mediated through the 5-HT₃ receptor in clonal (NCB-20) neuroblastoma cells (Lovinger, 1991). In addition to the potentiation recorded in these cells, ethanol produced similar effects in isolated adult rat neurons (Lovinger and White, 1991). For example, 25 and 50-100 mM ethanol potentiated 5-HT₃ receptor-mediated current by approximately 19 and 40%, respectively. Ethanol's potentiation decreased as the 5-HT agonist concentration increased, indicating that ethanol might alter ligand binding characteristics. However, ethanol (100 mM) has been shown to have little effect on 5-HT₃ antagonist binding or on agonist displacement of antagonist binding in membranes from NCB-20 cells or rat cortex plus hippocampus (Hellevuo et al., 1991). Other proposed mechanisms for the concentration dependence of ethanol sensitivity observed by Lovinger and White (1991) included an increased probability of channel opening by ethanol in the presence of low agonist concentrations. Because ethanol had no effect on 5-HT₃-mediated responses in approximately 20% of neurons tested, it is possible that subtypes of the 5-IIT₃ receptor exist which may be insensitive to ethanol. Ethanol demonstrated some selectivity in its actions on 5-HT₃ responses in that GABA$_A$ and voltage-sensitive Ca²⁺ currents in these neurons were not ethanol sensitive.

Grant and Barrett (1991) have shown that certain 5-HT₃ antagonists can interfere with the discriminative stimulus effects of ethanol. For instance, the 5-HT₃ receptor antagonists ICS 205-930 and MDL 72222 blocked ethanol appropriate responding in pigeons trained to discriminate ethanol (1.5 g/kg, intragastric) from water. The dose of ICS 205-930 which was effective at decreasing ethanol responding also produced nonspecific effects by decreasing motor performance. Nevertheless, there was a dose of MDL 72222 which inhibited ethanol responding without significantly altering response rate, providing support for a role of 5-HT₃ transmission in mediating ethanol's discriminative stimulus effects. Also, 5-HT₃ receptor antagonists have previously been reported to decrease ethanol consumption in humans (Sellers et al., 1988).

Voltage-sensitive ion channels

Calcium channels. Ethanol inhibits depolarization-dependent Ca²⁺ influx via voltage-gated Ca²⁺ channels in synaptosomes or presynaptic nerve terminals without affecting basal uptake (Harris & Hood, 1980; Leslie et al., 1983; Skattebol & Rabin, 1987). Acute ethanol exposure also reduces voltage-dependent Ca²⁺ influx in cultured neuronal cells (Messing et al., 1986; Skattebol & Rabin, 1987). Ethanol selectively inhibits Ca²⁺ entry which occurs in the first second(s) following depolarization, and this influx reportedly occurs through Ca²⁺ channels and does not involve other mechanisms such as Na⁺/Ca²⁺ exchange which may operate at later times and are less sensitive to ethanol (Leslie et al., 1983; Skattebol & Rabin, 1987). In PC12 cells, for example, 100 mM ethanol significantly inhibited fast-phase (1 s) Ca^{2+} entry whereas 400 mM was required to inhibit slow-phase uptake (Skattebol & Rabin, 1987). Ethanol appears to inhibit Ca^{2+} channels in synaptosomes from certain brain regions to a greater extent than other regions (see Leslie et al., 1990). Brain regions may also respond differently to ethanol inhibition depending on the time course of Ca^{2+} uptake (Leslie et al., 1983).

Calcium channel inhibition by ethanol has also been demonstrated electrophysiologically. Ethanol decreased the duration of action potentials which involve large inward Ca^{2+} currents in dorsal root ganglion cells whereas very low concentrations of ethanol increased action potential duration (Oaks & Pozos, 1982). Voltage sensitive calcium channels were initially classified into L, N, and T subtypes based on electrophysiological and pharmacological properties (Nowycky et al., 1985). The subtypes display different voltage dependence of activation, time course of inactivation, and sensitivity to drugs and neurotoxins. For example, L-type Ca^{2+} channels are slowly inactivating and are dihydropyridine (DHP) sensitive whereas T-type channels display transient inactivation. Ethanol (100 and 300 mM) blocked both type I (T) and type II (L) Ca^{2+} channel currents by approximately 15 and 40%, respectively (Twombly et al., 1990). Tolerance to ethanol's action on Ca^{2+} conductance resulted after culturing neurons in ethanol (Eskuri & Pozos, 1985). Following withdrawal of slices from chronic ethanol exposure *in vitro*, hyperexcitability such as increases in paired pulse potentiation of hippocampal slices was observed, and these patterns of hyperexcitability were decreased by coadministration of a DHP Ca^{2+} channel antagonist (Whittington & Little, 1991).

Chronic ethanol exposure also produced adaptive responses in biochemical studies of Ca^{2+} channels such as the development of tolerance to the inhibitory effects of ethanol on Ca^{2+} uptake (Harris and Hood, 1980; Leslie et al., 1983). Similar to the acute effects of ethanol in which certain Ca^{2+} channels were more sensitive to ethanol inhibition than others, Ca^{2+} channels from particular brain areas may be more sensitive to chronic ethanol treatment. For example, after chronic ethanol exposure, synaptosomes from cerebellum did not adapt to the *in vitro* inhibitory effect of ethanol, in contrast to Ca^{2+} uptake in hypothalamic synaptosomes, which demonstrated adaptation, in that ethanol *in vitro* no longer significantly inhibited uptake (Daniell and Leslie, 1986). Interestingly, synaptosomes from hypothalamus were also more sensitive to the acute inhibitory effects of ethanol than cerebellar synaptosomes. Although chronic ethanol did not alter the *in vitro* ethanol inhibition of Ca^{2+} uptake in striatal synaptosomes, it did affect the Ca^{2+}-stimulated release of dopamine measured simultaneously (Leslie et al., 1986).

The interaction between dihydropyridines (DHP) and ethanol has provided information on the effects of chronic ethanol on specific subtypes of voltage-sensitive Ca^{2+} channels. Exposure to 200 mM ethanol for several days increased Ca^{2+} uptake in PC12 cells, and an increased number of DHP Ca^{2+} channel binding sites was also demonstrated after chronic *in vitro* ethanol treatment (Messing et al., 1986). The increase in Ca^{2+} uptake occurred via DHP-sensitive Ca^{2+} channels (Greenberg et al., 1987). Chronic ethanol also increased DHP binding in rat brain (Dolin et al., 1987; Wu et al., 1987), and the enhanced effect of the DHP agonist Bay K 8644 after chronic ethanol treatment provides evidence for potential functional consequences of increased DHP binding (Dolin et al., 1987). Harper et al. (1989) showed that inhibition of protein synthesis blocked this increase in DHP binding, suggesting that de novo protein synthesis was responsible for the upregulation. However, studies in human alcoholics did not support alterations in DHP binding sites (Kril et al., 1989; Marks et al., 1989).

DHP Ca^{2+} channel antagonists potentiated the acute pharmacological effects of ethanol including ethanol-induced hypothermia, motor incoordination, and sedation, and nifedipine also decreased slightly the preference for ethanol (see Leslie et al., 1990 for review). The DHP agonist Bay K8644 decreased the anesthetic effect of ethanol (Dolin et al., 1988). DHP antagonists protected against mild ethanol withdrawal behavior, abolished spontaneous seizures, prevented or reduced audiogenic seizures, and prevented or reduced mortality during chronic ethanol withdrawal in rats (Little et al., 1986; Littleton et al., 1990). Furthermore, DHP antagonists given chronically during ethanol administration blocked development of tolerance and withdrawal and prevented the increase in DHP binding sites (Dolin & Little, 1989; Whittington et al., 1991; Wu et al., 1987). Chronic ethanol increased DHP binding sites to a significantly greater extent in WSP compared to WSR mice (Brennan et al., 1990). Thus, adaptation of subtypes of voltage sensitive calcium channels in response to chronic ethanol may be involved in ethanol dependence and development of withdrawal.

Sodium channels. The sodium current carried through voltage-dependent Na^+ channels, which is responsible for the generation of action potentials, has shown some slight sensitivity to ethanol. In rodent brain synaptosomes, ethanol, in a concentration-dependent and reversible manner, inhibited both batrachotoxin- and veratridine-stimulated $^{22}Na^+$ uptake without affecting basal uptake (Harris & Bruno, 1985; Mullin & Hunt, 1985). For a series of *n*-alkanols, the ability to partition into a hydrophobic region of the membrane correlated with their potency for inhibition of batrachotoxin-stimulated uptake (Mullin & Hunt, 1985), and other anesthetics also inhibited veratridine-stimulated sodium uptake (Harris & Bruno, 1985). Ethanol had no effect on the actions of scorpion venom, which binds at a site distinct from that of batrachotoxin and veratridine and has no effect on Na^+ flux alone but enhances batrachotoxin-stimulated $^{22}Na^+$ uptake (Mullin & Hunt, 1985). Ethanol also did not affect the inhibition of batrachotoxin-stimulated uptake produced by tetrodotoxin acting at another site on the sodium channel (Harris & Bruno, 1985; Mullin & Hunt, 1985). Although physiologically relevant concentrations of ethanol can significantly inhibit neurotoxin-mediated Na^+ uptake, the concentrations of ethanol required to produce approximately 50% inhibition of neurotoxin-stimulated Na^+ uptake were quite high, ranging from approximately 350 to over 500 mM depending on the neurotoxin and the brain region studied.

The effects of ethanol on neurotoxin binding were studied in rodent synaptosomes (Mullin & Hunt, 1987; Zimányi et al., 1988). The IC_{50}s for ethanol's inhibition of [^3H]batrachotoxin A 20-α-benzoate binding were above 300 mM. Ethanol increased the K_d without affecting the B_{max} and enhanced the dissociation rate constant, suggestive of an allosteric competitive inhibitor at the batrachotoxin site. In contrast, [^3H]saxitoxin binding (i.e., the tetrodotoxin site) was not affected by ethanol (Mullin & Hunt, 1987).

Chronic ethanol exposure did not alter veratridine-mediated Na^+ uptake or *in vitro* ethanol inhibition of this uptake in synaptosomes from ethanol-dependent and pair fed control mice (Harris & Bruno, 1985). However, later studies provided some evidence for alterations in Na^+ channel function following chronic ethanol treatment. Although a single intragastric dose of ethanol had no effect on batrachotoxin binding in the absence or presence of ethanol *in vitro*, and did not alter batrachotoxin-stimulated $^{22}Na^+$ uptake, it produced a dose- and time-dependent decrease in the *in vitro* ethanol inhibition of $^{22}Na^+$ uptake in synaptosomes (Mullin et al., 1987). This suggested that a single *in vivo* dose of ethanol could produce acute tolerance to ethanol's inhibition of uptake *in vitro*. When multiple daily doses of ethanol were administered, there was a decrease in batrachotoxin-stimulated uptake in synaptosomes from the ethanol-treated group in addition to a long-term diminished inhibition of uptake by ethanol *in vitro*; however, as observed with acute ethanol administration, chronic ethanol treatment did not alter batrachotoxin binding to its site in the channel (Mullin et al., 1987).

Potassium channels. Different types of K^+ currents have been identified in different species, but only the effects of ethanol on K^+ currents in mammalian tissues will be addressed here. For example, the ethanol-induced hyperpolarization of hippocampal neurons likely occurs via an increase in K^+ conductance (Carlen et al., 1985). Ethanol also increases a type of K^+ current resembling the anomalous rectifier which is observed when hyperpolarizing current is injected into locus coeruleus neurons (Shefner & Osmanovic, 1987). K^+ channel clones obtained from mammalian brain and expressed in *Xenopus* oocytes produced delayed rectifier currents which exhibited different sensitivities to ethanol, showing either no sensitivity or a slight inhibition in amplitude in the presence of 200 mM ethanol (Treistman et al., 1991). Low concentrations of ethanol have been shown to selectively inhibit a voltage-dependent K^+ current known as the M-current (a non-inactivating current) in CA1 hippocampal pyramidal neurons, whereas ethanol had little effect on other types of K^+ conductances in these cells (Moore et al., 1990). Increases in intracellular Ca^{2+} can activate a Ca^{2+}-dependent K^+ conductance, and ethanol enhanced Ca^{2+}-dependent K^+ flux in mouse brain synaptosomes (Yamamoto and Harris, 1983). Also, after-hyperpolarizations resulting from activation of Ca^{2+}-dependent K^+ conductances in the CA1 region of rat hippocampus were enhanced by ethanol (Carlen et al., 1985 but see Siggins et al., 1987). After chronic ethanol, these afterhyperpolarizations were decreased in amplitude and duration (Durand & Carlen, 1984). The transient outward K^+ current IA occurs in mammalian brain, but the effects of ethanol on this type of current have only been characterized in invertebrate neurons.

G-Protein Coupled Receptors

Stimulatory guanine nucleotide binding proteins (G_s) couple adenylate cyclase (AC) to an agonist-receptor complex causing activation of AC and increased production of cAMP which increases protein kinase A activity. Ethanol has been shown to increase basal and particularly agonist-stimulated AC activity in several brain regions *in vitro*. For example, ethanol enhanced dopamine- and isoproterenol-stimulated AC activity in striatum and in cortex and cerebellum, respectively (Luthin & Tabakoff, 1984; Rabin & Molinoff, 1981; Saito et al., 1985). Because the ethanol stimulation was not blocked by receptor antagonists, ethanol did not interact directly with dopamine or β-adrenergic receptors. Hoffman and Tabakoff (1982) reported that ethanol's stimulation of AC in striatum was not related to its actions on lipids surrounding the catalytic subunit of the enzyme. *In vitro* ethanol also increased prostaglandin E_1 (Stenstrom and Richelson, 1982) and adenosine (Gordon et al., 1986) receptor-mediated cAMP levels in clonal cell lines.

In experiments designed to determine the site(s) of action of ethanol on the adenylate cyclase system, it was reported that ethanol did not alter AC activity in lymphoma cells lacking a functional G_s protein, which pointed to G_s as a primary site of action for ethanol; furthermore, ethanol increased the maximum activity of dopamine-stimulated AC and the rate of enzyme activation by a non-hydrolyzable GTP analog (Gpp(NH)p) in striatum (Rabin & Molinoff, 1983). Luthin and Tabakoff (1984) found that lower concentrations of ethanol could be used to stimulate AC in striatum if Gpp(NH)p was present but that ethanol did not affect the affinity of the catalytic subunit of the enzyme. When G_s was irreversibly activated, ethanol was still able to increase AC activity (Luthin & Tabakoff, 1984; Rabin and Molinoff, 1983). These studies suggested that although ethanol had little effect on receptor or guanine nucleotide binding, ethanol favored the interaction of the nucleotide loaded-G_s-protein with the catalytic subunit of AC. In cortical membranes, ethanol potentiated the stimulatory effects of Gpp(NH)p and isoproterenol on AC activity, increased the rate of enzyme activation by guanine nucleotides, and directly affected the catalytic subunit of AC (Saito et al., 1985). Ethanol decreased the affinity for isoproterenol of the high-affinity (i.e. agonist-receptor-G_s complex) form of the cortical receptor (Valverius et al., 1987). While ethanol's site of action appears to involve the G_s-protein and/or G_s-protein-AC complex in both cortex and striatum, additional sites at the β-adrenergic receptor and the catalytic unit of AC were also indicated in cortex. It is also possible that ethanol could affect the inhibitory G-protein (G_i) pathway (Bauché et al., 1987 but see Hoffman & Tabakoff, 1986 and Rabin, 1985). Ethanol's inhibition of forskolin-stimulated AC activity may indicate an interaction with G_i because an inhibition of forskolin's direct actions on AC could result from activation of G_i (Stenstrom et al., 1985). However, in S49 lymphoma cells, ethanol inhibition of forskolin-stimulated AC activity was not blocked by treatment of the cells with pertussis toxin, a treatment that effectively eliminated the influence of G_i (Bode and Molinoff, 1988).

In a clonal neural cell line, chronic *in vitro* exposure of cells to ethanol resulted in tolerance to the acute ethanol-mediated increase in adenosine-stimulated cAMP levels (Gordon et al., 1986). Further evidence for development of cellular tolerance to ethanol came from a study showing that chronic exposure of clonal cells to ethanol decreased prostaglandin E_1-mediated AC activity and cAMP formation (Richelson et al., 1986). In studies of chronic ethanol exposure *in vivo*, there were decreases in receptor-stimulated AC activity in multiple brain regions (Lucchi et al., 1983; Saffey et al., 1988). Moreover, reduced basal and adenosine-stimulated cAMP levels and decreased *in vitro* ethanol stimulation of adenosine-mediated cAMP levels were reported in lymphocytes from alcoholics (Diamond et al., 1987), in addition to lower prostaglandin E_1-mediated AC activity in platelets from alcoholics (Tabakoff et al., 1988). In terms of mechanistic changes in the function of the cortical β-adrenergic receptor-coupled AC system after chronic ethanol treatment, Gpp(NH)p-mediated stimulation of AC activity was reduced in addition to reduced enhancement of Gpp(NH)p-stimulated AC by ethanol *in vitro*; furthermore, the EC_{50} for isoproterenol stimulation was increased in ethanol treated mice, indicating a decreased function or amount of the G_s protein and/or decreased interaction of the β-adrenergic receptor with G_s after chronic ethanol treatment (Saito et al., 1987). Additional support for this mechanism was indicated by the loss of high affinity cortical and hippocampal β-adrenergic agonist binding sites, but not the total number of receptors measured with antagonist binding. This change could reflect an uncoupling of β-adrenergic receptors with AC after chronic ethanol (Valverius et al., 1987; 1989). It was further shown that the reduction in both adenosine- and prostaglandin E_1-stimulated cAMP production after chronic ethanol exposure in NG108-15 cells may have resulted from a reduction in G_s alpha mRNA and protein levels (Mochly-Rosen et al., 1988).

Intracellular Calcium

In contrast to ethanol's acute inhibition of Ca^{2+} uptake, ethanol may increase free intracellular Ca^{2+} concentration ($[Ca^{2+}]_i$) in some neuronal preparations. Acute exposure to high concentrations of ethanol increased $[Ca^{2+}]_i$ in synaptosomes and PC12 cells and, in some cases, may have been due to effects of ethanol on intracellular regulatory mechanisms. Quin2 measurements in PC12 cells demonstrated increases in resting $[Ca^{2+}]_i$ in the presence of 400 mM ethanol (Rabe & Weight, 1988). Fura-2 measurements of $[Ca^{2+}]_i$ in mouse whole brain synaptosomes demonstrated that 350-700 mM ethanol increased resting $[Ca^{2+}]_i$, whereas lower ethanol concentrations of 50 and 100 mM had no effect (Daniell et al., 1987). A possible mechanism for ethanol-induced increases in resting $[Ca^{2+}]_i$ in synaptosomes was examined by varying the external Ca^{2+} concentration. Daniell et al. (1987) reported that ethanol's effects on $[Ca^{2+}]_i$ did not differ as the external Ca^{2+} concentration was increased from 0.01 to 1 mM when the increases were expressed as percent of control. High concentrations of ethanol (500-700 mM) were also required to elevate resting $[Ca^{2+}]_i$ in rat cortical synaptosomes resuspended in low Ca^{2+} buffer containing 0.1 mM Ca^{2+}, whereas slight increases in resting levels in the presence of lower ethanol concentrations (50-200 mM) were ob served in Ca^{2+}-free medium (Rezazadeh et al., 1989). Another report, using fura-2 loaded synaptosomes in zero Ca^{2+} buffer, observed slight increases in resting $[Ca^{2+}]_i$ with 100-500 mM ethanol (Davidson et al., 1988). These investigators also reported slight increases in resting levels produced by 50-500 mM ethanol in synaptosomes resuspended in 1 mM Ca^{2+} containing medium, whereas Ca^{2+} uptake was inhibited by 50-500 mM ethanol in these synaptosomes. Regardless of whether low or high ethanol concentrations can increase $[Ca^{2+}]_i$, the question remains as to how ethanol can inhibit Ca^{2+} uptake while increasing $[Ca^{2+}]_i$ in some preparations. Ethanol did not appear to inhibit the Na^+/Ca^{2+} exchange mechanism in synaptosomes (Daniell et al., 1987; Rezazadeh et al., 1989). Similar to ethanol's inhibition of external Ca^{2+} uptake, it is possible that ethanol could inhibit uptake of cytosolic Ca^{2+} into organelles. Alternatively, an increase in $[Ca^{2+}]_i$ by ethanol could inhibit, via negative feedfack, subsequent extracellular uptake of Ca^{2+}. Ethanol, at low and high concentrations, has been suggested to increase intracellular Ca^{2+} release based on studies in zero Ca^{2+} buffer, and 30-500 mM ethanol was reported to stimulate Ca^{2+} release from brain microsomes (Shah and Pant, 1988). Also, 250-750 mM ethanol increased release of Ca^{2+} from cortical and cerebellar microsomes, and the release was additive with that produced by inositol-1,4,5-trisphosphate (Machu et al., 1989). Further evidence for release of intracellularly bound Ca^{2+} by ethanol which was independent of inositol-1,4,5-trisphosphate-mediated release was reported in synaptosomes (Daniell and Harris, 1989). Ethanol has also been reported to activate a Ca^{2+}-dependent Cl^- conductance via release of intracellular Ca^{2+} in *Xenopus* oocytes (Wafford et al., 1989). Development of tolerance to ethanol's *in vitro* action on $[Ca^{2+}]_i$ was demonstrated in synaptosomes prepared from mice treated chronically with ethanol (Daniell & Harris, 1988). Although some evidence supports an action of ethanol on intracellular Ca^{2+} stores, either high concentrations of ethanol were required to increase $[Ca^{2+}]_i$ or stimulate intracellular release or lower ethanol concentrations produced only slight increases.

Brain Enzymes

Section IV on guanine nucleotide protein coupled receptors contains an overview of the effects of ethanol on adenylate cyclase activity. The reader is also referred to a review of ethanol actions on brain enzymes by Tabakoff et al. (1987).

Na+, K+-ATPase

Na+,K+-ATPase is a membrane bound enzyme which maintains the ionic gradient across cell membranes and thus regulates neuronal excitability and membrane transport. The activity of this enzyme is influenced by membrane lipid composition. For a review of ethanol actions on Na+,K+-ATPase see Swann (1987). *In vitro* concentrations of ethanol required to inhibit Na+,K+-ATPase are quite high. However, the *in vivo* effects of ethanol may be more pronounced, especially in the presence of catecholamine-stimulated Na+, K+-ATPase activity (Rangaraj et al., 1985), but these results were not replicated by Syapin et al. (1985). Moreover, conditions which increased internal Na+ or Ca^{2+} increased the ability of ethanol to inhibit Na+,K+-ATPase, suggesting that the ethanol sensitivity of this transport system may be increased during neuronal activity (Swann, 1990). Although the ability of alcohols to partition into the membrane is important for inhibition of Na+,K+-ATPase, there is some support for a direct effect of ethanol on the enzyme (Nhamburo et al., 1986; Swann, 1983). Slight increases in basal or stimulated Na+, K+-ATPase activity in some brain regions have been reported as evidence for development of tolerance following chronic ethanol exposure (Beauge et al., 1983; Keane & Leonard, 1983; Rao et al., 1985).

Choline acetyltransferase

In adult rats, in vivo ethanol exposure increased choline acetyltransferase activity (Soliman & Gabriel, 1985). Ethanol exposure during lactation via intake of the dam's milk increased striatal choline acetyltransferase in rat offspring (Lancaster et al., 1986), and increased activity was reported in cultured brain cells from rat fetuses of ethanol-treated dams; in addition ethanol *in vitro* increased enzyme activity (Okonmah et al., 1989).

Tyrosine hydroxylase

Tyrosine hydroxylase is the rate-limiting enzyme in the synthesis of catecholamines in the CNS, and central catecholamines may have roles in mediating ethanol consumption and pathophysiology. The specific activity of tyrosine hydroxylase was increased in rat pups exposed to ethanol postnatally via ingestion of milk from dams receiving ethanol (Detering et al., 1980). Ethanol administered *in ovo* also increased tyrosine hydroxylase activity in chick brain embryos (Kentroti and Vernadakis, 1990). Activity of this enzyme was higher in brains of alcohol-preferring (AA) than alcohol-nonpreferring (ANA) rats (Pispa et al., 1986).

Monoamine oxidase

Monoamine oxidase, a membrane-bound enzyme existing in two forms (MAO-A and MAO-B in brain), catalyzes the oxidative deamination of neurotransmitter amines. Diminished brain or platelet MAO activity was typically reported in human alcoholics but not in brains of rodents given alcohol chronically (see Tabakoff et al., 1987 for review). *In vitro* ethanol also inhibited brain and platelet MAO activity with the B form of the enzyme being selectively sensitive to inhibition by ethanol (Tabakoff et al., 1985).

Neuropeptides

Classifying certain neuropeptides as neurotransmiters is based on evidence for neuropeptide synthesis in neuronal cell bodies, transport to terminals, localization in vesicles, Ca^{2+}-dependent release during depolarization, and the existence of high affinity binding sites in brain. The interaction of ethanol with some neuropeptides has been reviewed by Deitrich et al. (1989).

Neurotensin

Centrally administered neurotensin enhanced the sedative effects of ethanol by lengthening ethanol-induced loss of righting reflex and increasing the hypothermic effects of ethanol (Frye et al., 1981; Lut-tinger et al., 1981). Low doses of neurotensin increased the sensitivity to ethanol-induced anesthesia in short-sleep (SS) but not long-sleep (LS) mice; higher doses increased ethanol-induced hypothermic ef-fects (Erwin et al., 1987). This action of neurotensin was relatively specific in that several other neuropeptides tested did not affect ethanol anesthesia in these lines. However, acute exposure to ethanol *in vitro* inhibited neurotensin-stimulated phospholipase C activity in neuroblastoma cells (Smith, 1991).

Opioids

The behavioral effects produced by neurotensin and opiates resem-ble those produced by ethanol. Similar to neurotensin, β-endorphin potentiated ethanol-induced loss of righting reflex and hypothermia (Frye et al., 1981; Luttinger et al., 1981). Likewise, β-endorphin en-hanced ethanol-induced anesthesia in SS and to a lesser extent in LS mice (Erwin et al., 1987). Evidence for increased β-endorphin and met-enkephalin levels following an acute dose of ethanol has been reported from rat brain or human plasma studies (Barret et al., 1987; Seizinger et al., 1983). Furthermore, the opiate antagonist naloxone attenuates some of ethanol's actions such as ethanol-induced analge-sia or hypothermia (Pillai & Ross, 1986; Pohorecky & Shah,1987). For an overview of the effects of chronic ethanol treatment on opiate ligand binding and function see Deitrich et al. (1989).

Thyrotropin releasing hormone

Thyrotropin releasing hormone produced a decreased sensitivity to the sedative and hypothermic effects of ethanol (Cott et al., 1976), and also decreased ethanol sleep time in SS and LS mice (see Deitrich et al., 1989). Thyrotropin releasing hormone reversed the decreased locomotor activity produced by ethanol, although the mechanism for this interaction is unknown (see Deitrich et al., 1989).

Overview and Conclusions

This chapter has focused on the interactions of ethanol with various neuronal processes in the mammalian CNS. Potential sites of action for ethanol can no longer be restricted to nonspecific actions on membrane lipids but can be extended to include specific lipid-pro-tein and protein interactions. Behavioral effects associated with acute ethanol exposure and adaptive changes following chronic ethanol have been linked with many of the systems discussed in this chapter. In particular, receptor-operated channels have demonstrated greater sensitivity to ethanol compared to voltage-operated channels and other systems discussed above. Low concentrations of ethanol have been shown to modulate GABA$_A$, EAA, and 5-HT$_3$ receptor-operated channels, suggesting that these receptor-operated channels may have roles in ethanol intoxication, tolerance, or dependence. Heterogeneity within a family of receptors or channels provides an explanation for differential sensitivities to ethanol depending on the particular subtype of receptor studied. The genetic approach using selected lines which differ in their sensitivity to ethanol should further improve understanding of how some of the behavioral effects of ethanol are related to specific neurochemical changes in the CNS.

References

Bauché, F., Bourdeaux-Jaubert, A.M., Giudicelli, Y., & Nordmann, R. (1987). Ethanol alters the adenosine receptor-N$_i$-mediated adenylate cyclase inhibitory response in rat brain cortex in vitro. *FEBS Letters, 219*: 296-300.

Barret, L., Bourhis, F., Danel, V., & Debru, J.L. (1987). Determination of β-endorphin in alcoholic patients in the acute stage of intoxication: relation with naloxone therapy. *Drug and Alcohol Dependence, 19*: 71-78.

Beauge, F., Stibler, H., & Kalant, H. (1983). Brain synaptosomal (Na$^+$ and K$^+$)-ATPase activity as an index of tolerance to ethanol. *Pharmacology, Biochemistry and Behavior, 18: Suppl. 1*: 519-524.

Bode, D.C. & Molinoff, P.B. (1988). Effects of ethanol in vitro on the beta adrenergic receptor-coupled adenylate cyclase system. *Journal of Pharmacology and Experimental Therapeutics, 246*:1040-1047.

Brennan, C.H., Crabbe, J., & Littleton, J.M. (1990). Genetic regulation of dihydropyridine-sensitive calcium channels in brain may determine susceptibility to physical dependence on alcohol. *Neuropharmacology, 29*: 429-432.

Brown, L. M., Gonzales, R.A., & Lesie, S.W. (1991). The effects of chronic ethanol exposure on N-methyl-D-aspartate-stimulated release of [^{3}H] catecholamines from rat brain. *Brain Research, 547*: 289-294.

Buck, K.J. & Harris, R.A. (1991). Neuroadaptive responses to chronic ethanol. *Alcoholism: Clinical and Experimental Research, 15*: 460-470.

Carlen, P.L., Gurevich, N., Davies, M.F., Blaxter, T.J., & O'Beirne, M. (1985). Enhanced neuronal K$^+$ conductance: a possible common mechanism for sedative-hypnotic drug action. *Canadian Journal of Physiology and Pharmacology, 63*: 831-837.

Cott, J.M., Breese, G.R., Cooper, B.R., Barlow, S., & Prange, A. J., Jr. (1976). Investigations into the mechanism of reduction of ethanol sleep by thyrotropin releasing hormone (TAN). *Journal of Pharmacology and Experimental Therapeutics, 196*: 594-604.

Daniell, L.C., Brass, E.P., & Harris, R. A. (1987). Effect of ethanol on intracellular ionized calcium concentration in synaptosomes and hepatocytes. *Molecular Pharmacology, 32*: 831-837.

Daniell, L.C. & Harris, R.A. (1988). Effect of chronic ethanol treatment and selective breeding for hypnotic sensitivity to ethanol on intracellular ionized calcium concentrations in synaptosomes. *Alcoholism: Clinical and Experimental Research, 12*: 179-183.

Daniell, L.C. & Harris, R.A. (1989). Ethanol and inositol 1,4,5-trisphosphate release calcium from separate stores of brain microsomes. *Journal of Pharmacology and Experimental Therapeutics, 250*: 875-881.

Daniell, L.C. & Leslie, S.W. (1986). Inhibition of fast phase calcium uptake and endogenous norepinephrine release in rat brain region synaptosomes by ethanol. *Brain Research, 377*: 18-28.

Davidson, M., Wilce, P., & Shanley, B. (1988). Ethanol increases synaptosomal free calcium concentration. *Neuroscience Letters, 89*: 165-169.

Deitrich, R.A., Dunwiddie, T.V., Harris, R.A., & Erwin, V. G. (1989). Mechanism of action of ethanol: Initial central nervous system actions. *Pharmacological Reviews, 41*: 489-537.

Detering, N., Edwards, E., Ozand, P., & Karahasan, A. (1980). Comparative effects of ethanol and malnutrition on the development of catecholamine neurons: Changes in specific activities of enzymes. *Journal of Neurochemistry, 34*: 297-304.

Diamond, I., Wrubel, B., Estrin, W., & Gordon, A. (1987). Basal and adenosine receptor-stimulated levels of cAMP are reduced in lymphocytes from alcoholic patients. *Proceedings of the National Academy of Sciences, 84*: 1413-1416.

Dildy-Mayfield, J.E. & Harris, R.A. (1992a). Acute and chronic ethanol exposure alters the function of hippocampal kainate receptors expressed in *Xenopus* oocytes. *Journal of Neurochemistry, 58*: 1569-1572.

Dildy-Mayfield, J.E. & Harris, R.A. (1992b). Comparison of ethanol sensitivity of rat brain kainate, DL-α-amino-3-hydroxy-5-methyl-

4-isoxolone propionic acid and N-methyl-D-aspartate receptors expressed in Xenopus oocytes. *Journal of Pharmacology and Experimental Therapeutics, 262:* 487-494.

Dildy-Mayfield, J.E. & Leslie, S.W. (1991). Mechanism of inhibition of N-methyl-D-aspartate-stimulated increases in free intracellular Ca^{2+} concentration by ethanol. *Journal of Neurochemistry, 56:* 1536-1543.

Dildy-Mayfield J.E., Sikela J.M., & Harris R.A. (1991). Evidence for kainate receptor subtypes based on differential ethanol sensitivity of brain and GluR3 receptors expressed in Xenopus oocytes. *Society for Neuroscience Abstract, 21:* 220.

Dolin, S.J. & Little, H.J. (1989). Are changes in neuronal calcium channels involved in ethanol tolerance? *Journal of Pharmacology and Experimental Therapeutics, 250:* 985-991.

Dolin, S., Little, H., Hudspith, M., Pagonis, C., & Littleton, J. (1987). Increased dihydropyridine-sensitive calcium channels in rat brain may underlie ethanol physical dependence. *Neuropharmacology, 26:* 275-279.

Dolin, S.J., Nalsey, M.J., & Little, H.J. (1988). Effects of the calcium channel activator Bay K 8644 on general anaesthetic potency in mice. *British Journal of Pharmacology, 94:* 413-422.

Durand, D. & Carlen, P.L. (1984). Decreased neuronal inhibition in vitro after long-term administration of ethanol. *Science, 224:* 1359-1361.

Erwin, V.G., Korte, A., & Marty, M. (1987). Neurotensin selectively alters ethanol-induced anesthesia in LS/Ibg and SS/Ibg lines of mice. *Brain Research, 400:* 80-90.

Eskuri, S. & Pozos, R. (1985). Development of ethanol tolerance in sensory neurones in culture. *Alcoholism: Clinical and Experimental Research, 9:* 197.

Farr, K.L., Montano, C.Y., Paxton, L.L., & Savage, D.D. (1988). Prenatal ethanol exposure decreases hippocampal ^{3}H-glutamate binding in 45-day-old rats. *Alcohol, 5:* 125-133.

Franklin, C.L. & Gruol, D.L. (1987). Acute ethanol alters the firing pattern and glutamate response of cerebellar Purkinje neurons in culture. *Brain Research, 416:* 205-218.

Freed, W.J. & Michaelis, E.K. (1978). Glutamic acid and ethanol dependence. *Pharmacology Biochemistry and Behavior, 8:* 509-514.

Frye, G.D., Luttinger, D., Nemeroff, C.B., Vogel, R.A., Prange, A.J., Jr., & Breese, G.R. (1981). Modification of the actions of ethanol by centrally acting peptides. *Peptides, 2* (suppl. 1): 99-106.

George, F. & Chin, H.S. (1984). Effects of ethanol on Purkinje cells recorded from cerebellar slices. *Alcohol, 1*: 353-358.

Gonzales, R.A. (1990). NMDA receptors excite alcohol research. *Trends in Pharmacological Sciences, 11*: 137-139.

Gonzales, R.A. & Woodward, J. J. (1990). Ethanol inhibits N-methyl-D-aspartate stimulated-[^{3}H]norepinephrine release from rat cortical slices. *Journal of Pharmacology and Experimental Therapeutics, 253*: 1138-1144.

Gordon, A.S., Collier, K., & Diamond, I. (1986). Ethanol regulation of adenosine receptor-stimulated cAMP levels in a clonal neural cell line: An *in vitro* model of cellular tolerance to ethanol. *Proceedings of the National Academy of Sciences, 83*: 2105-2108.

Grant, K.A. & Barrett, J. E. (1989). The role of the NMDA receptor in the discriminative stimulus effects of ethanol. *Alcoholism: Clinical and Experimental Therapeutics Abstract, 44*: 310.

Grant, K.A. & Barrett, J.E. (1991). Blockade of the discriminative stimulus effects of ethanol with-5-HT$_3$ receptor antagonists. *Psychopharmacology, 104*: 451-456.

Grant , K.A., Valverius, P., Hudspith, M., & Tabakoff, B. (1990). Ethanol withdrawal seizures and the NMDA receptor complex. *European Journal of Pharmacology, 176*: 289-296.

Greenberg, D.A., Carpenter, C.L., & Messing, R.O. (1987). Ethanol induced component of ^{45}Ca^{2+} uptake in PC12 cells is sensitive to Ca^{2+} channel modulating drugs. *Brain Research, 410*: 143-146.

Gulya, K., Grant, K.A., Valverius, P., Hoffman, P.L., & Tabakoff, B. (1991). Brain regional specificity and time-course of changes in the NMDA receptor-ionophore complex during ethanol withdrawal. *Brain Research, 547*: 129-134.

Harper, J.C., Brennan, C.H., & Littleton, J.M. (1989). Genetic up-regulation of calcium channels in a cellular model of ethanol dependence. *Neuropharmacology, 28*: 1299-1302.

Harris, R.A. & Allan, A. M. (1989). Alcohol intoxication: Ion channels and genetics. *FASEB Journal,* : 1689-1695.

Harris, R.A. & Bruno, P. (1985). Effects of ethanol and other intoxicant-anesthetics on voltage-dependent sodium channels of brain synaptosomes. *Journal of Pharmacology and Experimental Therapeutics, 232*: 401-406.

Harris, R.A. & Hood, W.F. (1980). Inhibition of synaptosomal calcium uptake by ethanol. *Journal of Pharmacology and Experimental Therapeutics, 213*: 562-568.

Hellevuo, K., Hoffman, P.L., & Tabakoff, B. (1991). Ethanol fails to modify [^{3}H]GR65630 binding to 5-HT$_3$ receptors in NCB-20 cells and in rat cerebral membranes. *Alcoholism: Clinical and Experimental Research, 15*: 775-778.

Hitzemann, R., Kreishman, G., Stout, J., & Schuler, H. (1991). Membranes and the genetics of ethanol response. *Annals New York Academy of Sciences, 625*: 515-523.

Hoffman, P.L., Rabe, C.S., Moses, F., & Tabakoff, B. (1989). N-methyl-D-aspartate receptors and ethanol: inhibition of calcium flux and cyclic GMP production. *Journal of Neurochemistry, 52*: 1937-1940.

Hoffman, P.L. & Tabakoff, B. (1982). Effects of ethanol on Arrhenius parameters and activity of mouse striatal adenylate cyclase. *Biochemical Pharmacology, 31*: 3101-3106.

Hoffman, P.L. & Tabakoff, B. (1986). Ethanol does not modify opiate-mediated inhibition of striatal adenylate cyclase. *Journal of Neuro chemistry, 46*: 812-816.

Hunt, W.A. (1985). Alcohol and Biological Membranes. In H. Bland and D. Goodwin (Eds.), *The Guilford Alcohol Studies Series*, The Guilford Press.

Iorio K.R., Reinlib L., Tabakoff B., & Hoffman P.L. (1992). Chronic exposure of cerebellar granule cells to ethanol results in increased N-methyl-D-aspartate receptor function. *Molecular Pharmacology, 41*: 1142-1148.

Keane, B. & Leonard, B.E. (1983). Changes in "open field" behaviour and in some membrane-bound enzymes following the chronic administration of ethanol to the rat. *Neuropharmacology, 22*: 555-557.

Kentroti, S. & Vernadakis, A. (1990). Neuronal plasticity in the developing chick brain: interaction of ethanol and neuropeptides. *Developmental Brain Research, 56*: 205-210.

Khanna, J.M., Kalant, H., Shah, G., & Chau, A. (1992). Effect of (+)MK-801 and ketamine on rapid tolerance to ethanol. *Brain Research Bulletin, 28*: 311-314.

Koob, G.F. (1992). Drugs of abuse: anatomy, pharmacology and function of reward pathways. *Trends in Pharmacological Sciences, 13*: 177-184.

Kril, J.J., Gundlach, A.L., Dodd, P. R., Johnston, G.A.R., & Harper, C. G. (1989). Cortical dihydropyridine binding sites are unaltered in human alcoholic brain. *Annals of Neurology, 26*: 395-397.

Kulkarni, S.K., Mehta, A.K., & Ticku, M.K. (1990). Comparison of anticonvulsant effect of ethanol against NMDA-, kainic acid-, and picrotoxin-induced convulsions in rats. *Life Sciences, 46*: 481-487.

Lancaster, F.E., Selvanayagam, P., & Hsu, L.L. (1986). Lactational ethanol exposure: Brain enzymes and [^{3}H]spiroperidol binding. *International Journal of Developmental Neuroscience, 4*: 151-160.

Leslie, S.W., Barr, E., Chandler, J., & Farrar, R.P. (1983). Inhibition of fast- and slow-phase depolarization-dependent synaptosomal calcium uptake by ethanol. *Journal of Pharmacology and Experimental Therapeutics, 225*: 571-575.

Leslie, S.W., Brown, L.M., Dildy, J.E., & Sims, J.S. (1990). Ethanol and neuronal calcium channels. *Alcohol, 7*: 233-236.

Leslie, S.W., Woodward, J.J., Wilcox, R.E., & Farrar, R.P. (1986). Chronic ethanol treatment uncouples striatal calcium entry and endogenous dopamine release. *Brain Research, 368*: 174-177.

Liljequist, S. (1991). The competitive NMDA receptor antagonist, CGP 39551, inhibits ethanol withdrawal seizures. *European Journal of Pharmacology, 192*: 197-198.

Lima-Landman, M.T.R. & Albuquerque, E.X. (1989). Ethanol potentiates and blocks NMDA-activated single-channel currents in rat hippocampal pyramidal cells. *FEBS Letters, 247*: 61-67.

Lin A.M.-Y., Freund, R.K., & Palmer, M.R. (1991). Ethanol potentiation of GABA-induced electrophysiological responses in cerebellum: requirement for catecholamine modulation. *Neuroscience Letters, 122*: 154-158.

Little, H.J., Dolin, S.J., & Halsey, M.J. (1986). Calcium channel antagonists decrease the ethanol withdrawal syndrome. *Life Sciences, 39*: 2059-2065.

Littleton, J.M., Little, H.J., & Whittington, M.A. (1990). Effects of dihydropyridine calcium channel antagonists in ethanol withdrawal: doses required, stereospecificity and actions of BAY K 8644. *Psychopharmacology, 100*: 387-392.

Lovinger, D.M. (1991). Ethanol potentiates 5-HT$_3$ receptor-mediated ion current in NCB-20 neuroblastoma cells. *Neuroscience Letters, 122*: 57-60.

Lovinger, D.M. & White, G. (1991). Ethanol potentiation of 5-hydroxytryptamine$_3$ receptor-mediated ion current in neuroblastoma cells and isolated adult mammalian neurons. *Molecular Pharmacology, 40*: 263-270.

Lovinger, D.M., White, G., & Weight, F.F. (1989). Ethanol inhibits NMDA-activated ion current in hippocampal neurons. *Science, 243*: 1721-1724.

Lovinger, D.M., White, G., & Weight, F.F. (1990). NMDA receptor-mediated synaptic excitation selectively inhibited by ethanol in hippocampal slice from adult rat. *Journal of Neuroscience, 10*: 1372-1379.

Lucchi, L., Covelli, V., Anthopoulou, H., Spano, P. F., & Trabucchi, M. (1983). Effect of chronic ethanol treatment on adenylate cyclase activity in rat striatum. *Neuroscience Letters, 40*: 187-192.

Luthin, G.R. & Tabakoff, B. (1984). Activation of adenylate cyclase by alcohols requires the nucleotide-binding protein. *Journal of Pharmacology and Experimental Therapeutics, 228*: 579-587.

Luttinger, D., Hemeroff, C.B., Mason, G.A., Frye, G.D., Breese, G.R., & Prange, A.J., Jr. (1981). Enhancement of ethanol-induced sedation and hypothermia by centrally administered neurotensin, β-endorphin, and bombesin. *Neuropharmacology, 20*: 305-309.

Machu, T., Woodward, J.J., & Leslie, S. W. (1989). Ethanol and inositol 1,4,5-trisphosphate mobilize calcium from rat brain microsomes. *Alcohol , 6*: 431-436.

Marks, S.S., Watson, D.L., Carpenter, C.L., Messing, R.O., & Greenberg, D. A. (1989). Comparative effects of chronic exposure to ethanol and calcium channel antagonists on calcium channel antagonist receptors in cultured neural (PC12) cells. *Journal of Neurochemistry, 53*: 168-172.

Martin, D., Morrisett, R.A., Bian, X-P., Wilson, W.A., & Swartzwelder, H. S. (1991). Ethanol inhibition of NMDA mediated depolarizations is increased in the presence of Mg^{2+}. *Brain Research, 546*: 227-234.

McLarnon, J.G., Wong, J.H.P., & Sawyer, D. (1991). The actions of intermediate and long-chain *n*-alkanols on unitary NMDA currents in hippocampal neurons. *Canadian Journal of Physiology and Pharmacology, 69*: 1422-1427.

Messing, R.O., Carpenter, C.L., Diamond, I., & Greenberg, D.A. (1986). Ethanol regulates calcium channels in clonal neural cells. *Proceedings National Academy of Sciences USA, 83*: 6213-6215.

Michaelis, E.K., Mulvaney, M.J., & Freed, W.J. (1978). Effects of acute and chronic ethanol intake on synaptosomal glutamate binding activity. *Biochemical Pharmacology, 27*: 1685-1691.

Mochly-Rosen, D., Chang, F-H., Cheevers, L., Kim, M., Diamond, I., & Gordon, A. S. (1988). Chronic ethanol causes heterologous desensitization of receptors by reducing α_s messenger RNA. *Nature*, 333: 848-850.

Moore, S.D., Madamba, S.G., & Siggins, G.R. (1990). Ethanol diminishes a voltage-dependent K^+ current, the M-current, in CA_1 hippocampal pyramidal neurons in vitro. *Brain Research, 516*: 222-228.

Morrisett , R.A., Martin, D., Oetting, T.A., Lewis, D.V., Wilson, W.A., & Swartzwelder, H.S. (1991). Ethanol and magnesium ions inhibit N-methyl-D-aspartate-mediated synaptic potentials in an interactive manner. *Neuropharmacology, 30*: 1173-1178.

Morrisett, R.A., Martin, D., Wilson, W.A., Savage, D.D., & Swartzwelder, H. S. (1989). Prenatal exposure to ethanol decreases the sensitivity of the adult rat hippocampus to N-methyl-D-aspartate. *Alcohol , 6*: 415-420.

Mulkeen, D., Anwyl, R., & Rowan, M.J. (1987). Enhancement of long-term potentiation by the calcium channel agonist Bayer K8644 in CA_1 of the rat hippocampus in vitro. *Neuroscience Letters, 80*: 351-355.

Mullin, M.J., Dalton, T.K., Hunt, W.A., Harris, R.A., & Majchrowicz, E. (1987). Actions of ethanol on voltage-sensitive sodium channels: Effects of acute and chronic ethanol treatment. *Journal of Pharmacology and Experimental Therapeutics, 242*: 541-547.

Mullin, M.J. & Hunt, W.A. (1985). Actions of ethanol on voltage-sensitive sodium channels: Effects on neurotoxin-stimulated sodium uptake in synaptosomes. *Journal of Pharmacology and Experimental Therapeutics, 232*: 413-419.

Mullin, M.J. & Hunt, W.A. (1987). Actions of ethanol on voltage-sensitive sodium channels: Effects on neurotoxin binding. *Journal of Pharmacology and Experimental Therapeutics, 242*: 536-540.

Nhamburo, P.T., Salafsky, B.P., Hoffman, P.L., & Tabakoff, B. (1986). Effects of short-chain alcohols and norepinephrine on brain (Na^+,K^+)ATPase activity. *Biochemical Pharmacology, 35*: 1987-1992.

Noble, E.P. & Ritchie, T. (1989). Prenatal ethanol exposure reduces the effects of excitatory amino acids in the rat hippocampus. *Life Sciences, 45*: 803-810.

Nowycky, M.C., Fox, A.P., & Tsien, R.W. (1985). Three types of neuronal calcium channel with different calcium agonist sensitivity. *Nature 316*: 440-443.

Oakes, S.G. & Pozos, R.S. (1982). Electrophysiological effects of acute ethanol exposure. I. Alterations in the action potentials of dorsal root ganglia neurons in dissociated culture. *Developmental Brain Research, 5*: 243-249.

Okonmah, A.D., Brown, J.W., Fishman, L.M., Carballeira, A., & Soliman, K.F.A. (1989). Influence of ethanol on fetal brain cholinergic enzyme activities. *Pharmacology, 39*: 367-372.

Olsen, R.W. & Tobin, A.J. (1990). Molecular biology of GABA$_A$ receptors. *FASEB Journal, 4*: 1469-1480.

Peoples, R.W. & Weight, F.F. (1992). Ethanol inhibition of N-methyl-D-aspartate-activated ion current in rat hippocampal neurons is not competitive with glycine. *Brain Research, 571*: 342-344.

Pillai, N.P. & Ross, D.N. (1986). Ethanol-induced hypothermia in rats: possible involvement of opiate kappa receptors. *Alcohol, 3*: 249-253.

Pispa, J.P., Huttunen, M.O., Sarviharju, M., & Ylikahri, R. (1986). Enzymes of catecholamine metabolism in the brains of rat strains differing in their preference for or tolerance of ethanol. *Alcohol and Alcoholism, 21*: 181-184.

Pohorecky, L.A. & Shah, P. (1987). Ethanol-induced analgesia. *Life Sciences, 41*: 1289-1295.

Rabe, C.S. & Tabakoff . B. (1990). Glycine site-directed agonists reverse the actions of ethanol at the N-methyl-D-aspartate receptor. *Molecular Pharmacology, 38*: 753-757.

Rabe, C.S. & Weight, F.F. (1988). Effects of ethanol on neurotransmitter release and intracellular free calcium in PC12 cells. *Jounal of Pharmacology and Experimental Therapeutics, 244*: 417-422.

Rabin, R.A. (1985). Effect of ethanol on inhibition of striatal adenylate cyclase activity. *Biochemical Pharmacology, 34*: 4329-4331.

Rabin, R.A. & Molinoff, P.B. (1981). Activation of adenylate cyclase by ethanol in mouse striatal tissue. *Journal of Pharmacology and Experimental Therapeutics, 216*: 129-134.

Rabin, R.A. & Molinoff, P.B. (1983). Multiple sites of action of ethanol on adenylate cyclase. *Journal of Pharmacology and Experimental Therapeutics, 227*: 551-556.

Rangaraj, N., Kalant, H., & Beauge, F. (1985). Alpha 1-adrenergic receptor involvement in norepinephrine-ethanol inhibition of rat brain Na^+-K^+ ATPase and in ethanol tolerance. *Canadian Journal of Physiology and Pharmacology, 63*: 1075-1079.

Rao, P.A., Kumari, C.L., & Sadasivudu, B. (1985). Acute and short term effects of ethanol on membrane enzymes in rat brain. *Neurochemical Research, 10*: 1577-1585.

Rezazadeh, S.M., Woodward, J.J., & Leslie, S.W. (1989). Fura-2 measurement of cytosolic free calcium in rat brain cortical synaptosomes and the influence of ethanol. *Alcohol, 6*: 341-345.

Richelson, E., Stenstrom, S., Forray, C., Enloe, L., & Pfenning, M. (1986). Effects of chronic exposure to ethanol on the prostaglandin E_1 receptor-mediated response and binding in a murine neuroblastoma clone (N1E-115). *Journal of Pharmacology and Experimental Therapeutics, 239*: 687-692.

Saffey, K., Gillman, M.A., & Cantrill, R.C. (1988). Chronic in vivo ethanol administration alters the sensitivity of adenylate cyclase coupling in homogenates of rat brain. *Neuroscience Letters, 84*: 317-322.

Saito, T., Lee, J.M., Hoffman, P.L., & Tabakoff, B. (1987). Effects of chronic ethanol treatment on the β-adrenergic receptor-coupled adenylate cyclase system of mouse cerebral cortex. *Journal of Neurochemistry, 48*: 1817-1822.

Saito, T., Lee, J.M., & Tabakoff, B. (1985). Ethanol's effects on cortical adenylate cyclase activity. *Journal of Neurochemistry, 44*: 1037-1044.

Seeman, P. (1972). The membrane actions of anesthetics and tranquilizers. *Pharmacological Reviews, 24*: 583-655.

Seizinger, B.R., Bovermann, K., Maysinger, D., Hollt, V., & Herz, A. (1983). Differential effects of acute and chronic ethanol treatment on particular opoid peptide systems in discrete regions of rat brain and pituitary. *Phamacology Biochemistry and Behavior, 18*: 361-369.

Sellers, E.M., Higgins, G.A., & Sobell, M.B. (1992). 5-HT and alcohol abuse. *Trends in Pharmacological Sciences, 13*: 69-75.

Sellers E.M., Kaplan, H.L., Lawrin, M.O., Somer, G., Naranjo, C.A., & Frecker, R.C. (1988). The 5-HT$_3$ antagonist GR38032F decreases alcohol consumption in rats. *Society for Neuroscience Abstract, 14*: 41.

Shah, J. & Pant, H.C. (1988). Spontaneous calcium release induced by ethanol in the isolated rat brain microsomes. *Brain Research, 474*: 94-99.

Shefner, S.A. & Osmanovic, S.S. (1987). Enhancement of anomalous rectification in rat locus coeruleus neurons by ethanol. *Society for Neuroscience Abstract, 13* : 534.

Siggins, G.R., Pittman, Q.J., & French, E.D. (1987). Effects of ethanol on CA1 and CA3 pyramidal cells in the hippocampal slice preparation: an intracellular study. *Brain Research, 414*: 22-34.

Simson, P.E., Criswell, H.E., Johnson, K.B., Hicks, R.E., & Breese, G.R. (1991). Ethanol inhibits NMDA-evoked electrophysiological activity in vivo. *Journal of Pharmacology and Experimental Therapeutics, 257*: 225-231.

Sinclair, J.G. & Lo, G F. (1986). Ethanol blocks tetanic and calcium-induced long-term potentiation in the hippocampal slice. *General Pharmacology, 17*: 231-233.

Skattebol, A. & Rabin, R.A. (1987). Effect of ethanol on $^{45}Ca^{2+}$ uptake in synaptosomes and PC12 cells. *Biochemical Pharmacology, 36*: 2227-2229.

Smith, T.L. (1991). Selective effects of acute and chronic ethanol exposure on neuropeptide and guanine nucleotide stimulated phospholipase C activity in intact N1E-115 neuroblastoma. *Journal of Pharmacology and Experimental Therapeutics, 258*: 410-415.

Soliman, K.F.A. & Gabriel, N.N. (1985). Brain cholinergic involvement in the rapid development of tolerance to the hypothermic action of ethanol. *General Pharmacology, 16*: 137-140.

Stenstrom, S. & Richelson, E. (1982). Acute effect of ethanol on prostaglandin E$_1$-mediated cyclic AMP formation by a murine neuroblastoma clone. *Journal of Pharmacology and Experimental Therapeutics, 221*: 334-341.

Stenstrom, S., Seppala, M., Pfenning, M., & Richelson, E. (1985). Inhibition by ethanol of forskolin-stimulated adenylate cyclase in a mruine neuroblastoma clone (N1E-115). *Biochemical Pharmacology, 34*: 3655-3659.

Swann, A.C. (1983). Brain (Na$^+$,K$^+$)-ATPase: Opposite effects of ethanol and dimethyl sulfoxide on temperature dependence of enzyme conformation and univalent cation binding. *The Journal of Biological Chemistry, 258*: 11780-11786.

Swann, A.C. (1987). Membrane effects of ethanol in excitable cells. *Review Clinical Basic Pharmacology, 6*: 213-248.

Swann, A.C. (1990). Ethanol inhibition of active [86]Rb$^+$ -transport: Evidence for enhancement by sodium or calcium influx. *Journal of Pharmacology and Experimental Therapeutics, 254*: 864-871.

Syapin, P. J., Chen, J., & Alkana, R.L. (1985). Effect of norepinephrine on inhibition of mouse brain (Na$^+$ K$^+$)-stimulated, (Mg$^+$ $^+$)-dependent, and (Ca$^+$ $^+$)-dependent ATPase activities by ethanol. *Alcohol, 2*: 145-148.

Tabakoff, B., Hoffman, P.L., Lee, J.M., Saito, T., Willard, B., & De Leon-Jones, F. (1988). Differences in platelet enzyme activity between alcoholics and nonalcoholics. *The New England Journal of Medicine, 318*: 134-139.

Tabakoff, B., Hoffman, P.L., & Liljequist, S. (1987). Effects of ethanol on the activity of brain enzymes. *Enzyme, 37*: 70-86.

Tabakoff, B., Lee, J.M., De Leon-Jones, F., & Hoffman, P. L. (1985). Ethanol inhibits the activity of the B form of monoamine oxidase in human platelet and brain tissue. *Psychopharmacology, 87*: 152-256.

Teichberg, V.I., Tal, N., Goldberg, O., & Luini, A. (1984). Barbiturates, alcohols and the CNS excitatory neurotransmission: specific effects on the kainate and quisqualate receptors. *Brain Research, 291*: 285-292.

Treistman, S.N., Bayley, H., Lemos, J.R., Wang, X., Nordmann, J.J., & Grant, A.J. (1991). Effects of ethanol on calcium channels, potassium channels, and vasopressin release. *Annals New York Academy of Sciences, 625*: 249-263.

Twombly, D.A., Herman, M.D., Kye, C.H., & Narahashi, T. (1990). Ethanol effects on two types of voltage-activated calcium channels. *Journal of Pharmacology and Experimental Therapeutics, 254*: 1029-1037.

Urrutia, A. & Gruol, D.L. (1992). Acute alcohol alters the excitability of cerebellar Purkinje neurons and hippocampal neurons in culture. *Brain Research, 569*: 26-37.

Valverius, P., Crabbe, J.C., Hoffman, P.L. & Tabakoff, B. (1990). NMDA receptors in mice bred to be prone or resistant to ethanol withdrawal seizures. *European Journal of Pharmacology, 184*:195-189.

Valverius, P., Hoffman, P.L., & Tabakoff, B. (1987). Effect of ethanol on mouse cerebral cortical β-adrenergic receptors. *Molecular Pharmacology, 32*: 217-222.

Valverius, P., Hoffman, P.L., & Tabakoff, B. (1989). Hippocampal and cerebellar β-adrenergic receptors and adenylate cyclase are differentially altered by chronic ethanol ingestion. *Journal of Neurochemistry, 52*: 492-497.

Wafford, K. A., Burnett, D.M., Leidenheimer, N.J., Burt, D.R., Wang, J.B., Kofuji, P., Dunwiddie, T. ., Harris, R.A. & Sikela, J.M. (1991). Ethanol sensitivity of the $GABA_A$ receptor expressed in Xenopus oocytes requires eight amino acids contained in the γ_{2L} subunit of the receptor complex. Neuron, 7: 27-33.

Wafford, K.A., Dunwiddie, T.V., & Harris, R.A. (1989). Calcium-dependent chloride currents elicited by injection of ethanol into Xenopus oocytes. *Brain Research, 505*: 215-219.

Wafford, K.A. & Whiting, P.J. (1992). Ethanol potentiation of $GABA_A$ receptors requires phosphorylation of the alternatively spliced variant of the γ2 subunit. *FEBS Letters, 313*:113-117.

White G., Lovinger D.M., & Grant, K.A. (1990a). Ethanol (EtOH) inhibition of NMDA activated current is not altered after chronic exposure of rats or neurons in culture. *Alcoholism: Clinical and Experimental Research Abstract , 14*: 352.

White, G., Lovinger, D.M., & Weight, F.F. (1990b). Ethanol inhibits NMDA-activated current but does not alter GABA-activated current in an isolated adult mammalian neuron. *Brain Research, 507*: 332-336.

Whittington, M.A., Dolin, S.J., Patch, T.L., Siarey, R.J., Butterworth, A. R., & Little, H. J. (1991). Chronic dihydropyridine treatment can reverse the behavioural consequences of and prevent adaptations to, chronic ethanol treatment. *British Journal of Pharmacology, 103*: 1669-1676.

Whittington, M.A., & Little, H.J. (1991). Nitrendipine, given during drinking, decreases the electrophysiological changes in the isolated hippocampal slice, seen during ethanol withdrawal. *British Journal of Pharmacology, 103*: 1677-1684.

Woodward, J.J. & Gonzales, R.A. (1990). Ethanol inhibition of N-methyl-D-aspartate-stimulated endogenous dopamine release from rat striatal slices: reversal by glycine. *Journal of Neurochemistry, 54*: 712-715.

Wu, P.H., Fan, T., & Naranjo, C.A. (1987). Increase in the brain regional depolarization-dependent Ca^{2+} uptake in rats preferring ethanol. *Pharmacology Biochemistry and Behavior, 27*: 355-357.

Yamamoto, H.A. & Harris, R.A. (1983). Calcium-dependent ^{86}Rb efflux and ethanol intoxication: studies of human red blood cells and rodent brain synaptosomes. *European Journal of Pharmacology, 88*: 357-363.

Zimányi, I., Lajtha, A., & Reith, M.E.A. (1988). The mode of action of ethanol on batrachotoxinin-A benzoate binding to sodium channels in mouse brain cortex. *European Journal of Pharmacology, 146*: 7-16.

The Psychobiology of Conditioning, Reinforcement and Craving

M. Vogel-Sprott
Department of Psychology, University of Waterloo
Waterloo, Ontario, Canada

This chapter presents an overview of contemporary learning theory and research on craving and addictive drinking. The first section provides some background history on the concept of craving and the observations that prompted an interest in the contribution of learning. This is followed by a description of some learning terms and concepts relevant to investigations of craving and drinking behavior. Classical conditioning and instrumental learning research in this area have tended to proceed independently. The findings, discussed in the sections on classical conditioning and instrumental learning, show that each has provided important evidence, but an understanding requires an integrated view. The final section offers a synthesis based upon contemporary theory that assumes learning is the process of acquiring information about the relationship between events.

Background

The concept of "craving" has often been invoked to account for addictive drinking. Craving was initially used loosely to refer to some pathognomic psychological or biological need that led to a loss of control over drinking so that "...every time the subjects starts drinking, he is compelled to continue until he reaches a state of severe intoxication." (Mardones, 1963, p.146).

The World Health Organization (WHO) was among the first to give serious consideration to the definition of craving (WHO, 1951, 1955). The WHO Expert Committee on Mental Health and on Alcohol concluded that "a physiological craving for alcohol, as indicated by withdrawal symptoms, is seen immediately following withdrawal of alcohol only after prolonged continuous and heavy use of alcohol; such a physiological craving cannot be postulated as the cause of the resumption of drinking after a considerable period of abstinence when withdrawal symptoms are no longer present." (WHO, 1955, p.63). However, the restriction of the term to physiological evidence of withdrawal symptoms became blurred in common practice. The pathological symptom of alcoholism, craving, was expanded to account for a loss of control over drinking that occurred both after a period of abstinence and during drinking. The popular acceptance of this view provided the basis for the slogan warning against a first drink, " One drink away from a drunk".

The proposal that craving mediated between initial consumption and subsequent loss of control (Jellinek, 1955, 1960), prompted numerous experiments during the 1960s and early 1970s. These studies found that alcoholics who were free to self-administer alcohol showed neither loss of control drinking, nor any tendency to drink "to oblivion" (Mello & Mendelson, 1970, 1972; Nathan, Lowenstein, Solomon, & Rossi 1970; Nathan, O'Brien, & Lowenstein, 1971). Alcoholics were able to drink according to rules prescribed for drinking (Paredes, Hood, Seymour, & Gollob, 1973). The amount of alcohol consumed was consistently shown to be a function of the amount of work required to obtain alcohol (Mello & Mendelson, 1972). When given the opportunity to drink alcohol continuously over a period of months, alcoholics spontaneously initiated and terminated several drinking episodes, and some deliberately diminished their consumption when the withdrawal of alcohol was anticipated (Mello & Mendelson, 1970, 1972; Nathan et al., 1970, 1971). No differences in alcoholics' reports of craving were observed on days when they repeatedly received breakfast drinks containing either alcohol or no alcohol (Merry, 1966). When groups of alcoholics rated their cravings after receiving a strongly flavoured drink that contained either alcohol or no alcohol, stronger cravings were reported *irrespective of the beverage*, if the alcoholics were told that the drink contained alcohol (Engle & Williams, 1972). Clinical reports also indicated that some ex-alcoholics could subsequently drink socially for continuous periods of as much as 11 years (Davies, 1962), and their overall adjustment and social functioning may have been better than that of ex-alcoholic abstainers (Pattison, 1966, 1968).

Such evidence clearly contradicted the notion of a fatalistic craving precipitating a drinking bout after one, or many drinks. It appeared that craving in alcoholics could not be reliably evoked by the consumption of alcohol per se. Although craving was inferred from, and purportedly explained, uncontrollable drinking, this loss of control could not be reliably demonstrated. Thus some investigators proposed that the concept of craving should be abandoned because it was basically untestable (e.g., Mello, 1972). Others recommended that craving should be restricted to the desire for alcohol experienced by addicts undergoing withdrawal (Marlatt, 1978). Others suggested that the problem rested with an incorrect definition of the loss of control that craving may cause (Glatt, 1967; Hodgson, Rankin, & Stockwell, 1978; Keller, 1972). It was argued that the loss of control did not mean that the first drink inevitably evoked uncontrolled drinking. Rather, loss of control by alcoholics referred to the gradual development of an impairment in the ability to *consistently* refrain from drinking, and to *consistently* stop drinking if drinking is started. This redefinition of the loss of control as a gradual loss of *predictable* control over drinking still left open the possibility that the erratic occurrence of craving triggered alcoholic drinking. However, it also implied that the inconsistent lapse to drinking binges must be influenced by some factor or events in addition to a drink of alcohol.

Glatt (1967) speculated that the additional determinants may involve an alcoholic's "state of mind", motivation for taking a drink, social circumstance, place of drinking, and possibly also a particular threshold blood alcohol concentration. A similar set of factors was considered by Keller (1972) to play a role in determining the plunge into alcoholic drinking. However Keller further speculated that the factors exert their influence through the process of learning. "The essence of the addiction is that, when the significant cue or signal impinges upon him, though he is unconscious of it, or conscious of it but unaware of its significance, he will reach out to drink... Addiction, in this conception is thought of as a form of learned or conditioned response."(Keller, 1972, p.160). This analysis did not indicate whether craving, or drinking, or both, were conditioned responses. The major emphasis concerned the helplessness of the addict to control drinking behavior owing to some sort of involuntary conditioned response that occurs erratically because it depends on the presence or absence of learned cues rather than alcohol consumption per se.

The utility of the concept of craving continues to be debated (see Koslowski & Wilkinson, 1987, and following commentaries). Some investigators argue that craving confuses the desire for a drug with the intention to use it. But others believe that craving is more than a "wooly scientific concept" (Rankin, 1987), and it may be a useful hypothetical construct in understanding alcoholism (Wilson, 1987). A similar debate has occurred in the area of learning. Under the influence of radical behaviorism, the postulation of "inner causes", such as cravings, was rejected on the grounds that there was no scientific means of determining if they were real or fictional (Skinner, 1953). However, interest in craving has revived with the development of more cognitively oriented learning theory (Bolles, 1972, 1975, 1979).

Contemporary research on the role of learning in craving and addictive drinking essentially attempts to explain the phenomena in terms of the principles that explain learned behavior in general. The approach is consistent with the widely held belief that motivation to use alcohol contributes to alcoholic drinking, but it is based upon the assumption that the learned motivational principles relevant to the pursuit of rewarding goals apply equally to the pursuit of nonpharmacological and pharmacological incentives. Because the research draws upon a common theoretical framework, a brief description of learning terms and principles precedes the discussion of the findings.

Terms and Principles

From a learning perspective, humans consume alcohol in a context involving environmental, physiological and behavioral events that permit the learning of drug self-administration as well as other activities. The opportunity for learning is provided whenever some event is reliably associated with another event. The events may be environmental stimuli or responses. In the simplest case, an acquired association may involve two paired events, such as two stimuli, or two responses, or a response and a stimulus. *Classical conditioning* and *instrumental learning* refer to two different training procedures that present relationships involving different types of events. Classical conditioning associates two environmental stimuli, whereas instrumental learning associates a subject's response with an environmental stimulus. Instrumental learning is also referred to as *operant conditioning*.

In classical conditioning, some neutral environmental stimulus is presented and is followed by some specific stimulus that reliably evokes a particular response. The two stimuli are referred to, respectively, as a *Conditioned Stimulus* (CS) and an *Unconditioned Stimulus* (UCS). The response to the UCS is called an *Unconditioned Response* (UCR). In repeated CS-UCS pairings, the CS serves as a predictive cue that signals the occurrence of the UCS. Evidence that this relationship has been learned is provided by presenting the CS alone and observing that it evokes a response that resembles the UCR. The response to the CS is termed a *Conditioned Response* (CR).

In instrumental learning, the display of a particular response by a subject is reliably followed by some specific stimulus outcome. Evidence that this response-outcome association has been learned is provided by demonstrating a reliable change in response frequency. If the association leads to an increased occurrence of the response, the stimulus consequence of the response is termed a *reinforcer*, and may be said to provide *reinforcement* for the response.

Reinforcers are considered to evoke a positive emotional state. Reinforcers that directly enhance pleasure are termed *positive* reinforcers, and those that terminate distress are termed *negative* reinforcers. Addictive drugs, like alcohol, may provide positive and negative reinforcement in the form of enhanced pleasure and relief from distress, respectively. These two sources of reinforcement have been thought to contribute to the addiction liability of a substance (Wise, 1988).

Incentive and motivational properties are attributed to reinforcers because their presence can instigate behavior as well as strengthen a response (Bindra, 1974: Bolles, 1972). When a reinforcer is used as a UCS in classical conditioning, the CS acquires incentive and motivational properties similar to the reinforcing UCS, and the CS is then referred to as a *conditioned incentive*. When such a CS is administered contingent upon the display of a response, the CS is referred to as a *secondary reinforcer* because it can increase the frequency of the response.

During the last decade, research on craving and addictive drinking has been pursued from the perspectives of classical conditioning and of instrumental learning. Each strategy has proceeded somewhat independently. The next sections describe the rationale of each approach and summarize the pertinent results.

Classical Conditioning: Cues and Craving

Rationale

An analysis of the role of classical conditioning in craving and re-lapse to drug use after a period of abstinence was initially offered for opiate addiction (e.g., Wikler,1965), and was subsequently extended to alcohol addiction (Ludwig, 1972; 1986; Ludwig & Stark 1974; Ludwig, Wikler, & Stark, 1974). This analysis emphasized *with-drawal-relief*. It was noted that particular environments could be consistently associated with periodic episodes of withdrawal symptoms. Thus these environmental stimuli could function like a CS and come to elicit a conditioned withdrawal response. Therefore, a "craving" for the drug after a period of abstinence was attributed to the presence of a CS that evokes "a correlate of a subclinical conditioned withdrawal symptom." (Ludwig et al., 1974, p.539).

The withdrawal-relief analysis initially identified stimuli associated with withdrawal as CSs that could come to evoke CRs resembling withdrawal. Subsequent research on classical conditioning of drug tolerance widened the range of stimuli evoking conditioned withdrawal to include events associated with drug administration (Poulos, Hinson, & Siegel, 1981; Siegel, 1983). This research indicated that a drug may evoke *drug-opposite* as well as drug-like responses. The occurrence of drug-opposite reactions ostensibly compensates for the pharmacological action of the drug, and is assumed to in-crease with drug use. Thus these reactions could account for toler-ance. In addition, because withdrawal symptoms often appear to oppose the effect of a drug, these compensatory reactions also could underlie withdrawal distress (Hinson & Siegel,1980). When toler-ance is established, events accompanying drug administrations could be regularly associated with the compensatory response. Thus a classical conditioning situation is created in which cues for the drug come to elicit a conditioned compensatory reaction resembling with-drawal.

A conditioned withdrawal-relief analysis assumes that a wide variety of stimuli associated with alcohol administration, and with withdrawal, come to elicit a conditioned reaction similar to that observed during actual drug withdrawal. In theory, these condi-tioned reactions are characterized by physiological states opposite to the initial effect of a drug, and by negative affect, indicated by self-reports of craving and distress. When a conditioned withdrawal reaction occurs, drug administration would reliably alleviate the distressing symptoms. Thus drug self-administration is viewed as a response maintained by the negative reinforcing effect of the drug, and relapse to drug use is attributed to conditioned stimuli evoking conditioned withdrawal symptoms.

A conditioned withdrawal-relief analysis only considers the negative reinforcing properties of addictive drugs. A *conditioned incentive* interpretation of craving and relapse to drug use has been offered by others who emphasize that many addictive drugs function as positive reinforcers, and have incentive motivational properties (Baker, Morse,& Sherman, 1987; Bozarth, 1987; Stewart & deWit, 1987; Stewart, deWit, & Eikelboom, 1984). Impetus for a conditioned incentive interpretation was provided by research with opiates and stimulants. These addictive drugs appeared to have the incentive and motivational properties of positive reinforcers because animals would learn to press a lever to receive the drug, and stimulus events that predicted drug availability could instigate lever pressing. Studies also showed that drug self-administration did not depend solely upon distress relief because animals would respond for drugs in the absence of deprivation, in the absence of acute withdrawal symptoms and in the absence of any experience of drug withdrawal. Converging evidence from biopsychology suggested that positive reinforcers and opiates activate a common central neural mechanism that evokes approach and appetitive behavior (Wise, 1988; Wise & Bozarth, 1987). Thus it seemed that addictive drugs could substitute for, or compete with biologially important reinforcers, such as food.

A conditioned incentive analysis proposes that environmental stimuli predicting drug administration can be associated with the activation of a central neural mechanism of positive reinforcement. Thus these environmental cues come to evoke a conditioned neuronal response resembling that activated by the drug. From this perspective, the drug itself, or cues predicting the drug, or even other positive reinforcers could prime the reinitiation of drug use by activating the positive reinforcing neural mechanism that evokes approach and consummatory behavior. To the extent that alcohol functions as a positive reinforcer, the conditioned incentive interpretation implies that cues predicting positive reinforcement, that is pleasurable emotional states, should evoke reports of craving, alcohol-seeking and drinking behavior.

The incentive and the withdrawal-relief analyses differ in emphasizing the positive and the negative reinforcing properties of addictive drugs. However, the interpretations agree that events associated with alcohol administration become learned cues for the reinforcing

effect of a drug, and the presentation of cues should increase alcoholics' reports of craving and drug-taking. Thus in classical conditioning interpretations, "craving" is evoked by the presentation of these
cues. The use of the term by alcoholics presumably describes their
subjective experience of these cues. This has prompted many investigations of the sorts of cues that lead alcoholics to report craving and
relapse.

Evidence

Laboratory studies have found that the presentation of environmental cues for alcohol increases alcoholics' self- reports of craving.
Some experiments have compared the effect of salient cues (sight
and smell of alcohol) to cues not commonly associated with drinking
(e.g.,Ludwig, Wikler, & Stark, 1974). Others have allowed alcoholics
to drink, and measured their ratings of craving and speed of drinking (Hodgson, Rankin,& Stockwell, 1979; Rankin, Hodgson, & Stockwell, 1979). Other experiments have adopted a balanced placebo
design (Rohsenow & Marlatt, 1981) to separate the pharmacological
action of the drug from the cues predicting alcohol administration.
In these experiments, half of the subjects are presented with cues for
alcohol when they are served either an alcoholic or a nonalcoholic
(placebo) beverage. The remainder are presented with cues unrelated to alcohol when their alcohol or placebo beverages are served.
This research has demonstrated that cues for alcohol per se have a
powerful effect. When these cues are present, alcoholics report
higher craving and drink alcohol or placebo at a higher rate (Berg,
Laberg, Skutle, & Ohman, 1981; Maisto, Lauerman, & Adesso, 1977:
Marlatt, Demming, & Reid, 1973; Stockwell, Hodgson, Rankin, &
Taylor, 1982).

The results of such alcohol experiments are in general accord with
the proposition that events associated with a reinforcer come to elicit
conditioned reactions that enhance the incentive value of the reinforcer. However, the laboratory findings do not clearly indicate whether
the craving evoked by these cues is for the positive or the negative
reinforcing effect of the drug. The hedonic nature of the cues is of
interest because the withdrawal-relief formulation predicts cues
evoke emotional distress and physical states resembling withdrawal,
whereas the conditioned incentive analysis predicts cues may elicit
pleasurable affective states.

Some information on this question has been obtained in retrospective studies of alcoholics' reports of the types of events and reactions

preceding craving or actual alcohol use. An extensive review of these findings (Niauria et al., 1988) concluded that increased craving and relapse were commonly reported in environments associated with drinking, but environments associated with withdrawal were seldom mentioned. Thus alcoholics' self-reports apparently failed to support the long standing proposition that craving for alcohol is evoked by environments paired with withdrawal. Niauria et al., (1988) also noted that alcoholics commonly reported craving and risk of relapse in the presence of cues evoking a variety of pleasurable *and* distressing emotional states, but the list rarely included the negative physical and emotional states associated with withdrawal. This evidence implies that a withdrawal-relief analysis is too narrow. A *general distress-relief* interpretation would be more consistent with the reports of numerous different distressing events preceding craving and actual drug use.

In sum, the self-reports of alcoholics suggest that craving and actual drug use may be little influenced by actual or conditioned withdrawal distress, and are more likely to occur in the presence of a wide variety of destabilizing emotional-provoking events, either positive or negative. In theory, actual pleasurable or distressing events can be identified as UCSs that should elicit specific positive or negative reinforcer approach/consummatory behavior. And the CSs associated with these UCSs should evoke CRs that resemble the reactions to the UCSs. Thus the presentation of these CSs should evoke reports of craving and overt alcohol-seeking and consumption because the drug could provide positive reinforcement (enhanced pleasure), and negative reinforcement (distress relief).

A classical conditioning interpretation implies that alcoholics' reports of increased craving should be associated with concordant increases in overt alcohol-seeking and consumption. Alcoholics' retrospective reports have provided much information about the types of cues and emotional reactions that may precede craving or actual alcohol use. But these data do not indicate whether the same cue, identified by an alcoholic as precipitating craving, also precipitates drinking.

The association between self-reports of craving and actual drug use has received comparatively little attention. Some investigators have suggested that alcoholics' reports of craving may not predict their alcohol administration (Marlatt & Gordon, 1980, 1985; Mathew, Claghorn, & Largen, 1979). A recent analysis of studies of alcoholics that reported correlations between measures of alcohol consumption and cravings indicated that the correlations could account for only

16%, and no more than 50% of the variance (Tiffany, 1990). The evidence of such weak relationships between self-reported craving and drinking led Tiffany to argue that drug use behavior may be only loosely coupled to verbal reports of craving. This possibility suggests that a classical conditioning analysis may only identify the conditions that allow environmental events to function as cues to elicit craving. To the extent that events that evoke craving do not reliably result in relapse to drug use, some additional factors must be influencing the re-emergence of drinking behavior. The possibility that environmental events play an important role here has been suggested by research on instrumental learning that examines response-reinforcer relationships to determine the conditions under which a particular response emerges to dominate activity.

Instrumental Learning: Reinforcement and Drinking

Rationale

In any environmental setting, a number of reinforcing activities are usually available for an individual to engage in. Research on behavioral choice has assessed the variation in behavior as a function of constraints and access to alternative reinforcers in the situation (e.g., Herrnstein, 1970; Premack, 1965). Behavior theories of choice have achieved considerable empirical success in accounting for a substantial portion of variability in animal and human behavior in a variety of situations (e.g.,Pierce & Epling, 1983; Rachlin et al., 1986). This work has also identified some general principles that lead to the emergence of one dominant response.

One important generalization is that when constraints are imposed on the access to a particular reinforcer, the response for this reinforcer diminishes, and responding is reallocated to other reinforcers available in the situation. Similarly, when constraints are placed on all but one reinforcer, all activity is allocated to this reinforcer. Vuchinich and Tucker (1988) have proposed that this generalization applies to the conditions under which alcohol consumption emerges as a highly preferred activity from among a set of available activities. This proposal implies that the availability and constraints on alcohol and on alternative reinforcers in a situation should determine whether alcoholics will resume drinking.

Evidence

Ethical considerations preclude the use of alcoholics in experiments on factors that may induce relapse to drinking. Thus studies using alcoholics have not tested the hypothesis that access to alcohol and constraints on other reinforcers result in a resumption of drinking. However, many observations consistent with this prediction have been obtained in earlier experiments that demonstrated alcoholics' drinking behavior altered as a function of constraints on the access to alcohol (e.g.,Bigelow & Liebson, 1972; Griffiths, Bigelow & Liebson, 1978: Mello. 1972; Mello & Mendelson, 1972). These studies found that alcohol self-administration by alcoholics decreased when the work required to obtain alcohol was increased, and when penalties for drinking were increased.

Animal studies have investigated alcohol self-administration as a function of the availability of other reinforcers. In this choice situation, subjects are given access to multiple reinforcers, and their consumption of each is measured. Because the animals are tested in a setting containing the cues that have been associated with drug self-administration, the test conditions may be analogous to those in which alcoholics are confronted by cues that evoke craving. Reviews of this research (e.g., Johanson & Schuster, 1981) support the conclusion that the behavior reinforced by alcohol is similar to behavior maintained by other reinforcers. A preference for alcohol self-administration increases and decreases respectively, as a function of the constraints and availability of other reinforcers in the situation.

Analogous choice behavior experiments have been conducted with nonalcoholic humans to examine alcohol consumption as a function of alternative reinforcers. Although cues for self-administration would not be expected to elicit reports of craving in nonalcoholics, their alcohol consumption also increased and decreased as a function of restriction and access to alternative reinforcers. These findings have been reviewed in detail elsewhere (Vuchinich & Tucker, 1988).

From the perspective of choice behavior theory, alcohol consumption can be construed as a learned response whose occurrence depends upon the availability of alcohol and of other reinforcers. The specific condition in which the drinking response should emerge as dominant is one where alcohol is available and access to alternative reinforcers by other behaviors is constrained.

Behavioral theories of choice have proceeded inductively, using an instrumental training paradigm to determine empirical response-reinforcer relationships. The evidence from these studies clearly identifies important environmental determinants of drug self-administration that seem pertinent to understanding the role of learning in craving and addictive drinking. However, because the empirical orientation of the work implicitly questions the need to postulate intervening inner causes like craving, the evidence is somewhat difficult to relate to that obtained in classical conditioning studies. The next section proposes an integrated learning interpretation of craving and addictive drinking based upon contemporary learning theory.

An Integration

Theory

Research in classical conditioning and in instrumental learning began as separate domains of inquiry. The findings were traditionally considered to pertain to different learning processes, possibly because the two training procedures differ: classical conditioning associates two environmental stimuli whereas instrumental training associates a subject's response with a stimulus. Nonetheless, the interpretation of the learning resulting from each training procedure tended to be mechanistic. Thus "a CS evoked a CR", and " a response was strengthened by a reinforcer".

In contrast, contemporary learning theory is inclined to a less mechanistic interpretation. It assumes that learning is the process of acquiring information about the association of events. Because the events that are related under classical conditioning are different from those that are related under instrumental training, the learned associations each provide different information. But the same learning *process* is involved because both the training procedures provide an opportunity to associate events.

Bolles (1972,1975,1979) has been a leading advocate of this theory. He assumes that learning is the process of associating events, and the learned information about associations is retained as "expectancies". Thus the classical conditioning procedure of associating two stimulus events provides an opportunity to acquire a "stimulus-outcome" expectancy, and the association of a response with a stimulus event during instrumental training results in the acquisition of a "response-outcome" expectancy. Bolles has argued persuasively that the acquisition and retention of expectancies instigate and guide behavior appropriate to the expected outcome. Thus the properties of incentive motivation attributed to expectancies are similar to those attributed to conditioned incentives and secondary reinforcers. For example, cues signalling emotional-provoking events result in a stimulus-outcome expectancy that enhances the incentive to seek reinforcement. And response-outcome expectancies determine the display of a particular response that is expected to yield the reinforcing outcome.

The use of expectancy terminology reflects a shift in the assumption about the nature of the learning process. In contemporary theory, the concept of expectancy represents an unobservable mental state. It has the status of an intervening variable because the environmental events influencing the state are specified, and the predictions concerning the behavioral effect of expectancies can be tested experimentally. Contemporary learning theory has led to research showing that the expectancies acquired under classical conditioning and under instrumental training are required to account for behavioral tolerance to alcohol (Vogel-Sprott, 1992; Vogel-Sprott & Sdao-Jarvie, 1989).

Craving and relapse to drinking occur after alcoholics have had extensive opportunity to associate events preceding drinking (stimulus-outcome), and to associate the reinforcing effect of alcohol with this response (response-outcome). Because each association involves different events, different information is acquired from each. Thus the learned information governing drinking behavior could be independent of that governing reports of craving. Stimulus-outcome expectancies may determine reports of craving, and response-outcome expectancies may determine the drinking behavior. The implications of these assumptions are discussed below.

Implications

One implication of the theory is that craving need not necessarily lead to alcohol use because craving and drinking each depend upon different, independent, expectancies. Reports of craving in the presence of cues signalling destabilizing emotional states result in the acquisition of stimulus-outcome expectancies that enhance the incentive value of reinforcers providing either pleasure or relief of distress. But the response-outcome expectancies acquired by an individual will determine the particular response that is expected to yield these desired outcomes. The re-emergence of drinking should occur only when an alcoholic expects the most desirable outcome to be obtained by drinking. In the absence of this particular response-outcome expectancy, craving may not predict a relapse to drinking. Thus, in order for craving to be followed by a resumption of drinking, the requisite stimulus-outcome *and* response-outcome expectancies are *both* needed.

In contrast to the usual notion that craving precedes a return to drinking, the theory implies that craving need not be a prerequisite. This implication could account for the evidence from instrumental learning studies showing that alcohol self-administration by addicted and nonaddicted subjects can emerge as a dominant response when the drug is the only available reinforcer. Such conditions provide opportunities to learn that the outcome of drinking is more desirable than the outcome of alternative responses. This expectancy could also be learned in real life circumstances that provide few alternative reinforcers other than alcohol. Such situations at the outset of a drinking career may play a role in determining which drinkers advance to alcoholism. In other words, response-outcome expectancies may be an important factor both in setting the stage for the development of alcoholism, and in determining whether an alcoholic resumes drinking.

Many interpretations of alcoholism have stressed the helplessness of the individual to control the addiction. Learning theory suggests that an alcoholic might appear to be a hapless victim of craving because it is based upon the presence of particular stimulus events in the environment. The encounter of such events in real life situations is not completely under an individual's control. Thus the occurrence of craving by alcoholics may be difficult to predict, and appear to be involuntary.

A distinction between craving and drinking behavior in terms of learned expectancies is consistent with some interpretations of addictive drinking that refer to cravings as "urges", and consider that urges do not necessarily lead to alcohol consumption (e.g., Baker et al., 1987; Niaura et al., 1988; Tiffany, 1990). There is currently considerable interest in factors that may prevent alcoholics from acting on the urge for alcohol. Research on the relation of relapse to the expected outcomes of drinking (Goldman, Brown, & Christiansen, 1987), and on relapse prevention treatment that endeavours to change expectancies (Marlatt & Gordon, 1985) are two important examples of such work. These investigations have identified a number of conditions that diminish the likelihood of drinking by alcoholics. Some of these, such as the expectation of penalizing consequences of drinking, appear to be specific instances of circumstances in which some response other than drinking is expected to yield a more desirable outcome. Thus clinical research appears to be validating the application of the learning theory assumptions about response-outcome expectancies.

One merit of using the term "urge" for craving is that urge has less pathological connotations, and it leads to hitherto unasked questions about the urges of nonalcoholics. In principle, stimulus-outcome expectancies concerning emotional-provoking states should also induce nonalcoholics to seek appropriate reinforcement and to report urges for these reinforcers. It may be that the interpretation and label of such urges depend upon expectation of what suitable reinforcement is attainable. Studies of alcoholics have identified a number of events leading to the expectation of pleasure or distress that result in reports of urges for alcohol. Investigations of the types of urges reported by nonalcoholics to these same emotional-provoking events appear to be an important area for future research.

Summary

A continuing central issue regarding alcoholism concerns questions about the craving for alcohol, why only some drinkers use it to extreme, and why only some of these relapse while attempting to maintain sobriety. This chapter considered the answers to these questions provided by contemporary learning theory. By assuming that learning is an information-gathering process that is retained in the form of expectancies, the theory integrates the evidence from both classical conditioning and instrumental learning. Thus it presents an interpretation of the role of learning in craving, and in the resumption of drinking. In addition, the theory offers testable predictions about the association of specific events leading to stimulus-outcome expectancies that affect craving, and to response-outcome expectancies that influence the occurrence of drinking.

Research and theory on alcoholism have expanded rapidly during the last 10 years. Work on the psychobiological effects of addictive drugs suggests that the concept of alcohol craving may someday be identified by its activation of basic brain mechanisms of reinforcement. But evidence that alcohol activates such a basic biological process common to all individuals still would not address the question of why only some drinkers abuse alcohol, or why only some alcoholics relapse. Learning, as discussed in the present chapter, offers an explanation of these individual differences. Investigations of genetic markers and special groups, such as women and families, represent some of the many other current explanatory approaches. It will be interesting indeed to follow the fate of these various theoretical explanations during the next decade of research.

References

Baker, T.B., Morse, E., & Sherman, J.E. (1987). Motivation to use drugs: A psychobiological analysis of urges. In C. P. Rivers (Ed.) *Nebraska Symposium on Motivation, 1986 Volume 34* (pp. 257-323). Lincoln: University of Nebraska Press.

Berg, G., Laberg, J.C., Skutle, A., & Ohman, A. (1981). Instructed versus pharmacological effects of alcohol in alcoholics and social drinkers. *Behavior Research and Therapy*, 19: 55-66.

Bigelow, G., & Liebson, I. (1972). Cost factors controlling alcoholic drinking. *Psychological Record*, 22: 305-314.

Bindra, D. (1974). A motivational view of learning, performance and behavior modification. *Psychological Review*, 81: 199-213.

Bolles, R.C. (1972). Reinforcement, expectancy and learning. *Psychological Review*, 79: 394-409.

Bolles, R.C. (1975). *Theory of Motivation* (2nd ed.). New York: Harper & Row.

Bolles, R.C. (1979). *Learning Theory* (2nd ed.). New York: Holt, Reinhart and Winston.

Bozarth, M.A. (Ed.) (1987). *Methods of assessing the reinforcing properties of abused drugs.* New York: Springer-Verlag.

Davies, D.L., (1962). Normal drinking in recovered alcoholics. *Quarterly Journal of Studies on Alcohol*, 23: 94-104.

Engle, K.B., & Williams, T.K. (1972). Effect of an ounce of vodka on alcoholics' desire for alcohol. *Quarterly Journal of Studies on Alcohol*, 33: 1099-1105.

Glatt, M.M., (1967). The question of moderate drinking despite "loss of control". *British Journal of Addiction*, 62: 267-274.

Goldman, M., Brown, S., & Christiansen, B. (1987). Expectancy theory: Thinking about drinking. In H. Blane & K. Leonard (Eds.), *Psychological Theories of Drinking and Alcoholism* (pp. 181-226). New York: Guilford.

Griffith, R.R., Bigelow, G.E., & Liebson, I. (1978). Relationship of social factors to ethanol self-administration in alcoholics. In P. Nathan, G.A. Marlatt, & T. Loberg (Eds.) *Alcoholism: New directions in behavioral research and treatment* (pp. 351-379). New York: Plenum.

Herrnstein, R.J. (1970). On the law of effect. *Journal of the Experimental Analysis of Behavior*, 13: 243-266.

Hinson, R.E., & Siegel, S. (1980). The contribution of Pavlovian conditioning to ethanol tolerance and dependence. In H. Rigter & J. C. Crabbe (Eds.), *Alcohol Tolerance and Dependence* (pp.179-197). Amsterdam: Elsevier/North Holland Biomedical Press.

Hodgson, R., Rankin, H., & Stockwell, T. (1978). Craving and loss of control. In P. Nathan, G. A. Marlatt, & T. Loberg (Eds.) *Alcoholism: New directions in behavioral research and treatment* (pp. 341-349). New York: Plenum.

Hodgson, R., Rankin, H., & Stockwell, T. (1979). Alcohol dependence and the priming effect. *Behavior Research and Therapy*, 17: 379-387.

Jellinek, E.M. (1960). *The disease concept of alcoholism*. New Brunswick, NJ: Hillhouse Press.

Jellinek, E.M. (1955). The "craving" for alcohol. *Quarterly Journal of Studies on Alcohol*, 16: 34-66.

Johanson, C.E., & Schuster, C.R. (1981). Animal models of drug self-administration. In N. K. Mello (Ed.) *Advances in substance abuse: Behavioral and biological research* (Vol. 2, pp.219-298) Greenwich, CT: JAI Press.

Keller, M. (1972). On the Loss-of-control phenomenon in alcoholism. *British Journal of Addiction*, 67: 153-166.

Kozlowski, L.T., & Wilkinson, D.A. (1987). Use and misuse of the concept of craving by alcohol, tobacco, and drug researchers. *British Journal of Addiction*, 82: 31-36.

Ludwig, A.M. (1972). On and off the wagon. *Quarterly Journal of Studies on Alcohol*, 33: 91-96.

Ludwig, A.M. (1986). Pavlov's "bells" and alcohol craving. *Addictive Behaviors*, 11: 87-91.

Ludwig, A.M., & Stark, L.H. (1974). Alcohol craving. *Quarterly Journal of Studies on Alcohol*, 35: 899-905.

Ludwig, A.M., Wickler, A., & Stark, L.H. (1974). The first drink: Psychobiological aspects of craving. *Archives of General Psychiatry*, 30: 539-547.

Maisto, S.A., Lauerman, R., & Adesso, V.J. (1977). A comparison of two experimental studies of the role of cognitive factors in alcoholics' drinking. *Journal of Studies on Alcohol*, 38: 145-149.

Mardones, J. (1963). The alcohols. In W. S. Root, & F. G. Hoffman (Eds.) *Physiological Pharmacology* (pp. 99-183). New York: Academic Press.

Marlatt, G.A. (1978). Craving for alcohol, loss of control and relapse: A cognitive-behavioral analysis. In P. Nathan, G.A. Marlatt, & T.

Loberg (Eds.) *Alcoholism: New directions in behavioral research and treatment* (pp. 271-314). New York: Plenum.

Marlatt, G.A., Demming, B., & Reid, J. (1973). Loss of control drinking in alcoholics: An experimental analogue. *Journal of Abnormal Psychology*, 81: 233-241.

Marlatt, G.A., & Gordon, J.R. (1980). Determinants of relapse: Implications for the maintenance of behavior change. In P. O. Davidson, & S.M. Davidson (Eds.) *Behavioral Medicine: Changing health lifestyles* (pp. 410-452). New York: Brunner/Mazel.

Marlatt, G.A., & Gordon, J.R. (1985). *Relapse Prevention.* New York: Guilford Press.

Mathew, R.J., Claghorn, J.L., & Largen, J. (1979). Craving for alcohol in sober alcoholics. *American Journal of Psychiatry*, 136: 603-606.

Mello, N.K. (1972). Behavioral studies of alcoholism. In B. Kissin, & H. Begleiter (Eds.) *The Biology of Alcoholism*, vol. 2 (pp. 219-291), New York: Plenum.

Mello, N.K., & Mendelson, J.H. (1970). Experimentally induced intoxication in alcoholics: A comparison between programed and spontaneous drinking. *Journal of Pharmacology and Experimental Therapeutics*, 173: 101-116.

Mello, N.K., & Mendelson, J.H. (1972). Drinking patterns during work-contingent and noncontingent alcohol acquisition. *Psychosomatic Medicine*, 34: 139-164.

Merry, J. (1966). The "loss of control" myth. *Lancet, 1*: 1257-1258.

Nathan, P.E., Lowenstein, L.M., Solomon, P., & Rossi, A.M. (1970). Behavioral analysis of chronic alcoholism. *Archives of General Psychiatry*, 22: 419-430.

Nathan, P.E., O'Brien, J.S., & Lowenstein, L.M. (1971). Operant studies of chronic alcoholism: Interaction of alcohol and alcoholics. In P.J. Creaven, & M.K. Roach (Eds.) *Biological aspects of alcohol.* Austin: University of Texas Press.

Niaura, R.S., Rohsenow, D.J., Binkoff, J.A., Monti, P.M., Pedraza, M., & Abrams, D. B. (1988) Relevance of cue reactivity to understanding alcohol and smoking relapse. *Journal of Abnormal Psychology*, 97:133-152.

Paredes, A., Hood, W.R., Seymour, H., & Gollob, M. (1973). Loss of control in alcoholism. *Quarterly Journal of Studies on Alcohol*, 34: 1146-1161.

Pattison, E.M. (1966). A critique of alcoholism treatment concepts with special reference to abstinence. *Quarterly Journal of Studies on Alcohol*, 27: 49-71.

Pattison, E.M. (1968). Abstinence criteria: A critique of abstinence criteria in the treatment of alcoholism. *International Journal of Social Psychiatry*, 14: 268-276.

Pierce, W.D., & Epling, W.F. (1983). Choice, matching and human behavior: A review of the literature. *The Behavior Analyst*, 6: 57-76.

Poulos, C.X., Hinson, R.E., & Siegel, S. (1981). The role of Pavlovian processes in drug tolerance and dependence: Implications for treatment. *Addictive Behaviors*, 6: 205-211.

Premack, D. (1965). Reinforcement theory. In D. Levine (Ed.) *Nebraska Symposium on Motivation* (pp. 123-180). Lincoln: University of Nebraska Press.

Rachlin, H., Logue, A.W., Gibbon, J., & Frankel, M. (1986). Cognition and behavior in studies of choice. *Psychological Review*, 93:33-45.

Rankin, H. (1987). Some comments on the "Use and misuse of the concept of craving" by Kozlowski and Wilkinson: Craving is more than a wooly scientific concept. *British Journal of Addiction*, 82: 981.

Rankin, H. Hodgson, R., & Stockwell, T. (1979). The concept of craving and its measurement. *Behavior Research and Therapy*, 17: 389-396.

Rohsenow, D.J., & Marlatt, G.A. (1981). The balanced placebo design: Methodological considerations. *Addictive Behaviors*, 6:107-122.

Siegel, S. (1983). Classical conditioning, drug tolerance and drug dependence. In Y. Israel, B.F. Glasser, H. Kalant, R.E. Popham, W. Schmidt, & R.G. Smart (Eds.) *Research advances in alcohol and drug problems*. (Vol. 7. pp. 207-246). New York: Plenum Press.

Skinner, B.F. (1953). *Science and human behavior*. London: Collier-MacMillan.

Stewart, J., & deWit, H. (1987). Reinstatement of drug-taking behavior as a method of assessing incentive motivational properties of drugs. In M.A. Bozarth (Ed.) *Method of assessing the reinforcing properties of abused drugs*. (pp.211-227). New York: Springer-Verlag.

Stewart, J., deWit, H., & Eikelboom, R. (1984). The role of unconditioned and conditioned drug effects in the self-administration of opiates and stimulants. *Psychological Review*, 91: 251-268.

Stockwell, T.R., Hodgson, R.J., Rankin, H.J., & Taylor, C. (1982). Alcohol dependence, beliefs and the priming effect. *Behavior Research and Therapy*, 20: 513-522.

Tiffany, S.T. (1990). A cognitive model of drug urges and drug-use behavior: Role of automatic and nonautomatic processes. *Psychological Review*, 97: 147-168.

Vogel-Sprott, M. (1992). *Alcohol tolerance and social drinking: Learning the consequences*. New York: Guilford Press.

Vogel-Sprott, M., & Sdao-Jarvie, K. (1989). Learning alcohol tolerance. The contribution of response expectancies. *Psychopharmacology*, 98: 289-296.

Vuchinich, R.E., & Tucker, J. A. (1988). Contributions from behavioral
theories of choice to an analysis of alcohol abuse. *Journal of Abnormal Psychology*, 97: 181-195.

WHO (1951). Report on the first session of the alcoholism subcom-
mittee of the expert committee on mental health. *World Health
Organization technical report series*, 42: 3-24.

WHO Expert Committee on Mental Health and on Alcohol (1955).
Symposium on the "craving" for alcohol. *Quarterly Journal of Studies on Alcohol, 16*, 34-66.

Wikler, A. (1965). Conditioning factors in opiate addiction and relapse. In D.I. Wilner, & G.G. Kassenbaum (Eds.) *Narcotics* (pp.85-
100). New York: McGraw-Hill.

Wilson, G.T. (1987). Cognitive studies in alcoholism. *Journal of Con-
sulting and Clinical Psychology*, 55: 325-331.

Wise, R.A. (1988). The neurobiology of craving: Implications for the
understanding and treatment of addiction. *Journal of Abnormal
Psychology*, 97: 118-132.

Wise, R.A., & Bozarth, M.A. (1987). A psychomotor stimulant theory
of addiction. *Psychological Review*, 94: 469-492.

Neurologic Pathology of Alcohol Abuse

Peter L. Carlen and Enrique Menzano
Neuropharmacology Program, Addiction Research Foundation and
The Playfair Neuroscience Unit, Toronto Hospital Research Institute
University of Toronto, Canada

Alcohol is the most abused drug in the world. It is taken for its effects on the central nervous system (CNS). There are no specific alcohol receptors and the reasons for the addictive properties of ethanol are not as yet completely understood. It has CNS effects at 5 to 100 mM concentrations, 10^3 to 10^6 times higher than most other psychoactive drugs. Hence, at these relatively high concentrations, it is not unexpected that deleterious CNS pathological consequences could occur with prolonged high intake. This review will briefly mention the acute effects and focus on topical aspects of the chronic neurologic and neuropathologic consequences of alcohol abuse. A summary of the neurological complications of alcoholism is presented in Table 1. There are several other recent related review articles (Victor, 1982; Thomas, 1986; Charness, Simon & Greenberg, 1989; Lishman, 1990).

Table 1
Neurological Complications of Alcoholism

Acute effects
- Acute intoxication
- Alcoholic blackouts
- Pathological alcoholic intoxication

Tolerance
- Cross-tolerance: e.g. sedatives, general anesthetics
- Loss of tolerance: elderly, brain damage

Withdrawal
- Tremulousness
- Seizures
- Hallucinations
- Confusion
- Delirium tremens

Chronic syndromes
- Probably nutritionally related:
  - Wernicke's encephalopathy
  - Korsakoff's syndrome
  - Alcoholic cerebellar degeneration
  - Alcoholic pellagra encephalopathy
  - Vitamin B6 deficiency
  - Tobacco-alcohol amblyopia
  - Alcoholic neuropathy
- Possibly nutritionally related:
  - Alcoholic cerebral atrophy
  - Marchiafava-Bignami disease
  - Central pontine myelinolysis
  - Alcoholic myopathy
- Miscellaneous
  - Parkinsonism (transient)
  - Other movement disorders: postural tremor, transient chorea/orolingual dyskinesias, akathisia
  - Liver disease: Portosystemic encephalopathy, myelopathy, non-Wilsonian hepatocerebral degeneration
  - Sleep apnoea
  - Subdural and other intracerebral hematomas
  - Strokes in young adults
  - Pressure palsies

Acute Intoxication

Severe acute intoxication can rarely result in an unexplained cerebral oedema. Intoxication is commonly associated with traumatic injuries. Alcohol intoxication is the most frequent concomitant of fatal motor vehicle accidents. Traumatic brain injuries including subdural, epidural, and intracerebral hematomas, are often associated with alcoholism.

Tolerance

Even after one drink, acute tolerance can develop to the behavioral effects of alcohol. Habitual drinkers characteristically manifest less evidence of intoxication than occasional drinkers and they are usually less sensitive to other CNS depressant drugs because of cross-tolerance. This cross-tolerance includes most general anaesthetics, such as barbiturates, which is important, because if an alcoholic requires emergency surgery, often much higher doses of general anaesthetic are required. Loss of tolerance to alcohol occurs in the elderly and in chronic alcoholics who have developed cognitive impairments (personal observation). Finally, alcoholics do not apparently develop tolerance to the neurotoxicological effects of long-term alcohol abuse.

Withdrawal Syndromes

Following heavy drinking, many alcoholics experience a tremulous-hyperexcitable withdrawal syndrome. This syndrome, well-described by Victor (1982), has several features including postural tremor, agitation, confusion, ataxia and, in some cases, seizures (Victor & Brausch, 1967). The seizures are usually generalized, but can be partial, most likely due to a focal lesion in an epileptogenic area. Epileptiform EEG abnormalities are common in epileptic patients, but uncommon in alcoholics with withdrawal seizures. Alcoholics who experience withdrawal seizures rarely complain of an aura, whereas epileptics, particularly those with complex partial seizures, often note preconvulsive auras. The alcohol withdrawal state is a hyperexcitable brain state which can, however, evoke seizures in patients with epilepsy. Alcohol withdrawal is one of the commonest causes of status epilepticus. It is hypothesized that long-term alcohol intoxication actually establishes an epileptogenic state of the brain which becomes manifest upon alcohol withdrawal (Carlen, Rougier-Naquet, Reynolds, 1990).

In addition to the acute withdrawal syndrome, delirium tremens (DTs) can occur. The DTs usually follow by a few days, a severe acute withdrawal syndrome and is characterized by delirium, hallucinations, and a hyperautonomic state including sweating and tachycardia. Unfortunately, there can be up to a 15% mortality associated with this syndrome, possibly from hyperadrenergic-mediated ischemic myocardial necrosis and dehydration (Victor, 1982).

Chronic and Miscellaneous Syndromes

Alcohol related dementias

It is estimated that the lifetime prevalence of alcoholism in the USA is 13% (DSM III R, 1987). The prevalence of alcohol-related dementia in community studies ranges from 1 to 3% (Evans et al, 1989; Schoenberg, Kokmen & Okazaki, 1987; Copeland et al, 1992) compared to the prevalence of Alzheimer's dementia which is usually over 50% of dementia patients. However, in a recent epidemiological study of a sample of 130 subjects drawn from over 800 institutionalized elderly in a rural community (North Bay, Ontario, Canada) of about 55,000 population, it was found that 84% had significant cognitive deficits, and of these, alcoholism was the primary factor for cognitive impairment in 24% (Carlen et al., 1994). The alcohol group were on an average 10 years younger and had been institutionalized almost twice as long (7.5 years) as the other groups (Alzheimer's, vascular, and other miscellaneous causes of dementia).

Wernicke-Korsakoff syndrome

Victor and his colleagues made the definitive studies of the Wernicke-Korsakoff syndrome (WKS) which has a characteristic pathology and clinical presentation (Victor, Adams & Collins, 1989). Wernicke's encephalopathy (WE) is characterized by ophthalmoplegia, mental dysfunction, and ataxia, and is due to a thiamine (vitamin B_1) deficiency. It often coexists with the alcohol withdrawal syndrome and may be missed since ataxia, confusion and nystagmus are seen in both syndromes. The ophthalmoplegia may include any of the oculomotor nerves or an internuclear ophthalmoplegia. However, if clear-cut ophthalmoplegia is not apparent, then nystagmus is usually noted. Mental dysfunction includes apathy, short attention span, confusion and drowsiness, all of which can merge into an amnestic state. The ataxia is usually truncal, without ataxia of the limbs. Autonomic dysfunction is also frequent, characterized by orthostatic hypotension and hypothermia. A peripheral neuropathy is usually present, which could be due to the alcoholism per se in addition to the characteristic thiamine deficiency. In alcoholics, this deficiency can be due to several factors including: decreased vitamin B_1 in the diet, alcohol intake increasing the metabolic need for thiamine, decreased absorption of thiamine because of alcohol-related gastrointestinal disorders, and decreased utilization of thiamine at the cellular level. WE also appears in other disease states characterized by decreased nutritional intake or utilization; i.e. renal failure, chronic renal dialysis, chronic bowel disease, persistent vomiting, or with intravenous hyperalimentation.

WE is classified as a medical emergency, since not to treat with thiamine can lead to the development of the more permanent Korsakoff's Syndrome (KS). This syndrome may occur without a prior documented episode of WE. Superficially, patients can appear to converse and reason normally. However, they have limited insight into their condition, which is characterized by a profound anterograde and retrograde amnesia. They are unable to learn new information and sometimes confabulate. They usually have no memory of prior events from the time that they developed the Korsakoff's syndrome. Some patients with the KS may also have a co-existing dementia.

Both WE and KS have the same distribution of neuropathological lesions, except that acute cases have a wider and more caudal distribution of lesions, whereas chronic cases are more restricted and rostral (Torvik, 1987). The medial nucleus of the mammillary bodies is always involved. Also, lesions are characteristically seen in the thalamus, especially the dorsomedial nucleus, hypothalamus periaqueductal gray of the mesencephalon (floor of the fourth ventricle, locus ceruleus, abducens nucleus), medulla (vestibular nuclei, dorsal motor nucleus of the vagus, tractus solitarius), cerebellar vermis, cerebral cortex, hippocampus, spinal cord, and peripheral nerves (Victor et al, 1989). The central nervous system lesions are noteworthy for their consistent and bilateral localization, and usually their proximity to the ventricular system. Most damaged structures are gray matter where neuronal loss is prominent, with the exception of the basis pontis and the fornix where demyelination is prominent. Loss of cholinergic neurons in the nucleus basalis of

Meynert is seen both in Alzheimer's disease and in Korsakoff's syndrome (Arendt et al, 1983).

Modern imaging techniques permit *in vivo* examination of the neuropathology of the WKS. CT scans sometimes show low-density diencephalic abnormalities in acute WE (McDowell & LeBlanc, 1985). Significant cerebral atrophy is seen in alcoholics with a marked amnestic syndrome (Wilkinson & Carlen, 1980). MRI scanning, which permits greater spatial resolution, has demonstrated smaller mammillary bodies in subjects with a recent history of classic WE compared to presumed Alzheimer's and control subjects (Charness and De LaPaz, 1987). Three-dimensional measurements of local cerebral blood flow (LCBF), using xenon contrast computed tomography in chronic alcoholics, showed that Wernicke-Korsakoff patients had more severe reductions in LCBF diffusely in gray and white matter, especially in the hypothalamus and basal forebrain (Hata et al, 1987). Single photon emission tomography using the lipophilic blood flow marker, ^{99m}Tc-HMPAO, showed reduced blood flow in the posterior temporal and parietal areas in Alzheimer subjects and present temporal blood flow with reduction in other brain areas in Korsakoff's patients (Hunter et al, 1989). Furthermore, these authors showed that reduced frontal lobe blood flow was correlated with neuropsychological impairments in KS patients. Frontal lobe dysfunction has recently been demonstrated to produce a disorganization of retrieval processes in both Alzheimer's disease and alcoholic KS (Kopelman, 1991).

On the other hand, positron emission tomography (PET) studies, using the glucose analogue fluoro-deoxyglucose (FDG) found that localized cerebral glucose utilization at rest is not significantly affected by chronic ethanol consumption (Kessler et al, 1984; Eckardt MJ et al, 1988). Only subtle changes were observed in comparison to more striking alterations in neuropathology, neurophysiology and neuropsychological studies. Isotopes with briefer uptake time and receptor-specific ligands as well as cognitive challenges probably will better disclose functional abnormalities (Eckardt et al, 1990).

The diagnosis of the Wernicke-Korsakoff syndrome is often missed during life. In an autopsy study of 131 cases of WE, only 26 cases had been correctly diagnosed antemortem (Harper, 1983). Similarly, another autopsy study reported that only 1 of 22 patients with WE had been identified antemortem (Torvik, Lindlow, Rogde, 1982).

Alcoholic dementia

Many investigators differentiate alcoholic dementia from the KS. There certainly is a significant group of alcoholics who have a dementia syndrome which comprises a more global impairment than the characteristic amnestic syndrome of the KS. Whether alcoholic dementia is merely an extension of the KS is still unclear. The P300, a cognitive evoked potential which is characteristically slowed in dementias, is delayed as expected in Alzheimer's disease (Blackwood, St. Clair, Blackburn, Tyrer, 1987). Porjesz, Begleiter and Samuelly (1980) showed that chronic alcoholics (not specifically demented) had low amplitude P300 waves with identical latencies to both target and non-target stimuli. In neuropsychologically diagnosed KS patients, the P300 is of normal latency, whereas in alcoholic dementia, the P300 is delayed (Noldy et al, 1991). Alcoholic dementia is associated with CT scan-measured cerebral atrophy which is not very closely related to the degree of cognitive impairment (Carlen et al, 1981). Alcoholics with a significant amnestic syndrome (KS) have as much or more cerebral atrophy on CT scan as those without the amnestic syndrome (Wilkinson & Carlen, 1980). However, cerebral atrophy is also seen in alcoholics without significant neurocognitive deficits (Carlen et al, 1981). Autopsy studies of chronic alcoholics demonstrate cerebral atrophy (Courville, 1966) and lower brain weight than age-matched controls (Torvik, 1987; Harper and Blumbergs, 1982). Even in "moderate" drinkers, autopsy data suggest a loss of cerebral tissue (Harper, Kril & Daly, 1988) Some of the decreased brain volume is attributed to white matter loss (Harper, Kril & Holloway, 1984; De La Monte, 1988) which could be due to direct axonal damage or secondarily to neuronal loss.

In fact, selective neuronal loss has been demonstrated in an autopsy study of the human alcoholic cerebral cortex. The neuronal count in the superior frontal cortex, but not in the motor cortex, was significantly reduced, compared to sex- and age-matched controls (Harper, Kril & Daly, 1987). This was found to be due to loss of the larger neurons in the frontal cortex along with an increase in glia (Harper & Kril, 1989). Similar neuronal loss is seen in aging (Terry, DeTeresa & Hansen, 1987) and in Alzheimer's disease (Terry, Peck, DeTeresa, Schechter & Horoupian, 1981). Studies in animal models of chronic alcoholism have also demonstrated neuronal loss in hippocampus and cerebellum (Riley & Walker, 1978), as well as decreased dendritic arborization in hippocampal CA1 neurons

(McMullen, Saint-Cyr, Carlen, 1984) and cerebellar Purkinje neurons (Pentney, 1982; Tavares, Paula-Barbosa, Gray, 1983).

Reversibility

When alcoholics stop drinking, their presenting dementia (or encephalopathy) can sometimes show a marked recovery over weeks to months with maintained abstinence. Initially, alcohol withdrawal symptoms and signs may predominate. Thereafter, a devolution of their cognitive impairments, and motor disabilities, such as ataxia or tremor, may ensue. In the series of Wernicke-Korsakoff patients studied by Victor et al (1989), of 104 patients who had an amnestic syndrome and received thiamine and dietary treatment, 46% showed significant or complete recovery. Onset of recovery occurred rarely within a few days, occasionally within a few weeks, and usually within one to three months. Recovery took place over a few months.

This type of recovery was also noted in the more global alcoholic dementia (Carlen & Wilkinson, 1986), which, as stated above, may merge with or be part of the KS. The fact that alcoholics were well known to demonstrate cerebral atrophy pathologically (Courville, 1966) and on CT scans (Fox, Ramsey, Huckman, Proscke, 1976; Cala, Jones, Mastaglia, Wiley, 1978), and that they sometimes demonstrated marked clinical improvement with maintained abstinence, led us to speculate that this cerebral atrophy might be reversible.

Repeated CT scans initially in a small group of 8 alcoholics (Carlen, Wortzman, Holgate, Wilkinson, Rankin, 1978) and later in a larger group of 20 alcoholics (Carlen, Wilkinson, Wortzman, Holgate, 1984) showed that the measured cerebral atrophy was partially reversible with maintained abstinence. Those alcoholics who continued to drink in the interscan interval showed no decreased atrophy. Computerized estimations of CSF volume and brain density showed a negative correlation with each other, indicating that those alcoholics with the greatest measured cerebral atrophy had less radiodense brains (Carlen et al, 1986). The change in cerebral atrophy correlated weakly but significantly with some neurological change scores. The greater the reversibility of the cerebral atrophy, the greater was the increase in brain density, suggesting that recovery or reversibility of cerebral atrophy was associated with a decrease in brain water, possibly due to increased protein synthesis. Noble and Tewari (1973) showed that chronic ethanol administration decreased brain protein synthesis in mice by 50%. With two weeks of abstinence, brain protein synthesis significantly increased.

Neuropsychological testing of functional improvement over a three-month period in 38 recently abstinent alcoholics and 14 alcoholics who continued drinking, showed increases in verbal IQ up to 22 points, performance IQ up to 30 points, and memory quotient up to 40 points (Carlen et al, 1984). Computerized EEG measures of recently abstinent clinically impaired alcoholics showed increased alpha rhythm and decreased beta (20 to 30 Hz) power over four to six weeks (Zilm, Huszar, Carlen, Kaplan, Wilkinson, 1980). In another study of 80 alcoholics admitted to a treatment facility, a significant cerebrospinal fluid acidosis was apparent for up to seven weeks after the last drink. Repeated CSF measures showed decreased acidosis over a few weeks (Carlen et al, 1980).

The biological basis for the functional and morphological recovery are not clear. Certainly, there are many biochemical abnormalities which reverse during withdrawal, such as CSF acidosis (Carlen et al, 1980). From a cellular morphological perspective, McMullen, Carlen & St. Cyr (1984) showed in a rat model of chronic alcoholic brain damage, that CA1 dendrites were attenuated after 4 months of ethanol diet compared to pair-fed controls. This dendritic attenuation reversed following 2 months of alcohol abstinence, suggesting dendritic regrowth.

Theories of pathogenesis of alcohol-related brain damage

Cellular and molecular neuroscience is presently producing an explosion in knowledge, leading to new concepts of the pathogenesis of alcohol-related brain dysfunction. It is well accepted that vitamin B1 deficiency plays a major causative role in the Wernicke-Korsakoff syndrome. Other B vitamin deficiencies such as niacin (Serdaru et al, 1988) may also play a role, as well as malnutrition per se. Also CNS trauma has been implicated. Alcoholics are known to snore a great deal. Snoring is usually part of the sleep apnoea syndrome. Alcohol intoxication contributes to sleep apnoea, which can cause significant brain dysfunction (Issa & Sullivan, 1982). Alcoholic liver disease can also cause an encephalopathy which can be overt or subclinical. Chronic alcohol intake has been shown to decrease CNS protein synthesis as mentioned earlier (Noble, Tewari, 1973), and also is hypothesized to impair intracellular calcium homeostasis leading to calcium-mediated neurotoxicity (Carlen & Wu, 1988).

More recently, the role of zinc (Zn) deficiency has been hypothesized to be an important causative factor for alcoholic brain dysfunction (Menzano & Carlen, 1994). Zn deficiency is well recognized in chronic alcoholism (McDonald, Sullivan, Sturner, 1981) and is often associated with liver disease (Prasad, 1988). Zn deficiency is associated with hyperadreno-corticolism (Quaterman, 1972), and, conversely, hypercorticolism, is associated with low serum Zn (Etzell, Shapiro, Cousins, 1979). Alcoholism per se is also associated with high serum corticoids (Merry, Marks, 1969). Tying the above observations together, we hypothesized that Zn deficiency in alcoholics could be an important cause for hyperadrenocorticolism and brain damage (Menzano & Carlen, 1994). Steroids can cause cerebral atrophy (Bentson, Reza, Winter, Wilson, 1978) and treated Cushing's syndrome is associated with reversible cerebral atrophy (Heinz, Martinez, Haenggeli, 1977). Hence, alcoholism is associated with low Zn and high corticoids. The raised corticoids could then be the cause of the "reversible" cerebral atrophy seen in recently abstinent alcoholics.

Glutamate is the major cerebral excitatory neurotransmitter. Too much glutamatergic action can cause neuronal toxicity ("excitotoxicity"). This excitotoxicity is mediated in large part through activation of one of the glutamate receptor subtypes, the NMDA (N-methyl-D-aspartate) receptor, which when activated, can cause neuronal death via an intracellular Ca^{2+} dependent mechanism, and can be blocked by Zn (Peters, Koh & Choi, 1987). Glucocorticoids damage neurons by an NMDA-receptor mediated mechanism (Armanini, Hutchins, Stein, Sapolsky, 1990). Acutely, ethanol inhibits NMDA receptor activation (Lovinger, White, Weight, 1989). Chronic exposure to ethanol results in an up-regulation of the number of recognition sites of the NMDA receptor system (Grant, Valverius, Hudspith, Tabakoff, 1990; Gulya, Grant, Valverius, Hoffman, Tabakoff, 1991). Conversely, the NMDA receptor antagonist, MK-801, inhibits ethanol withdrawal seizures in rats (Grant et al, 1990; Morrisett et al, 1990). Zn blocks NMDA toxicity in cortical neurons (Peters, Koh, Choi, 1987). Therefore, the Zn deficiency and increased glucocorticoids associated with chronic alcoholism are two related factors which enhance NMDA (glutamate)-mediated excitotoxicity in CNS neurons (Menzano, Carlen, submitted).

Oxygen derived free radicals are well known to cause cell damage (Halliwell, Gutteridge, 1985) and are also implicated in the genesis of alcoholic brain damage (Pratt, Rooprai, Shaw, Thomson, 1990). Superoxide dismutase (SOD), which helps to eliminate free radicals, is decreased in the rat brain following chronic ethanol administration (Ledig et al, 1981). Sustained Zn deficiency per se also decreases SOD activity (Erdo, Michler, Wolff, 1991).

The role of thiamine deficiency in the development of the Wernicke-Korsakoff syndrome and alcoholic brain damage has recently been extensively discussed in an excellent review by Martin, McCool and Singleton (1992). Thiamine deficiency increases voluntary ethanol consumption in a rat animal model (Eriksson, Pekkanen, Rusi, 1980), and concomitant ethanol administration accelerates the neurological deficits due to thiamine deficiency (Zimitat, Kril, Harper, Nixon, 1990). Thiamine deficiency increases liver alcohol dehydrogenase activity, but has no effect on liver acetaldehyde dehydrogenase activity (Martin, Impeduglia, Rathna Giri, Karanian, 1988). This leads to increased ethanol metabolism permitting greater amounts of ethanol to be consumed chronically. Because liver acetaldehyde dehydrogenase activity is not concomitantly increased, the same amount of consumed ethanol produces more acetaldehyde, which damages cells, thereby enhancing the neurotoxicity of ethanol (Pratt, Rooprai, Shaw, Thomson, 1990).

Prolonged thiamine deficiency is associated with decreased transketolase, alpha-ketoglutarate dehydrogenase, and the pyruvate dehydrogenase complex, all enzymes involved in carbohydrate metabolism (Martin et al, 1992). Transketolase activity is a very sensitive measure of thiamine deficiency (Thomson, Ryle, Shaw, 1983). Decreased transketolase activity would be predicted to impair cellular synthesis of reducing equivalents (NADPH) and pentoses, both of which are necessary for various CNS synthetic pathways.

Transketolase may also act as an intracellular thiamine storage site. Active transport of thiamine across the membrane is postulated to involve an antiport with H^+ ions (Brown, 1990) such that in thiamine deficiency, intracellular acidosis should result along with increased intracellular Ca^{2+} (Vogel, Hakim, 1988). Intracellular acidosis could result in decreased cellular reuptake of glutamate (Poolma, Hellingwerf, Konings, 1987) leading to excitotoxicity. The NMDA antagonist, MK-801, prevents pyrithamine-induced lesions and amino acid changes in rat brain (Langlais, Mair, 1990).

Alcoholic cerebellar degeneration

Gait ataxia is a common finding in chronic alcoholics, even when sober. Usually there is little if any limb ataxia or dysarthria. Midline cerebellar degeneration, particularly of the anterior and superior vermis, is the primary lesion (Victor, Adams & Mancall, 1959). This pattern and syndrome is also seen in the WKS (Victor, Adams & Collins, 1989). Histologically, a significant loss of Purkinje cells is noted along with shrinkage of the granular and especially the molecular layers (Phillips, Harper & Kril, 1987). There is a poor correlation between the degree of cerebellar atrophy seen on prior CT scanning and the amount of histologically measured Purkinje cell loss (Phillips et al, 1987). Also, MRI or CT assessed cerebellar cortical atrophy correlates poorly with the clinical syndrome of ataxia in alcoholics (Hillbom, Muuronen, Holm & Hindmarsh, 1986). However, functional metabolic assessment of the brains of alcoholics using positron emission tomography (PET) scans showed that subjects with cerebellar ataxia had hypometabolism in the superior cerebellar vermis, but not necessarily cerebellar atrophy on CT scan (Gilman et al, 1990). Alcoholics with and without cerebellar signs had hypometabolism in the medial frontal cerebral cortex which correlated with the degree of CT scan-assessed cerebral frontal atrophy.

Central pontine myelinolysis

This is a rare syndrome characterized pathologically by non-inflammatory demyelination of the base of the pons (Adams, Victor and Mancall, 1959). About 10% of patients can have extrapontine lesions (Wright, Laurens & Victor, 1979). It often occurs in association with other alcoholism-related encephalopathies such as Wernicke's encephalopathy, pellagra encephalopathy or withdrawal seizures. Also, non-alcoholism-related conditions, including malnutrition, anorexia, burns, cancer, Addison's disease, and non-alcoholic (as well as alcoholic) liver disease can cause this syndrome. Recently, electrolyte changes have been implicated in the causation of this syndrome. Rapid correction of hyponatremia is now a recognized risk factor (Burcar, Norenberg & Yarnell, 1977; Slager, 1986). Hypokalemia may also be a risk factor in alcoholics (Bahr, Sommer, Petersen, Wietholter & Dichgans, 1990).

Patients with this lesion detected by CT scan, MRI scan, or at autopsy, may be asymptomatic, or may have a syndrome characterized by coma, lethargy or confusion, paraparesis or quadriparesis, dysarthria, and dysphagia. Serial MRI scans, can, in some cases, show resolution of the pontine lesion along with clinical recovery (Miller, Baker, Okazaki & Whisnant, 1988).

Alcoholic pellagra encephalopathy

Niacin deficiency causes the pellagra syndrome characterized by dermatitis, diarrhea, and dementia. In alcoholics, it can co-exist with other alcohol-related encephalopathies (Serdaru et al, 1988). Pathological lesions include swollen neurons with eccentric nuclei and loss of Nissl particles in the cerebral cortex, reticular formation, pontine nuclei and dentate nuclei. Clinically one observes a fluctuating confusional state that can progress to coma, increased tone, and startle myoclonus. Often in alcoholics, there is no evidence of pellagra dermatitis or diarrhea.

Vitamin B6 deficiency

Lack of pyridoxine (Vitamin B6) can occur in alcoholics, especially those with liver disease. Pyridoxine is converted to pyridoxal 5-phosphate in the liver and its deficiency is associated with a peripheral neuropathy, neuromuscular irritability, and seizures as well as stomatitis, dermatitis, immune suppression, and asideroblastic anemia. Vitamin B6 deficiency is usually associated with other nutritional deficiencies in alcoholics.

Marchiafava Bignami disease

This is a rare disease characterized pathologically by demyelination of the corpus callosum and clinically by confusion and coma in chronic alcoholics. The prognosis is poor and those patients that survive have a dementia.

Cerebral trauma and alcoholism

This subjects deserves special mention since it is so common, yet so little studied. Alcoholics have a tendency to fall and suffer head injuries because of intoxication and cerebellar ataxia. Alcoholics have cerebral atrophy, thereby exposing their subdural bridging veins to shearing forces which can result in a subdural hematoma. Also, alcoholics frequently have a low platelet count, predisposing them to easy bleeding. Alcohol abuse is the condition most frequently associated with fatal motor vehicle accidents. In a retrospective study of 100 consecutive intracranial hematomas requiring operation (acute and chronic subdurals, epidurals, and intracerebral hemorrhages), 50% of all patients were either alcoholics or were intoxicated on admission (Jacob, Fleming, Carlen, unpublished observations).

Movement disorders

Movement disorders, especially alcoholic postural tremor, are common in alcoholics (reviewed by Neiman, Lang, Fornazzari & Carlen, 1990). Alcoholic tremor resembles the benign essential postural tremor seen in non-alcoholics. This tremor is most marked in the acute alcohol withdrawal phase. The underlying pathophysiological mechanisms are not well understood. Although no pharmacological intervention is usually indicated since the tremor subsides along with the withdrawal syndrome, it is responsive to the ß-blocker, propranolol.

Asterixis is a disorder of motor control characterized by brief irregular lapses of posture best seen as coarse flexion-extension movements (flap) of the extended wrists in outstretched hands. These involuntary lapses are associated with EMG electrical silence in the arm muscles which are usually tonically active. It is part of the syndrome of hepatic encephalopathy which also includes a more rapid metabolic tremor.

A 3-Hz leg tremor, best seen with posturing of the foot over the contralateral knee, has been described in alcoholic cerebellar degeneration (Silverskiold, 1977). The underlying pathophysiology is not known.

Transient Parkinsonism has recently been recognized as occurring in alcoholics over 50 years of age (Carlen, Lee, Jacob, Livshits, 1981; Lang, Marsden, Obeso, & Parkes, 1982). Patients can show all the signs characteristic of idiopathic Parkinson's disease; i.e. bradykinesia, stooped posture, shuffling gait, lack of associated movements, expressionless face, and a coarse resting tremor. These patients often have, in addition, signs of alcohol withdrawal including postural tremor, ataxia and confusion. All patients improved with maintained abstinence, without antiparkinsonian medication. Several had repeated episodes of transient parkinsonism with repeated episodes of alcohol intoxication and withdrawal.

More rarely, transient dyskinesias have been reported during alcohol withdrawal. This condition can affect patients younger than age 50, and is more common in women. More often the dyskinesias occur 10 to 14 days after alcohol withdrawal (Fornazzari & Carlen, 1982). The following dyskinesias have been reported: lingual-oral dyskinesias, athetotic movements, choreiform movements.

Acquired hepatolenticular (non-Wilsonian) degeneration from severe alcoholic or nonalcoholic liver disease with portosystemic shunts is another condition producing persistent choreiform movements (Victor, Adams & Cole, 1965). Also, a rare myelopathy can develop in alcoholics, usually, but not always, in association with severe alcoholic liver disease.

Strokes in alcoholics

Alcohol abuse is a risk factor for both ischemic and hemorrhagic stroke (Hillbom, 1987). Strokes in alcoholics are more likely to occur during heavy alcohol intoxication, and this is particularly evident in the under 50 population. Alcohol alters platelet reactivity, but whether this is the cause for alcoholism-induced strokes is still unclear.

Alcoholic neuropathy

Most chronic alcoholics have subtle evidence of decreased temperature and vibration sensation in the peripheral lower limbs compared to the hands, and depressed ankle deep tendon reflexes. Sometimes this symmetrical peripheral neuropathy can become symptomatic with dysesthesia in the feet (burning foot syndrome), muscle cramps, distal weakness, gait (sensory) ataxia, skin atrophic changes, and occasionally autonomic disturbances.

The cause of the alcoholic polyneuropathy is thought to be nutritional deficiency, especially of thiamine and other B vitamins (Victor, Adams & Collins, 1989). Pathologically, one sees axonal degeneration, and in advanced cases, demyelination secondary to the axonal degeneration. With abstinence, clinical improvement, if it occurs, is slow, over many months.

Pressure neuropathies are associated with alcohol-induced stupor or coma and a prolonged abnormal limb position causing a compression neuropathy ("Saturday night palsy"). Radial and peroneal nerves are most frequently affected. Pressure palsies are usually demyelinating, giving rise to a favorable prognosis.

Alcoholic myopathy

Alcohol abuse can cause an acute or chronic skeletal myopathy, or a cardiomyopathy. Many chronic alcoholics have mild to moderate proximal muscle weakness which is not symptomatic. This chronic myopathy is actually present on muscle biopsy in about half of alcoholic outpatients (Urbano-Marques, Estruch, Navarro-Lopez, Gran, Mont & Rubin, 1989). Preferential atrophy of Type II fibers is noted on muscle biopsy. Maintained abstinence usually leads to improvement.

Rarely, an acute alcoholic myopathy may develop over hours to days during an alcoholic binge. The clinical presentation includes myalgia, proximal muscle weakness, myoglobinuria, and sometimes acute renal insufficiency secondary to the myoglobinuria. Muscle enzymes such as creatine phosphokinase are elevated. This is an acute necrotizing myopathy associated with rhabdomyolysis. Acute deficits in glycogen catabolic pathways are suspected to cause the rhabdomyolysis, but hypophosphatemia and hypokalemia may also be important. Sometimes, alcoholics in coma can also develop rhabdomyolysis from a "crush syndrome" wherein they lie for a prolonged time on a muscle, causing compression-ischemic damage.

Conclusion

It is clear that there are a myriad of neurological complications from alcohol abuse. It is important that clinicians be aware of these syndromes. The tremendous developments presently occurring in neuroscience research will provide important insights into the pathogenesis and treatment of these disorders.

References

Adams, R.D., Victor, M., Mancall, E.L. (1959). Central pontine myelinolysis: a hitherto undescribed disease occurring in alcoholic and malnourished patients. *Arch. Neurol. Psychiatry*, 81:154-72.

Arendt, T., Bigl, V., Arendt, A., Tennstedt, A. (1983). Loss of neurons in the nucleus basalis of Meynert in Alzheimer's disease, paralysis agitans and Korsakoff's disease. *Acta Neuropathol.* 61: 101-108.

Armanini, M.P., Hutchins, C., Stein, B.A., Sapolsky, R. (1990). Glucocorticoid endangerment of hippocampal neurons is NMDA-receptor dependent. *Brain Res.*, 532:7-12.

Bahr, M., Sommer, N., Petersen, D., Wietholter, H., Dichgans, J. (1990). Central pontine myelinolysis associated with low potassium levels in alcoholism. *J. Neurol*, 237:275-276.

Bentson, J., Reza, M., Winte,r J., Wilson, G. (1978). Steroids and apparent cerebral atrophy on computed tomography scans. *J. Comput. Assist. Tomogr.*, 2:16-23.

Blackwood, D.H., St. Clair, D.M., Blackburn, J.M., Tyrer, G.M. (1987). Cognitive brain potentials and psychological deficits in Alzheimer's dementia and Korsakoff's amnesic syndrome. *Psychological Medicine*, 17:349-358.

Brown, R.D., (1990). The proton channel blocking agent omeprazole is an inhibitor of the thiamine shuttle. *J .Theor. Biol.*, 143:565-573.

Burcar, P.J, Norenberg, M.D., Yarnell, P.R. (1982). Hyponatremia and central pontine myelinolysis, *Neurology*, 27:223-6.

Carlen, P.L., Wortzman, G., Holgate, R.C., Wilkinson, D.A., Rankin, J.G. (1978). Reversible cerebral atrophy in recently abstinent chronic alcoholics. *Science*, 200: 1076-78.

Carlen, P.L., Kapur, B., Huszar, L.A., Lee, M.A., Moddell, G., Singh, R., Wilkinson, D.A. (1980). Prolonged cerebrospinal fluid acidosis in recently abstinent chronic alcoholics. Neurology, 30:956 62.

Carlen, P.L., Lee, M.A., Jacob, M., Livshits, O. (1981). Parkinsonism provoked by alcoholism. *Ann. Neurol.*, 9: 84 86.

Carle, P.L., Wilkinson, D.A., Wortzman, G., Holgate, R., Lee, M.A., Cordingley, J., Rankin, J.G.R., Huszar, L.A., Moddel, G., Singh, R., Kiraly, L. (1981). Cerebral atrophy and function deficits in chronic alcoholics without clinically evident liver disease. *Neurology*, 31: 377-385.

Carlen, P.L., Wilkinson, D.A., Wortzman, G., Holgate, R.C. (1984). Partially reversible cerebral atrophy and functional improvement in recently abstinent alcoholics. *Can. J. Neurol. Sci.*, 11: 441-46.

Carlen, P.L., Penn, R.D., Fornazzari, L., Bennett, J., Wilkinson, D.A., Wortzman, G. (1986). CT scan assessment of alcoholic brain damage and its potential reversibility. *Alcoholism: Clin. Exp. Res.*, 10(3): 226-32.

Carlen, P.L., Wilkinson, D.A. (1986). Reversibility of alcohol-related brain damage: clinical and experimental observations. *Acta Medica. Scand.*, (Suppl. 717): 13-19.

Carlen, P.L., Wu, P.H. (1988). Calcium and sedative-hypnotic drug actions. *International Review of Neurobiology*, 29: 161-189.

Carlen, P.L., Rougier-Naquet, I., Reynolds, J. (1990). Alterations of neuronal calcium and potassium ionic currents during alcohol administration and withdrawal. *Alcohol and Seizures: Basic Mechanisms and Clinical Concepts*. Ed.s R.J. Porter, R.H., Mattson, J.A., Cramer, I., Diamond, F.A., Davis, Co., Philadelphia, 68-78.

Carlen, P.L., McAndrews, M.P., Weis,s R.T., Dongier, M., Hill, J.M., Menzano, E., Farcnik, K., Abarbanel, H.M., Eastwood, M.R. (1994) Hidden alcohol-related dementia in the institutionalized elderly. Alcoholism: Clin. Exp. Res., in press.

Charness, M.E., De LaPaz, R.L. (1987). Mammillary body atrophy in Wernicke's encephalopathy: antemortem identification using magnetic resonance imaging. *Ann. Neurol.*, 22: 595-600.

Copeland, J.R.M., Davidson, I.A., Dewey, M.E., Gilmore, C., Larkin, B.A., McWilliam, C., Saunders, P.A., Scott, A., Sharma, V., Sullivan, C. (1992). Alzheimer's disease, other dementias, depression and pseudo-dementia: prevalence, incidence and three-year outcome in Liverpool. *British J. of Psychiatry*, 161: 230-239.

Courville, C.B. (1966). *Effects of alcohol on the nervous system of man.* Second Edition. Los Angeles: San Lucas Press.

DeLaMonte, S.M. (1988). Disproportionate atrophy of cerebral white matter in chronic alcoholics. *Arch Neurol*, 45:990-92.

Diagnostic and Statistical Manual of Mental Disorders. (1987). (Third Edition-Revised), American Psychiatric Association, Washington, DC.

Eckardt, M.J., Rohrbaugh, J.W., Rio, D.A., Martin, P. (1990). Positron emission tomography as a technique for studying the chronic effects of alcohol on the human brain. *Ann Medicine*, 22:341-345.

Eriksson, K., Pekkanen, L., Rusi, M. (1980). The effects of dietary thiamine on voluntary ethanol drinking and ethanol metabolism in the rat. *Br. J. Nutr.*, 43: 1-13.

Erdo, S., Michler, A., Wolff, J.R. (1991). GABA accelerates excitotoxic cell death in cortical cultures: protection by blockers of GABA-gated chloride channels. *Brain Res.*, 254-258.

Etzell, K.R., Shapiro, S.G., Cousins, R.J. (1979). Regulation of liver metallothionein and plasma Zn by the glucocorticoid dexamethasone. *Biochem Biophys Res Commun*, 89:1120-1126.

Evans, D.A., Funkenstein, H., Albert, M.S., Scherr, P.A., Gok, N.R., Chown, M.D., Herbert, L.E., Hennikens, C.H., Taylor, D.O. (1989). Prevalence of Alzheimer's disease in a community population of older persons. *JAMA*, 262: 2551-2556.

Faraj, B.A., Lenton, J.D., Jutner, M. et. al. (1987). Prevalence of low monoamine oxidase function in alcoholism. *Alcoholism (NY)* 11: 464-467.

Fornazzari, L, Carlen, P.L. (1982). Transient dyskinesias during alcohol withdrawal. *Can. J. Neurol. Sci.* 9: 89-90.

Gilman, S., Adams, K., Koepp,e R.A., Berent, S., Kluin, K.J., Modell, J.G., Kroll, P., Brunberg, J.A. (1990). Cerebellar and frontal hypometabolism in alcoholic cerebellar degeneration studied with positron emission tomography. *Ann. Neurol.*, 28: 75-785.

Grant, K.A., Valverius, P., Hudspith, M., Tabakoff, B. (1990). Ethanol withdrawal seizures and the NMDA receptor complex. *Eur. J. Pharmacol.*, 176: 289-296.

Gulya, K., Grant, K.A., Valverius, P., Hoffman, P., Tabakoff, B. (1991). Brain regional specificity and time course of changes in the NMDA receptor-ionophere complex during ethanol withdrawal. *Brain Res.*, 547: 129-134.

Halliwell, B., Gutteridge, J. (1985). The importance of free radicals and catalytic metal ions in human diseases. *Molec. Aspects. Med.*, 8:89-193.

Harper C.G., Blumbergs, P.C. (1982). Brain weights in alcoholics. *J. Neurol. Neurosurg. Psychiatry*, 45: 838-840.

Harper, C. (1983). The incidence of Wernicke's encephalopathy in Australia — a neuropathological study of 131 cases. J. Neurol. Neurosurg. Psychiatry, 46: 593-98.

Harper, C.G., Kril, J.J., Holloway, R.L. (1984). Brain shrinkage in chronic alcoholics: a pathological study. *Br. Med. J.*, 290: 501-504.

Harpe, C., Kril, J., Daly, J. (1987). Are we drinking our neurones away? *Br. Med. J.*, 294: 534-536.

Harper, C., Kril, J., Daly, J. (1988). Does a "moderate" alcohol intake damage the brain? *Neurol. Neurosurg. Psychiatry*, 51:909-913.

Hata, T., Stirling Meyer, J., Tanahashi, N., Ishikawa, Y., Imai, A., Shinohara, T., Melex, M., Fann, W.E., Kandula, P., Sakai, F. (1987). Three-dimensional mapping of local cerebral perfusion in alcoholic encephalopathy with and without Wernicke-Korsakoff syndrome. *J. of Cerebral Blood Flow and Metabolism*, 7: 35-43.

Heinz, E.R., Martinez, J., Haenggeli, A. (1977). Reversibility of cerebral atrophy in anorexia nervosa and Cushing's syndrome. *J. Comput. Assist. Tomogr.*, 1: 415-418.

Hillbom, M., Muuronen, A., Holm, L., Hindmarsh, T. (1986). The clinical versus radiological diagnosis of alcoholic cerebellar degeneration. *J. Neurol.*, 231: 258-262.

Hillbom, M.E. (1987). What supports the role of alcohol as a risk factor for stroke? *Acta Med. Scand., Suppl.*, 717: 93-106.

Hunter, R., McLuskie, R., Wyper, D., Patterson, J., Christie, J.E., Brooks, D.N., McCulloch, J., Fink, G., Goodwin, G.M. (1989). The pattern of function-related regional cerebral blood flow investigated by single photon emission tomography with [99mTC]-HMPAO in patients with presenile Alzheimer's Disease and Korsakoff's psychosis. *Psychological Medicine*, 19: 847-855.

Issa, F.G., Sullivan, C.E. (1982). Alcohol, snoring and sleep apnoea. *J. Neurol. Neurosurg. & Psychiatry*, 45: 353-359.

Kessler, R.M., Parker, E.S., Clark, C.M., Martin, P.R., George, D.T., Weingartner, H. (1984). Regional cerebral glucose metabolism in patients with alcoholic Korsakoff's syndrome. *Soc. Neuroscience Abstr.*, 10: 541.

Kopelman, M.D. (1991). Frontal dysfunction and memory deficits in the alcoholic Korsakoff syndrome and Alzheimer-type dementia. *Brain*, 114: 117-137.

Lang, A.E., Marsden, C.D., Obeso, J.A., Parkes, J.D. (1982). Alcohol and Parkinson's Disease. *Ann. Neurol.*, 12: 254-256.

Langlais, P.J., Mair, R.G. (1990). Protective effects of the glutamate antagonist MK-801 on pyrithiamine-induced lesions and amino acid changes in rat brain. *Neuroscience*, 10: 1664-1674.

Laposata, E.A., Lange, L.G. (1986). Presence of nonoxidative ethanol metabolism in human organs commonly damaged by ethanol abuse. *Science*, 231: 497-499.

Ledig, M. et al. (1981). Superoxide dismutase activity in rat brain during acute and chronic alcohol intoxication. *Neurochem. Res.*, 6(4): 3858-390.

Lieber, C.S. (1988). Biochemical and molecular basis of alcohol-induced injury to liver and other tissues. *N. Engl. J. Med.*, 319: 1639-1650.

Lishman, W.A. (1990). Alcohol and the brain. *British J. of Psychiatry*, 156: 635-644.

Lovinger, D.M., White, G., Weight, F.F. (1989). Ethanol inhibits NMDA-activated ion current in hippocampal neurons. *Science*, 243: 1721-1724.

Martin, P.R., Impeduglia, G., Rathna Giri, P., Karanian, J. (1989). Acceleration of ethanol metabolism by past thiamine deficiency. *Alcohol Clin. Exp. Res.*, 13: 457-460.

Martin, P.R., McCool, B.A., Singleton, C.K. (1993). Genetic sensitivity to thiamine deficiency and development of alcoholic brain disease. *Alcoholism: Clin Exp Res.*, in press.

McDonald, L., Sullivan, A., Sturner, W.P. (1981). Zn concentrations in vitreous humor: a postmortem study comparing alcoholic and other patients. *J. Forensic Sci.* 26: 476-479.

McDowell, J.R., LeBlanc, H.J. (1984). Computed tomographic findings in Wernicke-Korsakoff syndrome. *Arch. Neurol.*, 41:453-454.

McMullen, P.A., Saint-Cyr, J.A., Carlen, P.L. (1984). Morphological alterations in rat hippocampal pyramidal cell dendrites resulting from chronic ethanol consumptions and withdrawal. *J. Comp. Neurol.*, 225: 111-118.

Menzano, E., Carlen, P.L. (1994). Zinc deficiency and corticosteroids in the pathogenesis of alcoholic brain dysfunction. Alcoholism: Clin. Exp. Res., in press.

Merry, J., Marks, V. (1969). Plasma hydrocortisone response to ethanol in chronic alcoholics. *Lancet*, i: 921-923.

Miller, G.M., Baker, H.L. Jr., Okazaki, H., Whisnant, J.P. (1988). Central pontine myelinolysis and imitators: MR findings. *Radiology*, 168: 795-802.

Morrisett, R.A., Rezvani, A., Overstreet, D., Janoswsky, .DS., Wilson, W., Swartzwelder, S. (1990). MK-801 potently inhibits alcohol withdrawal seizures in rats. *Eur. J. Pharm.*, 176:103-105.

Neiman, J., Lang, A.E., Fornazzari, L., Carlen, P.L. (1990). Movement disorders in alcoholism; a review. *Neurology*, 40(5): 741-746.

Noble, E.P., Tewari, S. (1973). Protein and ribonucleic acid metabolism in brains of mice following chronic alcohol consumption. In Eds: F.A. Scxias, S. Eggleston. *Alcoholism and the Central Nervous System*. 333-345, New York: NY Acad. of Sci. .

Noldy, N.E., McAndrews, M.P., Carlen, P.L. (1991). P300 in Korsakoff's and other alcoholics with cognitive impairments. *Psychophysiology*, 28 (Suppl): 541.

Pentney, R.J. (1982). Quantative effects of ethanol of Purkinje cell dendritic tree. *Bran. Res.*, 249:397-401.

Peters, S., Koh, J., Choi, D.W. (1987). Zn selectively blocks the action of N-methyl-D-Aspartate on cortical neurons. *Science*, 236:589-593.

Phillips, S.C., Harper, C.G., and Kril, J. (1987). A quantitative histological study of the cerebellar vermis in alcoholic patients. *Brain*, 110: 301-314.

Poolman, B., Hellingwerf, K.J., Konings, W.N. (1987). Regulation of the glutamate-glutamine transport system by intracellular pH in Streptococcus lactis. *J. Bacteriol.*, 169: 2272-2276.

Porjesz, B., Begleiter, B., Samuelly, I. (1980). Cognitive deficits in chronic alcoholics and elderly subjects assessed by evoked brain potentials. *Acta Psychiat. Scandianavica*, 286: 15-29.

Prasad, A.S. (1988). Clinical spectrum and diagnostic aspects of human Zn deficiency, In *Essential and Toxic Trace Elements in Human Health and Disease*, Alan R. Liss, New York.

Pratt, O., Rooprai, H., Shaw, G., Thomson, A. (1990). The genesis of alcoholic brain tissue injury. *Alcohol and Alcoholism*, 25(2/3): 217-230.

Quaterman, J. (1972). The effect of Zn deficiency on the activity of adrenal glands. *Proc Nutri. Soc*, 31: 74A-75A.

Riley, J.N., Walker, D.W. (1978). Morphological alterations in hippocampus after long-term alcohol consumption in mice. *Science*, 201: 646-648.

Schoenberg, B.S., Kokmen, E., Okazaki, H. (1987). Alzheimer's disease and other dementing illnesses in a defined United States population: incidence rates and clinical features. *Annals of Neurology*, 22: 724-729.

Serdaru, M., Hanssen-Hauw, C., Laplane, D., Buge, A., Castaigne, P., Goulon, M., Lhermitte, F., Hauw, J.J. (1988). The clinical spectrum of alcoholic pellagra encephalopathy, *Brain*, 111: 829-842.

Silverskiold, B.P. (1977). Cortical cerebellar degeneration associated with a specific disorder of standing and locomotion. *Acta Neurol. Scand.*, 55: 257-272.

Singleton, C.K., McCool, B.A., Harvey, A.J., Martin, P.R. (1990). Cloning and characterization of the human transketolase gene. *Alcohol Clin Exp Res*, 14: 264.

Slager, U.T. (1986). Central pontine myelinolysis and abnormalities in serum sodium. *Clin Neuropath*, 5: No. 6-252-256.

Tavares, M.A., Paula-Barbosa M.M., Gray, E.G. (1983). A morphometric Golgi analysis of the Purkinje cell dendritic tree after long-term alcohol consumption in the adult rat. *Neurocytol*, 12: 929-948.

Terry, R.D., Pack, A., DeTeresa, R., Schechter, R., Horoupian, D.S. (1981). Some morphometric aspects of the brain in senile dementia of the Alzheimer type. *Ann Neurol*, 10: 184-192.

Terry, R.D., DeTeresa, R., Hansen, L. (1987). Neocortical cell counts in normal human adult aging. *Ann Neurol.* 21: 530-539.

Thomas, P.K. (1986). Alcohol and disease: central nervous system. *Acta Med. Scand.* (suppl) 703: 251-264.

Thomson, A.D., Ryle, P.R., Shaw, G.K. (1983). Ethanol, thiamine and brain damage. *Alcohol & Alcoholism*, 18: 27-43.

Torvik, A., Lindboe, C.F., Rogde, S. (1982). Brain lesions in alcoholics: a neuropathological study with clinical correlations. J. *Neurol. Sci.* 56: 233-248.

Torvik, A. (1987). Brain lesions in alcoholics: neuropathological observations. *Acta Med. Scand.* Suppl, 717: 47-54.

Urbano-Marquez, A., Estruch, R., Navarro-Lopez, F., Grau, J.M., Mont, L., Rubin, E. (1989). The effects of alcoholism on skeletal and cardiac muscle. *N. Engl. J. Med.*, 320: 409-415.

Victor, M., Adams, R.D., Mancall, E.L. (1959). A restricted form of cerebellar cortical degeneration occurring in alcoholic patients. *Arch. Neurol.*, 71: 579-688.

Victor, M., Adams, R.D., Cole, M. (1965). The acquired (non-Wilsonian) type of chronic hepatocerebral degeneration. *Medicine*, 44: 345-396.

Victor, M., Brausch, C. (1967). The rose of abstinence in the genesis of alcoholic epilepsy. *Epilepsia*, 8:1-20.

Victor, M. (1982). Neurologic disorders due to alcoholism. A.B. Baker, L. Baker (Eds.), *Clinical Neurology*, Vol 2 (revised edition). pp. 1-83, Philadelphia: J.B. Lippincott.

Victor, M., Adams, R.D., Collins, G.H. (1989). The Wernicke-Korsakoff syndrome and related neurologic disorders due to alcoholism and malnutrition. *Contemporary neurology series*, 3:1-231. Philadelphia: F.A. Davis.

Vogel, S., Hakim, A.M. (1988). Effect of nimodipine of the regional cerebral acidosis accompanying thiamine deficiency in the rat. *J. Neurochem.*, 51: 1102-1110.

Wilkinson, D.A., Carlen, P.L. (1980). Relationship of neuropsychological test performance to brain morphology in amnesic and non-amnesic chronic alcoholics. *Acta Psychiat. Scan.*, 62 (Suppl 286): 89-103.

Wright, D.G., Laureno, R., Victor, M. (1979). Pontine and extrapontine myelinolysis. *Brain*, 102: 361-385.

Zilm, D.H., Huszar, L.A., Carlen, P.L., Kaplan, H.L., Wilkinson, D.A. (1980). EEG correlates of alcohol-induced organic brain syndrome in man. *Clin. Toxicol.*,16(3): 345-358.

Zimitat, C., Kril, J., Harper, C.G., Nixon, P.F. (1990). Progression of neurological disease in thiamine-deficient rats is enhanced by ethanol. *Alcohol*, 7: 493-501.

Emerging Approaches to Pharmacotherapy of Alcohol Abuse and Dependence

Peter Valverius and Stefan Borg
Section of Psychiatry at St. Göran's Hospital
Department of Clinical Neurosciences, Karolinska Institute
Stockholm, Sweden

Various drugs are currently used to alleviate the ethanol withdrawal syndrome (e.g., anxiolytics, sedatives), prevent high consumption of ethanol by producing an adverse reaction (e.g. disulfiram) or to prevent the development of medical complications of ethanol dependence (e.g., Vitamin B_1 for Wernicke's encephalopathy). However, pharmacotherapies for the treatment of ethanol intoxication and for reduction or prevention of "psychologic" dependence or "craving" for ethanol in man need to be developed.

The introduction of "new" drugs for treatment of certain aspects of alcoholism such as the alcohol withdrawal syndrome is based many times on the known effects of the drug on signs and symptoms which occur in relationship with the alcoholism related syndrome: e.g. anxiety, seizures, tachycardia, changes in blood pressure, etc., which accompany alcohol withdrawal in a physically dependent individual. One example is carbamazepine (Tegretol), which was known for its antiepileptic and psychotropic properties before it was used to treat symptoms of the alcohol withdrawal syndrome (for review see: Butler and Messiha, 1986).

Thus, established drugs may be used or may be modified to increase their efficacy in the treatment of different manifestations of alcoholism. For example, the development of new benzodiazepines with new and more efficient pharmacokinetic profiles may alleviate the anxiety of the alcohol withdrawal syndrome, or the development of a depot-preparation of disulfiram may help to attenuate high ethanol consumption.

The major criticism of these drugs is that they do not act on specific mechanisms that underlie high ethanol consumption or dependence. That is, the use of such drugs is directed against signs and symptoms and not against the specific pathological causes of ethanol consumption and/or dependence. Furthermore, disulfiram, which in many patients decreases ethanol consumption (Fuller et al., 1986), does this by causing fear of the effects of the drug-ethanol interactions and not by attenuation of the craving for ethanol.

However, as knowledge of the basic mechanisms of ethanol at the molecular and cellular levels increases, new candidate drugs should emerge. These drugs will intervene with some specific aspect of the mechanisms resulting in, e.g., ethanol intoxication, dependence or the withdrawal syndrome, and will thus be useful for treating different manifestations of alcohol use, abuse and dependence such as the euphorigenic and sedative effects of ethanol, tolerance, physical dependence, withdrawal symptoms, craving and drug seeking behavior.

From the clinical point of view, pharmacotherapeutic intervention in processes related to ethanol consumption can be divided into four main groups:

1. Drugs blocking different manifestations of ethanol intoxication (e.g., euphoria and sedation, reinforcing properties),
2. Drugs affecting ethanol consumption, drinking behavior and craving for ethanol,
3. Drugs alleviating different signs of physical dependence (e.g., ethanol withdrawal symptoms, withdrawal seizures, long term withdrawal),
4. Drugs for the treatment of medical consequences of high ethanol consumption (e.g. ethanol- induced neuropathy and other ethanol-related medical disorders).

This grouping does not reflect on the central neuronal systems involved in the manifestation of the various clinical states. Findings from both animal models and human studies indicate that many different central neurotransmitter systems are involved in drinking behavior, and in the clinical manifestations of ethanol tolerance or dependence. For example, ethanol consumption is thought to be affected by adrenergic, serotonergic and opioid transmitter systems; some manifestations of ethanol induced intoxication are dependent on the GABAergic transmitter system; dependence on ethanol (and thus the withdrawal syndrome) may be regulated by the opioid transmitter system, receptor regulated ion channels, and/or activity of the receptor regulated adenylate cyclase system (for references see below). These findings suggest that one transmitter system may affect several different manifestations or clinical stages of ethanol intoxication, dependence or withdrawal. In this paper we will review the clinical application of current pharmacological research in the treatment of alcohol abuse and dependence.

Drugs Affecting Different Manifestations of Ethanol Intoxication

Ethanol intoxication comprises excitatory, euphorigenic, sedative and depressant symptoms (DSM-III-R, 1987). Furthermore, it is believed that during ethanol intoxication the reinforcing properties of ethanol are important for the maintenance of ethanol consumption and the development of ethanol dependence (Kalant, 1989). Our society accepts and even desires some of the manifestations of ethanol intoxication while others are rejected. Therefore, one rationale for pharmacotherapy may be to abolish the reinforcing properties of ethanol (if this is at all possible without eliminating all the pleasurable effects) and to treat intoxications that threaten life.

The adrenergic transmitter system: alpha-methyl-para-tyrosine

The adrenergic transmitter system in the human brain is a key regulator of heart rate, blood pressure, fluid intake, diaphoresis and sleep (Ricardo and Koh, 1978; Bradford, 1986), and plays a central role in self-stimulation behavior, anxiety and aggression (Charney and Redmont, 1983; Crow, 1976). Alpha-methyl-para-tyrosine (AMPT) is a specific inhibitor of tyrosine hydroxylase, a key enzyme in the synthesis of catecholamines (Bradford, 1986). When AMPT was administered together with ethanol the central stimulatory effect of ethanol was blocked or decreased in animals (Strömbom and Svensson,1979; Muñoz et al., 1986) and in men (Ahlenius et al., 1973). AMPT inhibits the synthesis of *all* catecholamines (Bradford, 1986), and the cause of the observed inhibition of the stimulatory effect of ethanol may thus be mediated by the adrenergic transmitter systems alone or together with the dopaminergic transmitter system (see below). However,

AMPT has very diverse pharmacological effects (e.g., general depression and akinesia [Bradford, 1986]) and may therefore not be usable in practical therapy.

The GABAergic transmitter system: RO15-4513

GABA (γ-aminobutyric acid) is the most ubiquitous inhibitory neurotransmitter in the brain. GABA affects many processes of the CNS, among others the regulation of anxiety and sleep (Bradford, 1986). Ethanol (in pharmacologically relevant concentrations) has been reported to affect the function of the (GABA)$_A$ receptor-modulated chloride channel. At lower concentrations (20-70 mM) ethanol stimulates the influx of chloride ions into synaptoneurosomes (Suzdak et al.,1986a; Suzdak et al, 1987); higher concentrations of ethanol decrease the influx of these ions (for review see: Morrow et al, 1988). RO15-4513 is an imidazobenzodiazepine which is a partial inverse agonist binding to the (GABA)$_A$-receptor modulated chloride channel (Suzdak et al., 1986b). This compound antagonizes the effects of ethanol on the (GABA)$_A$-receptor regulated chloride channel (Suzdak et al., 1986b) and also blocks the anticonflict, anticonvulsant, motor impairment and other behavioral effects of acute ethanol ingestion (Koob et al., 1988; Nutt and Lister, 1987; Hoffman et al., 1987; Lister and Durcan, 1989) and, if administered after ethanol, reverses ethanol-induced intoxication (Suzdak et al., 1986b). However, RO15-4513 did not affect the other effects of acute ethanol ingestion such as hypothermia (Hoffman et al., 1987; Nutt et al., 1988). These findings suggest that only certain symptoms of acute ethanol intoxication are mediated through the (GABA)$_A$-receptor. Drugs which interact with the GABA receptor may therefore affect those intoxication symptoms.

NMDA-receptor regulated ion channels: glutamate

Glutamate is the major stimulatory neurotransmitter in the mammalian CNS and affects multiple functions, including learning, memory (neuronal plasticity) and neuronal development. It has been shown in dissociated hippocampal neurons , that ethanol inhibited the NMDA-activated ion currents (Lovinger et al., 1989). In cerebellar granule cells, ethanol inhibited the NMDA effect on calcium uptake and on production of cGMP (Hoffman et al., 1989). NMDA affects the release of noradrenaline, dopamine and acetylcholine in different brain regions (Göthert and Fink, 1989; Woodward and Gonzales,1990) and it has been shown that ethanol inhibits the NMDA-activated release of these neurotransmitters (for review see: Tabakoff et al., 1991). These findings suggest a pivotal interaction of ethanol with the NMDA-receptor regulated ion channels and demonstrate that this ion channel is very sensitive to ethanol. Discriminative stimulus studies have shown that animals perceive the subjective effects of non-competitive NMDA-receptor antagonists (such as MK-801 or PCP) as being similar to those of ethanol (Grant et al., 1991). This suggests that ethanol induced inhibition of NMDA receptor function occurs *in vivo*. As yet, no *in vivo* studies have been published on drugs which may modify the acute effects of ethanol on this ion channel. It is, however, interesting that *in vitro* studies have demonstrated that high concentrations of the amino acid glycine (which acts as a co-agonist at the NMDA receptor) reverse ethanol's actions at the NMDA-receptor regulated ion channel (Rabe and Tabakoff, 1990).

To date no effective drug treatment exists to modify the reinforcing and euphorigenic properties of ethanol. This may be due to lack of knowledge about the reinforcing and euphorigenic mechanisms of ethanol's actions. The preliminary findings that AMPT decreased ethanol's CNS stimulating effect and that RO15-4513 antagonizes certain manifestations of ethanol intoxication, as well as the finding of the high ethanol sensitivity of NMDA-receptor regulated ion channels, may provide the necessary information to develop efficient drugs to modify some reinforcing actions of ethanol.

Drugs Affecting Ethanol Consumption, Drinking Behavior and Craving

Serotonergic transmitter system: serotonin uptake Inhibitors

The effect of serotonin (5-hydroxytryptamine, 5-HT) on ethanol preference and ingestion was first proposed two decades ago (Myers and Veale, 1968; Hill, 1974). Since then a large number of findings support the hypothesis that agents which decrease the function of the 5-HT-transmitter system in the brain increase ethanol intake and, conversely, agents that enhance 5-HT function decrease ethanol ingestion (for review: Engel et al., 1992;Naranjo et al., 1986). This effect has been shown for precursors of 5-HT, 5-HT releasers (fenfluramine), 5-HT uptake inhibitors (e.g. zimelidine, citalopram, viqualine and others), 5-HT receptor agonists (both unselective, e.g.

5-HT and quipazine; and selective, e.g. ipsapirone and 8-OH-DPAT) in rodents (Engel et al., 1992;Naranjo et al., 1986).

The increasing number of double-blind, cross-over, placebo-controlled human studies involving 5-HT uptake blockers and 5-HT releasers suggests that manipulation of the serotonergic transmitter system may affect different aspects of ethanol consumption. The 5-HT uptake inhibitors, citalopram, fluoxetine, viqualine and zimelidine, have been shown to reduce reported ethanol ingestion by 10-20% below that of placebo in both alcohol dependent men and in social drinkers (Naranjo et al., 1984; Naranjo et al., 1987; Gorelick, 1986; Naranjo et al, 1989). Some of these compounds decreased the amount of ethanol ingested (fluoxetine, viqualine), while other compounds (citalopram, zimelidine) increased the number of days when no ethanol was ingested (Naranjo and Bremner, 1992). An interesting "side effect" of 5-HT uptake inhibitors was the reversal of ethanol-induced memory impairment in heavily drinking alcoholics (Weingartner et al., 1983) and the reduction of ethanol-induced cognitive impairment (Linnoila et al., 1987).

The main criticism of the above discussed studies is the low number of subjects: in most reports the different groups consisted of less than 25 subjects; in some studies the total number of subjects was less than 50. Also the drop-out rates seemed to be high (25-34%). These studies give some indication of the effect of the drugs investigated but lack statistical power, and are less than adequate for the detection of side-effects.

The 5-HT2 antagonist ritanserin and the 5-HT3 antagonist odansetron are two new compounds whose effect on ethanol ingestion is being investigated in animal models and clinical trials. Ritanserin reduced both alcohol intake and preference in rats and increased water intake without affecting total fluid intake (Meert, 1993, Meert et al., 1994). Odansetron reduced ethanol intake in medium and high alcohol preferring rats without affecting alcohol preference or total fluid intake (Meert, 1993). Clinical studies of ritanserin in alcohol dependent patients are ongoing in several centers (Meert et al., 1994).

Dopaminergic transmitter systems: bromocriptine

The catecholaminergic transmitter systems have been implicated in the regulation of ethanol consumption since the middle of the 1970s. Results from behavioral studies hinted at dopaminergic involvement in ethanol intoxication and suggested that adrenergic mechanisms may contribute more to the regulation of ethanol ingestion than dopamine (Kiianmaa et al., 1975; Brown and Amit, 1977; Kiianmaa et al., 1979; Corcoran et al., 1983). Other findings suggest, however, that the long-acting non-selective dopaminergic agonist bromocriptine and the mixed D1/D2 agonist SDZ 5-152 may modify the reinforcing properties of ethanol. Both compounds reversed ethanol preference and decreased ethanol intake in rats without affecting water ingestion (Weiss et al., 1990; Rassnick et al., 1989). The dopamine D_2 antagonist sulpiride increased ethanol ingestion in alcohol preferring rats when injected into the nucleus accumbens, whereas the dopamine D_1 antagonist SCH 23390 had no such effect (Mardones et al., 1992). These findings seem to support the hypothesis that the dopaminergic transmitter system modulates some of the reinforcing properties of ethanol and affects ethanol consumption.

Similarly, in a double-blind placebo controlled study of alcoholic men, bromocriptine decreased ethanol craving, reduced drinking behavior, reduced depressive reactions and improved social function (Borg, 1983).

The issue of whether the dopaminergic neurotransmitter system is involved in the regulation of ethanol ingestion is not settled. It is possible that the observed effects of dopaminergic agonists and antagonists result from downstream activity of other neurotransmitter systems.

Opioid transmitter system: naltrexone and naloxone

The endogenous opioid peptides (such as β-endorphin, met-enkephalin and leu-enkephalin) and opiates (e.g. morphine, heroin, methadone) interact differentially with the opioid receptors (mu-, delta- and kappa-opioid receptors). These receptors have many functions among which are the regulation of muscle tension, sedation, analgesia, locomotor activity, seizure activity, stereotyped behavior, eating and drinking behavior and core body temperature. All of these functions are also affected by ethanol ingestion and dependence. Opiates and opioid peptides also modulate the function of the noradrenergic, dopaminergic and cholinergic neurotransmitter systems as well as the release of glutamate (for review see: Bradford, 1986).

Opioid receptor agonists (e.g. morphine or methadone), when given in small doses (e.g. <3 mg/kg or <2 mg/kg bodyweight, respectively), increase intake of ethanol in animals (Reid and Hubbell, 1992). Higher doses of morphine or methadone (>10 mg/kg or >4mg/kg bodyweight, respectively) decrease ethanol consumption

(Reid and Hubbell, 1992). The effect of opiates on ethanol ingestion seems not to be related to analgesia, narcosis or catatonia (Reid and Hubbell, 1992). Studies in both humans and animals suggest that opioid receptor antagonists (naloxone and naltrexone) significantly decrease ethanol ingestion (Hubbell et al., 1986; Volpicelli et al., 1986; Myers et al., 1986; Volpicelli et al., 1990). Furthermore, animal studies suggest that the blockade of the delta-opioid receptor with a specific antagonist (e.g., ICI 174864 or naltrindole HCL) suppresses voluntary ethanol drinking by up to 78%, without effect on water intake (Froehlich et al., 1991).

Naltrexone is a non-selective, long acting (compared to naloxone) opioid receptor antagonist whose effect on ethanol drinking, relapse rate and craving has been examined in ethanol-dependent men (Volpicelli et al., 1990; O'Malley, 1992). The naltrexone treated subjects showed a reduced mean number of days/week in which ethanol was sampled, a large reduction in relapse rate, and lower scores on craving. These studies suggested that naltrexone did not affect the initiation of ethanol consumption but rather decreased the amount of ethanol consumed (O'Malley, 1992). These studies had a small number of subjects but the subjects all met the DSM-III-R criteria for alcohol dependence. The findings are promising and should encourage further research. It is also necessary to investigate the effect of opioid antagonists in non-ethanol dependent consumers with high and low intake of ethanol.

Opioid regulation of ethanol drinking seems to depend on the timing of opiate administration and ethanol ingestion. If ethanol is offered during morphine intoxication, a morphine dose dependent *decrease* (compared to not morphine treated animals) in ethanol drinking is observed (Ho and Chen, 1975; Volpicelli and Ulm, 1991). If, however, ethanol is available during the opiate withdrawal phase, then a morphine dose dependent *increase* (compared to not morphine treated animals) in ethanol consumption is seen (Ho and Chen, 1975; Volpicelli et al., 1991). These experiments suggest that ethanol consumption may be regulated by the amount of endogenous opioid peptides or the activity of the opioid receptors. However, the stress of morphine withdrawal may also confound these results.

GABAergic or excitatory amino acid transmitter systems: calcium acetylhomotaurinate

Calcium acetylhomotaurinate (acamprosate, Ca-AOTAL) is structurally related to glutamate and GABA (Lhuintre et al., 1990). There is some evidence that acamprosate affects GABAergic function and displaces GABA from its binding site (Chabenat et al., 1988; Boismare et al., 1984; Daoust et al., 1987). Other evidence indicates the action of acamprosate on NMDA-regulated ion channels (Zeise et al, 1990; Zeise et al., 1992). Whether acamprosate acts directly on these transmitter systems or through other (neuro)-mediators is still not known.

Acamprosate reduced voluntary ethanol ingestion in ethanol dependent rats by up to 70% in a dose dependent way (Le Magnen et al., 1987; Gewiss et al., 1991). However, these animal studies are open to methodological critique. Studies using animals genetically selected for high or low ethanol sensitivity (e.g. Alcohol Non-Tolerant (ANT) and Alcohol Tolerant (AT) rats, Rusi et al., 1977); or for high or low ethanol preference (e.g. Alko-Alcohol (AA) or Alko-Non-Alcohol (ANA) rats, Lê and Kiianmaa, 1989) would be interesting because many behavioral and neurochemical differences between the different animal lines are known. This approach could give a hint of the mechanism of action of acamprosate.

Several placebo controlled, double-blind, multicenter human studies using acamprosate have been performed. The results suggest that acamprosate decreases plasma γ-glutamyltranferase (GGT), a marker of heavy ethanol consumption, ethanol ingestion and relapse rate in ethanol dependent individuals (Lhuintre et al., 1990; Pelc et al., 1992). The first study (Lhuintre et al., 1990) contained a total of 569 alcohol-dependent men and women. A number of clinical (e.g. alcohol consumption, number of weaning attempts) and biochemical measurements (e.g. GGT and mean corpuscular volume) were used as end-point criteria. The GGT measurement was significantly lower in the treatment group compared with the placebo group after 60 and 90 days of therapy. Oral and glossal tremor were significantly reduced in the treatment group. Evaluation of adverse reactions indicated that diarrhea was the only side effect of acamprosate. The second study (102 subjects who met the DSM-III-R criteria for alcohol dependence) measured compliance to treatment, number of abstaining patients and mean number of days without alcohol (Pelc et al., 1992). In this study, all of these parameters were improved by acamprosate. The side-effects observed included gastralgia, diarrhea, headache, paresthesia and diaphoresis. However, the subjects investigated in these two studies were all heavy drinkers and severely ethanol dependent. The effect of acamprosate on individuals with a lesser degree of ethanol dependence and/or lower ethanol consumption (i.e., the patient group most prevalent, but not most visible in society) was not investigated. The effects of acamprosate on ethanol consumption by non-ethanol dependent humans is also not known.

The findings of the effects of acamprosate on ethanol consumption and relapse rate in humans is very promising. The main problem is that no accurate objective measure of ethanol consumption was used and that self-reports of ethanol consumption and number of ethanol-free days are notoriously unreliable. Therefore, while the inclusion of biochemical measurements such as GGT (which is not specific for ethanol consumption) adds to the reliability of these studies, other markers of high ethanol use and or relapse into long term ethanol consumption (see below for discussion) are necessary for accurate evaluation of these drugs. More research in clinical settings and, especially, on acamprosate's mechanism of action may not only be important for the use of the drug but may also become a tool for understanding the control mechanisms of ethanol ingestion.

Aversives: disulfiram and calcium carbimide

Disulfiram and calcium carbimide both inhibit aldehyde dehydro-genase (ALDH) (for review see: Marchner, 1984). The inhibition of ALDH raises acetaldehyde concentrations in blood and tissues, which in turn results in adverse reactions consisting of flushing, increased heart rate, nausea, dizziness, etc. (Christensen et al., 1991; Johansson et al., 1991). Disulfiram inhibits ALDH in an irreversible manner, the onset of inhibition is slow (12 hours), and the duration is long since restoration of ALDH activity requires *de novo* synthesis of the enzyme (Marchner, 1984). Calcium carbimide inhibits ALDH in a reversible manner, the onset is faster (approx. 1 hour) and the duration is shorter (approx. 12 hours) (Marchner, 1984).

It is assumed that most alcohol dependent individuals develop a conditioned aversive response sufficient to deter them from drinking during drug therapy, after they have been informed about the nature and risks of the drug-ethanol interaction (for review see: Peachey, 1984). The patients that drink during therapy experience the result-ing acetaldehyde intoxication and are thus strengthened in the over-all conditioned aversion. This aversion is assumed to decrease ethanol consumption or to increase the period of sobriety.

The success of aversive therapy is dependent on several factors: patient compliance, appropriate selection of ethanol-dependent pa-tients and the combination with counseling or other forms of treat-ment (Peachey, 1984). Those patients who have a stable social situation with good support from family, friends and collaborators and who have little co-morbidity (i.e., do not show signs of depression, anxiety or somatic symptoms) are expected to do best with this treatment (Peachey, 1984). These patients are more likely to attend appointments and to take part in other therapeutic approaches. However, some ethanol-dependent patients are able to drink alcohol during drug therapy, which may result in enhanced ethanol craving during the drug-ethanol reaction (Mellor and Sims, 1971).

The long term efficacy of aversive therapy has not been established (Fuller et al., 1986; Wright and Moore, 1988), although in one study some beneficial effect of long-term (2 years) disulfiram treatment on drinking was seen (Öjehagen et al., 1991). Over short periods of time (up to 3-6 months) aversive drug treatment seems to be efficient in reducing ethanol consumption and/or in increasing the number of total abstinent days (Wright and Moore, 1988, Öjehagen et al., 1991).

Since compliance is one of the key factors, the administration of disulfiram in other forms than tablets may provide better results, especially if drug administration could be performed at long intervals (e.g., once a week). Implantation of disulfiram subcutaneously has not proven successful (Johnsen and Mørland, 1990; Johnsen and Mørland, 1991) since often the drug-ethanol reaction did not occur (Johnsen and Mørland, 1991), possibly due to lack of sufficient absorption of disulfiram. Other preparation, such as depot-disulfiram or controlled release formulations of disulfiram, have been examined in animals (Faiman et al., 1992) or in small clinical studies (Phillips, 1992). The findings suggest that this approach may be promising, but research is far from completed.

Other neurotransmitter systems

Several other putative neuromodulators and hormones have been suggested to affect the consumption of or the craving for ethanol. Cholecystokinin, a neuropeptide, has been shown to reduce ethanol consumption in rats through an action on the satiety centers in the brain (Kulkosky et al., 1989). Melatonin, an important regulator of circadian rhythms, has been suggested to affect ethanol consumption in rats (Smith et al.,1980). On the other hand, ethanol has been shown to enhance the release of melatonin from cultured pineal glands (Chung et al., 1989). Dihydropyridine sensitive calcium channels may be of importance in the development of physical dependence and/or tolerance to ethanol (see below). Engel et al. (1988) made the interesting observation that nifedipine, a calcium channel antagonist, decreased both ethanol preference and consumption in rats without affecting the total fluid intake.

These findings, as preliminary as they are, offer new ways to understand the regulation of ethanol ingestion in animals and later in humans and may thus open new avenues for the development of drugs to decrease ethanol consumption.

Drugs Affecting Physical Dependence on Ethanol and the Ethanol Withdrawal Syndrome

Physical dependence is a consequence of high ethanol consumption (i.e., chronic ethanol intoxication) over a sufficiently long period of time. The development of physical dependence is the adaptation of different bodily functions (such as temperature and blood pressure regulation) to the effects of ethanol intoxication.

The ethanol withdrawal syndrome is the clinical manifestation of physical dependence. It consists of a number of symptoms, such as anxiety, hallucinations, disorientation, tremor, hyperthermia, sweating, tachycardia, dysregulation of blood pressure, seizures, etc. upon cessation of ethanol intake and elimination of ethanol. The symptoms may vary in degree. A modest withdrawal syndrome may consist of slight anxiety and a barely noticeable tremor of the hands. A severe ethanol withdrawal syndrome is the delirium tremens (DT), a life threatening state with most of the above named symptoms.

The range of symptoms of the ethanol withdrawal syndrome suggests that most of the neurotransmitter systems of the brain are involved in the manifestation of this state. For example, the NMDA-receptor regulated ion channel may be involved in the pathogenesis of alcohol withdrawal seizures (Grant et al., 1990); the adrenergic transmitter system may be involved in the changes of blood pressure regulation or heart rate (Kwast et al., 1987) and the GABAergic transmitter system in anxiety (Roy et al., 1990). In the following section we will review possible pharmacological manipulations of the different transmitter systems involved in physical dependence and the ethanol withdrawal syndrome.

GABAergic transmitter system: benzodiazepines

Traditionally barbiturates and benzodiazepines have been used to alleviate the ethanol withdrawal syndrome (for review see: Nutt et al., 1989). These compounds bind to the GABA-benzodiazepine receptor-regulated chloride channel and have been used for several decades as safe, efficient and inexpensive medication. The side effects of memory impairment, drowsiness and lethargy as well as the potential for the development of dependence on benzodiazepines necessitate a reduction of the overall dosage, since the drugs themselves may interfere with other therapeutic approaches dealing with stress management, coping behavior or drinking behavior modification.

Evidence suggests that benzodiazepines act through $GABA_A$-receptors on the noradrenergic transmitter system to decrease noradrenaline release (Corrodi et al., 1971; Yoshishige et al., 1985); and on the hypothalamic-pituitary-adrenal axis (Merry and Marks, 1972; Wilkins and Gorelick, 1986) possibly by decreasing stress-induced elevations in ACTH and cortisone levels (Bizzi et al., 1984). These findings suggests that benzodiazepines may affect, at least in part, ethanol withdrawal related mental confusion, depression, fatigue etc.

Benzodiazepines have serious side effects, and, as stated above, have a high potential for the development of dependence. Therefore the development of drugs that act on the GABA receptor regulated chloride channel, and that do not have the disadvantages of the benzodiazepines, is a very important endeavor.

NMDA-receptor regulated ion channels: MK-801

Chronic ethanol consumption has been shown to increase the number of [³H]MK-801 binding sites, which represent the functional form of the NMDA-receptor regulated ion channel, in different regions of the mouse brain (Grant et al., 1990; Gulya et al., 1991). Maximum increases in MK-801 binding were observed approximately 8 - 10 hours after ethanol withdrawal, i.e. at the height of the ethanol withdrawal syndrome. At this time the withdrawal seizure score was maximal and no ethanol could be detected in the blood (Gulya et al., 1991). Administration of MK-801 (a non-competitive antagonist of the NMDA-receptor) to ethanol dependent mice (Grant et al., 1990) and rats (Morrisett et al., 1990) decreased the occurrence and severity of handling-induced and audiogenic ethanol withdrawal seizures in a dose dependent way. In contrast, NMDA, an agonist at the NMDA-receptor, exacerbated handling-induced withdrawal seizures (Grant et al., 1990). One other non-competitive antagonist, ADCI, was shown to decrease ethanol withdrawal seizures as well as whole-body tremors in ethanol dependent mice (Grant et al., 1991). These findings suggest that the NMDA-receptor regulated ion channels are associated with ethanol withdrawal seizures and possibly with other manifestations of physical dependence.

In the frontal cortex of deceased sober and intoxicated ethanol dependent men, the number of [³H]MK-801 binding sites was decreased by approximately 32% (Laestadius and Valverius, 1992). These findings contrast those observed in C57BL mice (see above). However, in sober alcoholics the EC_{50} for glutamate to increase [³H]MK-801 binding was significantly lower compared to that of controls (Laestadius and Valverius, 1992), suggesting a higher glutamate sensitivity of the NMDA-receptor regulated ion channel. These findings suggest an important role for the NMDA-receptor regulated ion channel in the regulation of some aspects of physical dependence, e.g. ethanol withdrawal seizures. Today, however, drugs that affect NMDA-receptor function have severe side-effects, such as hallucinations and possibly phencyclidine-like dissociative anesthesia (Littleton and Bouchenafa, 1992). It seems promising to develop drugs which act on this ion channel but do not have these side effects and to test whether these drugs could become more specific anti-ethanol-withdrawal agents.

Dihydropyridine (DHP) sensitive calcium channels: nitrendipine

Many studies support the findings that chronic ethanol ingestion increases the number of DHP binding sites in the brains of ethanol-dependent rats and in cells grown in ethanol solution (Dolin et al.1987; Brennan et al.,1989). Other evidence suggests that in the brains of mice selectively bred to be withdrawal seizure prone (WSP), the increase in the number of DHP binding sites induced by chronic ethanol ingestion is much larger than that in those mice, that were selectively bred to be withdrawal seizure resistant (WSR) (Brennan et al., 1990).

In animals nitrendipine, verapamil and flunarizine (calcium channel antagonists) decreased ethanol withdrawal seizure incidence and mortality (Little et al., 1986; Little et al., 1988). In humans calcium channel blockers are used in the treatment of angina pectoris and other cardiac disorders. Thus the existing drugs are cardioselective (or non-selective) and would have severe cardiovascular "side effects" if used in sufficiently high doses for treatment of ethanol withdrawal. However, the continued development of more CNS-specific compounds, which pass the blood brain barrier, could be of great interest for treatment of physical dependence on ethanol.

Adrenergic transmitter system: atenolol and clonidine

Chronic ingestion of ethanol has been shown to decrease the efficacy of the interaction of β-adrenergic receptors with their effector, adenylate cyclase, in both mouse and human brain, as well as in platelets (Saito et al., 1987; Valverius et al., 1989; Tabakoff et al., 1988). During ethanol withdrawal, the coupling of the receptor to adenylate cyclase returns to normal while the ethanol induced increase in noradrenaline turnover (Pohorecky, 1974; Valverius et al. 1987) persists. This noradrenergic hyperactivity may result in at least some ethanol withdrawal signs. β-adrenergic blockers such as atenolol and propranolol have been used to attenuate the ethanol withdrawal syndrome in humans (Kraus et al., 1985). The results of a double blind, placebo controlled study suggest that atenolol resolved ethanol withdrawal symptoms more rapidly than placebo, shortened hospital stay, decreased anxiety and hallucinations and reduced subjective feelings of craving (Horwitz et al., 1989) in patients with a moderate or mild ethanol withdrawal syndrome.

These drugs have not been used for long-term treatment and in patients suffering a severe withdrawal syndrome. It has also been reported that propranolol may have side effects such as hallucinations and delirium in alcoholics with an acute ethanol withdrawal syndrome (Jacob et al.,1983).

α-Adrenergic agonists (such as clonidine and lofexidine) are believed to cause an inhibition of noradrenaline release in the brain through effects on the noradrenergic neurons in the locus coeruleus (Björkqvist, 1975). These compounds have been shown to be effective in the treatment of ethanol withdrawal-related tremor, tachycardia and hypertension (Björkqvist, 1975; Wilkins et al., 1983). In patient suffering Korsakoff's psychosis, clonidine significantly reduced anterograde amnesia (Mair and McEntee, 1986). Other symptoms of withdrawal (e.g. insomnia, restlessness) were not affected and the concomitant use of anticonvulsant drugs was necessary (Cushman,1988).

Dopaminergic transmitter system: bromocriptine

The dopaminergic transmitter system is affected by chronic ethanol ingestion in alcohol dependent men. For example, the maximum growth hormone responses to dopaminergic agonist (apomorphine) stimulation were significantly increased in early ethanol withdrawal (Annunziate et al., 1983). After two months of sobriety, the maximum growth hormone responses to apomorphine was significantly reduced in alcoholics compared to controls (Balldin et al., 1992). It is also thought that the dopaminergic transmitter system may be involved in the pathogenesis of ethanol withdrawal hallucination (e.g. in delirium tremens)(Balldin et al., 1992). Thus haloperidol (together with anti-convulsants) is one of the drugs of choice in treatment of delirium tremens (Naranjo and Sellers, 1986). Bromocriptine and apomorphine have been used to alleviate the ethanol withdrawal syndrome (Borg and Weinholdt, 1982; Anokhina, 1984) but these agonists did not affect the whole withdrawal syndrome and were more efficient in decreasing the craving for ethanol than in alleviating the ethanol withdrawal syndrome.

Drugs Affecting Tolerance to Ethanol

Functional tolerance to ethanol, e.g. the tolerance to the hypnotic or hypothermic effects of ethanol, is not well understood. It is thought that at least three neuronal regulatory systems are involved in the development and maintenance of tolerance: the noradrenergic and serotonergic transmitter systems and the neuropeptide arginine vasopressin (AVP) (for review see: Hoffman et al., 1990). The manipulation of one or more of these regulators may affect the development or dissipation of functional ethanol tolerance. However, until now, no such drugs have been investigated in humans.

Several promising lines of research have been followed. Vasopressin, a hormone responsible for the regulation of osmolality in the mammalian body, has been shown to maintain ethanol tolerance in animals by stimulating V_1-receptors (Szabó et al., 1988a). A V_1- selective antagonist blocked the effect of AVP on the maintenance of functional tolerance to ethanol. Thus, by analogy, the dissipation of functional tolerance may be modulated using drugs acting on this receptor.

The partial depletion of the noradrenergic transmitter system in the brain has been shown to prevent the development of functional tolerance. Intracerebroventricular injections of forskolin, an adenylate cyclase stimulator which increases the concentration of cAMP in brain, has been shown to reverse the blockade of ethanol tolerance in 6-hydroxydopamine treated mice (Szabó et al., 1988b).

These findings suggest that the development of functional tolerance to the effects of ethanol may become a target for pharmacological interaction when the mechanisms of the development of tolerance are better known. As yet no compounds are available for human studies. Whether inhibition of the development of tolerance will be beneficial to an alcoholic (or developing alcoholic) remains to be seen.

Drugs Affecting Medical Complications of Ethanol Dependence

Since many ethanol-induced morphological changes (such as fatty liver, expansion of the ventricles in the brain) are reversible, the best treatment of medical complications of high ethanol consumption and ethanol dependence is a decrease in ethanol consumption or total abstinence from alcohol. However, it is the nature of alcohol dependence that abstinence and/or a decrease in alcohol consumption are difficult to maintain. This indicates a need for compounds which protect the brain, liver and other organs from ethanol induced organ damage. Many compounds have been tried. The only compound with a proven effect is thiamine (Vitamin B_1) in the prevention and treatment of Wernicke's encephalopathy (Victor and Adams, 1971). Many other drugs have been tried in animal models (e.g. hyperbaric oxygen, clofibrate, nicotinic acid, lipotrophic cocktail, different steroids, propylthiouracil, D-penicillamine, insulin with glucagon, colchicine etc.) but until now, none of these treatments has had any proven effect (for review see: Thomson et al., 1984).

Conclusions

Several new drug candidates have shown promising properties in the treatment of different aspects of the alcohol dependence syndrome: e.g., serotonin uptake inhibitors, opioid antagonists and acamprosate. A problem with most human studies of the treatment of ethanol dependence is the lack of an objective end-point criterion: what comprises a successful treatment outcome? It is therefore important first to define both the starting point (for example: define the subject's clinical stage of ethanol dependence) and the end point (e.g., objectively registered long term sobriety or lowered ethanol consumption) and then to relate the efficiency of a drug both to the start point and to the end point. For example, reported ethanol consumption is often used to measure the success of a treatment (sometimes together with scalar measurements of anxiety, craving etc.). Patients' reports are, however, approximations and as such often impaired by errors. Therefore new stringent and objective clinical protocols need to be developed for the evaluation of the effects of emerging drugs against craving for alcohol, relapse into alcohol abuse and high ethanol consumption. The use of biological markers for ethanol consumption such as carbohydrate deficient transferrin (CDT), for long term decrease in ethanol consumption (Stibler et al.(1986)) or the ratio of 5-HTOL/5-HIAA for short term sobriety (Voltaire et al.,1992) may help to better define the starting- and end points for treatment research. Further discussion of biologic markers for ethanol consumption can be found in the chapter by Salaspuro (this volume).

Most manifestations of high ethanol consumption, dependence on and tolerance to ethanol involve the interaction of many regulatory systems. The interactions of different neurotransmitter systems complicate the development of new drugs because no key system for all manifestations exists. Often changes in one neurotransmitter system affect other systems, e.g. the increase in the number of functional NMDA-receptor regulated ionophores will affect noradrenaline and dopamine release, which are important in the development of tolerance and dependence. As ethanol's actions on the molecular and cellular level of the CNS are understood, new drug candidates for the treatment of the different manifestations of alcohol dependence and abuse should emerge.

References

Ahlenius, S., Carlsson, A., Engel, J., Svensson, T. and Södersten, P. (1973). Antagonism by alpha methyltyrosine of the ethanol-induced stimulation and euphoria in man. *Clin. Pharmacol. Ther.,* 14(4). 586 - 591.

Annunziato, L., Amoroso, S., Di Renzo, G., Argenzio, F., Aurilio, C., Grella, A. and Quattrone, A. (1983). Increased GH responsiveness to dopamine receptor stimulation in alcohol addicts during the late withdrawal syndrome. *Life Sci.,* 33: 2651 - 2655.

Anokhina, I.P. Dopamine receptor agonists in the treatment of alcoholism. (1984). In: Edwards, G. and Littleton, J. (eds.). Pharmacological treatments for alcoholism, pp. 145 - 151, Croom Helm, London.

Balldin, J.I., Berggren, U.C. and Lindstedt, G. (1992). Neuroendocrine evidence for reduced dopamine receptor sensitivity in alcoholism. *Alcoholism: Clin. Exp. Res.,* 16(1). 71 - 74.

Bizzi, A., Ricci, M.R., Veneroni, E., Amato, M. and Garratini, S. (1984). Benzodiazepine receptor antagonists reverse the effect of diazepam on plasma corticosterone in stressed rats. *J. Pharm. Pharmacol.*, 36: 134 - 135.

Björkqvist, S.E. Clonidine in alcohol withdrawal. *(1975). Acta. Psychiatr. Scand.*, 52: 256 - 263.

Borg, V. and Weinholdt, T. (1980) A preliminary double-blind study of two dopaminergic drugs, apomorphine and bromocriptine (parlodel), in the treatment of the alcohol-withdrawal syndrome. *Curr. Ther. Res.*, 27: 170-177.

Borg, V. (1983). Bromocriptine in the prevention of alcohol abuse. *Acta Psychiatr. Scand.*, 68: 100 - 110.

Bradford, H.F. (1986). Chemical Neurobiology: An Introduction to Neurochemistry, pp. 179 - 210 and 229 - 246. New York: W. H. Freeman and Company.

Brennan, C.H., Crabbe, J. and Littleton, J.M. (1990). Genetic regulation of dihydropyridine-sensitive calcium channels in brain may determine susceptibility to physical dependence on alcohol. *Neuropharmacol.*, 29: 429 - 432.

Brennan, C.II., Lewis, A. and Littleton, J.M. (1989). Membrane receptors involved in up-regulation of calcium channels in bovine adrenal chromaffine cells chronically exposed to ethanol. *Neuropharmacol.*, 28: 1303 - 1307.

Brown, Z.W. and Amit, Z. (1977). The effects of selective catecholamine depletions by 6-hydroxydopamine on ethanol preference in rats. *Neurosci. Lett.*, 5: 333 - 336.

Butler, D. and Messiha, F.S. (1986). Alcohol withdrawal and carbamazepine. *Alcohol,* 3(2). 113 - 129.

Chabenat, C., Chretien, P., Daoust, M., Moore, N., André, D., Lhuintre, J.P., Saligaut, C., Boucly, P. and Boismare, F. (1988). Physicochemical, pharmacological and pharmacokinetic study of a new GABEergic compound, calcium acetylhomotaurinate. *Methods. Find. Exp. Clin. Pharmacol* (Spain), 10(5). 311 - 317.

Charney, D.S. and Redmont, D.E. Jr(1983). Neurobiological Mechanisms in Human Anxiety: Evidence Supporting Central Noradrenergic Hyperactivity. *Neuropharmacology,* 22(128). 1531 - 1536.

Christensen, J.K., Møller, I.W., Rønsted, P., Angelo, H.R. and Johansson, B. (1991). Dose-effect relationship of disulfiram in human volunteers. I: Clinical studies. *Pharmacol. Toxicol.*, 68(3). 163 - 165.

Chung, C.T., Tamarkin, L., Hoffman, P.L. and Tabakoff, B. (1989). Ethanol enhancement of isoproterenol-stimulated melatonin and cyclic AMP release from cultured pineal glands. *J. Pharmacol. Exp. Ther.*, 249: 16 - 22.

Corcoran, M.E., Lewis, J. and Fibiger, H.C. (1983). Forebrain noradrenaline and oral self-administration of ethanol by rats. *Behav. Brain Res.*, 8(1).1-21.

Corrodi, H., Fuxe, K., Ledbruck, P. and Olson, L. (1971). Minor tranquilizers, stress and central catecholamine neurons. *Brain Res.*, 29: 1 - 16.

Crow, T.J. Specific Monoamine Systems as Reward Pathways. (1976) In: Wauquier, A. and Rols, E.T. (Editors). *Brain Stimulation Reward*, pp. 211 - 237. Amsterdam-Oxford, United Kingdom: North Holland Publishing Company.

Cushman, P. Clonidine and alcohol withdrawal. *(1988). Adv. Alcohol Subst. Abuse, 7:* 17 - 28.

Daoust, M., Saligaut, C., Lhuintre, J.P., Moore, N., Flipo, J.L. and Boismare, F. (1987). GABA transmission, but not benzodiazepine receptor stimulation modulates ethanol intake by rats. *Alcohol, 4:* 469 - 472.

Dolin, S., Little, H., Hudspith, M., Pagonis, C. and Littleton, J.M. (1987). Increased dihydropyridine-sensitive calcium channels in rat brain may underlie ethanol physical dependence. *Neuropharmacology,* 26: 275 - 279.

DSM-III-R. (1987). American Psychiatric Association: *Diagnostic and statistical manual of mental disorders* (Third edition, revised), pp. 100 - 119, Washington DC, USA.

Engel, J.A., Enerback, C., Fahlke, C., Hulthe, P., Hård, E., Johannessen, K., Svensson, L. and Söderpalm, B. (1992). Serotoninergic and dopaminergic involvement in ethanol intake. In: Naranjo, C.A. and Sellers, E.M. (eds.). *Novel Pharmacological Interventions for Alcoholism.* pp. 68 - 82, New York: Springer Verlag.

Engel, J.A., Fahlke, C., Hulthe, P., Hård, E., Johannessen, K., Snape, B. and Svensson, L. (1988). Biochemical and behavioral evidence for an interaction between ethanol and calcium channel antagonists. *J. Neural. Transm.*, 74: 181 - 193.

Faiman, M.D., Thompson, K.E. and Smith, K.L. (1992). Controlled release disulfiram (DS) implant. In: Naranjo, C.A. and Sellers, E.M. (eds.). *Novel Pharmacological Interventions for Alcoholism, pp. 267 - 272, New York: Springer Verlag.*

Froehlich, J.C., Zweifel, M., Harts, J., Lumeng, L, and Li, T.K. (1991). Importance of delta opioid receptors in maintaining alcohol drinking. *Psychopharmacology* (Berl), 103(4).467-72.

Fuller, R. K., Branchey, L., Brightwell, D.R., Derman, R. M., Emrick, C. D., Iber, F. L., James, K. E., Lacoursiere, R. B., Lee, K. K., Lowenstam. I., et al. (1986). Disulfiram treatment of alcoholism. A

Veterans Administration cooperative study. *JAMA*, 256(11). 1449 - 1455.

Gewiss, M., Heidberger, Ch., Opsomer, L., Durbin, Ph. and De Witte, Ph. (1991). Acamprosate and diazepam differentially modulate alcohol-induced behavioral and cortical alterations in rats following chronic inhalation of ethanol vapour. *Alcohol & Alcoholism*, 26(2). 129 - 137.

Gorelick, D.A. (1986). Effect of fluoxetine on alcohol consumption in male alcoholics. *Alcohol Clin.Exp. Res.*, 10: 113.

Göthert, M. and Fink, K. (1989). Inhibition of N-methyl-D-aspartate (NMDA)- and L-glutamate-induced noradrenaline and acetylcholine release in the rat brain by ethanol. *Arch. Pharmacol.*, 340: 516 - 521.

Grant, K.A., Valverius, P., Hudspith, M. and Tabakoff, B. (1990). Ethanol withdrawal seizures and the NMDA receptor complex. *Eur. J. Pharmacol.*,176: 289 - 296.

Grant, K.A., Knisely, J.S., Tabakoff, B., Barrettt, J.E. and Balster, R.L. 1991. Ethanol-like discriminative stimulus effects of non-competitive N-methyl-D-aspartate antagonists. *Behav. Pharmacol.*, (submitted).

Gulya, K., Grant, K.A., Valverius, P., Hoffman, P.L. and Tabakoff, B. (1991). Brain regional specificity and time course of changes in the NMDA receptor-ionophore complex during ethanol withdrawal. *Brain Res.*, 547: 129 - 134.

Hellevuo, K., Kiianmaa, K. and Kim, C. (1990). Effect of ethanol on brain catecholamines in rat lines developed for differential ethanol induced motor impairment. *Alcohol*, 7(2). 159 - 163.

Hill, S.Y. (1974). Intraventricular injection of 5-hydroxytryptamine and alcohol consumption in rats. *Biol. Psychiatry*, 8: 151 - 158.

Ho, A.K.S. and Chen, C.A. Interactions of narcotics, narcotic antagonists, and ethanol during acute, chronic and withdrawal states. *Ann. New York Acad. Sci.*, 260: 247 - 310, 1975.

Hoffman, P.L., Ishizawa, H., Rathna Giri, P., Dave, J.R. Grant, K.A., Liu, L-I., Gulya, K. and Tabakoff, B. (1990). The role of arginine vasopressin in alcohol tolerance. *Ann. Med.*, 22: 269 - 274.

Hoffman, P.L., Rabe, C.S., Moses, F. and Tabakoff, B. (1989). NMDA receptors and ethanol: Inhibition of ethanol calcium flux and cyclic GMP production. *J. Neurochem*, 52: 1937 - 1940.

Hoffman, P.L., Tabakoff, B., Szabó, G., Suzdak, P.D. and Paul, S.M. (1987). Effect of an imidazobenzodiazepine, Ro 15-4513, on the incoordination and hypothermia produced by ethanol and pentobarbital. *Life Sci.*, 41: 611 - 619.

Horwitz, R.I., Gottlieb, L.D. and Kraus, M. (1989). The efficacy of atenolol in the outpatient management of the alcohol withdrawal syndrome. *Arch. Intern. Med.*, 149: 1089 - 1093.

Hubbell, C.L., Czirr, S.A., Hunter, G.A., Beaman, C.M., LeCann, N.C. and Reid, L.D. (1986). Consumption of ethanol solution is potentiated by morphine and attenuated by naloxone persistently across repeated daily administrations. *Alcohol*, 3: 39 - 54.

Jacob, M.S., Zilm, D.H., Macleod, S.M. and Sellers, E.M. (1983). Propranolol-associated confused states during alcohol withdrawal. *J. Clin. Psychopharmacol.*, 3: 185 - 187.

Johansson, B., Angelo, H.R., Christensen, J.K., Møller, I.W.,. and Rønsted, P. (1991). Dose-effect relationship of disulfiram in humna volunteers. II: A study of the relation between the disulfiram-alcohol reaction and plasma concentrations of acetaldehyde, diethyldithiocarbamic acid methyl ester, and erythrocyte aldehyde dehydrogenase activity. *Pharmacol. Toxicol.*, 68(3). 166 - 170.

Johnsen, J. and Mørland, J. (1990). Disulfiram implants: Lack of pharmacological and clinical effects. *Tidsskr. Nor. Laegeføren.*, 110(10). 1229 - 1230.

Johnsen, J. and Mørland, J. (1991). Disulfiram implant: a double-blind placebo controlled follow-up on treatment outcome. *Alcohol Clin. Exp. Res.*, 15(3). 532 - 536.

Kalant, H. (1989). The Nature of Addiction: An Analysis of the Problem. In: Goldstein, A. (Editor). *Molecular and Cellular Aspects of the Drug Addictions*. New York: Springer Verlag.

Kiianmaa, K., Andersson, K. and Fuxe, K. (1979). On the role of ascending dopamine systems in the control of voluntary ethanol intake and ethanol intoxication. *Pharmacol. Biochem. Behav.*, 10(4). 603 - 608.

Kiianmaa, K., Fuxe, K., Jonsson, G. and Ahtee, L. (1975). Evidence for the involvement of central NA neurons in alcohol intake: Increased alcohol consumption after degeneration of the NA pathways to the cortex. *Neurosci. Lett.*, 1: 41 - 45.

Koob, G.F., Percy,L. and Britton, K.T. (1988). The effects of Ro-15-4513 on the behavioral actions of ethanol in an operant reaction time test and a conflict test. *Pharmacol. Biochem. Behav.*, 31: 757 - 760.

Kraus, M., Gottlieb, L.D. and Kraus, M.L. (1985). Randomized clinical trial of atenolol in patients with alcohol withdrawal syndrome. *N. Engl. J. Med.*, 313: 905 - 909.

Kulkosky, P.J., Sanchez, M.R., Foderaro, M.A. and Chiu, N. (1989). Cholecystokinin and satiation with alcohol. *Alcohol*, 6: 395 - 402.

Kwast, M., Tabakoff, B. and Hoffman, P.L. (1987). Effect of ethanol on cardiac -adrenoceptors. *Eur. J. Pharmacol.*, 142: 441 - 445.

Laestadius, Å. and Valverius, P. (1992). NMDA receptor ionophore complex in brains of alcohol dependent humans. *Alcohol and Alcoholism*, 27(Suppl. 1). 56.

Le Magnen, J., Tran, G., Durlach, J. and Martin, C. (1987). Dose-dependent suppression of the high alcohol intake of chronically intoxicated rats by Ca-acetyl homotaurinate. *Alcohol*, 4(2). 97 - 102.

Lê, A.D. and Kiianmaa, K. (1989). Initial Sensitivity and the development of acute and rapid tolerance to ethanol in the AT and ANT Rats. In: Kiianmaa, K., Tabakoff, B. and Saito, T. (eds.). Genetic Aspects of Alcoholism, pp. 147 - 155, The Finnish Foundation for Alcohol Studies, Helsinki, Finland.

Lhuintre, J.P., Moore, N., Tran, G., Steru, L., Langrenon, S., Daoust, M., Parot, Ph., Ladure, Ph., Libert, C., Boismare, F. and Hillemand,B. Acamprosate appears to decrease alcohol intake in weaned alcoholics. *Alcohol and Alcoholism*, 25(6). 613 - 622(1990).

Linnoila, M., Eckardt, M., Durcan, M., Lister,R. and Martin, P. (1987). Interactions of serotonin with ethanol: Clinical and animal studies. *Psychopharmacol. Bull.*, 23: 452 - 457.

Lister, R.G. and Durcan, M.J. (1989). Antagonism of the intoxicating effects of ethanol by the potent benzodiazepine receptor ligand Ro 19-4603. *Brain Res.*, 482: 141 - 144.

Little, H.J., Dolin, S.J. and Whittington, M.A. (1988). Possible role of calcium channels in ethanol tolerance and dependence. Ann. N.Y. Acad. Sci. Vol. 560, Calcium Channels —Structure and Function. pp. 465 - 466.

Little, H.J., Dolin, S.J. and Halsey, M.J. (1986). Calcium channel antagonists decrease the ethanol withdrawal syndrome. *Life Sci.*, 39: 2059 - 2065.

Littleton, J. and Bouchenafa, O. (1992). Agents which modify channels as potential treatments in alcohol withdrawal. In: Naranjo, C.A. and Sellers, E.M. (eds.). Novel Pharmacological Interventions for Alcoholism. pp. 186 - 200, New York: Springer Verlag.

Lovinger, D.M., White, G. and Weight, F.F. (1989). Ethanol inhibits NMDA-activated ion current in hippocampal neurons. *Science*, 243: 387 - 393.

Mair, R.G. and McEntee, W.J. (1986). Cognitive enhancement in Korsakoff's psychosis by clonidine: a comparison with L-dopa and ephedrine. *Psychopharmacology*, 88: 374 - 380.

Marchner, H. (1984). The pharmacology of alcohol-sensitizing drugs. In: Edwards, G. and Littleton, J. (eds.). *Pharmacological treatments for alcoholism*, pp. 491 - 530, London: Croom Helm.

Mardones, J., Alvarado, R., Contreras, S. and Segovia-Riquelme, N. (1992). Drug-induced specific and non-specific changes in voluntary ethanol intake by rats. In: Naranjo, C.A. and Sellers, E.M. (eds.). Novel Pharmacological Interventions for Alcoholism. pp. 68 - 82, New York: Springer Verlag.

Meert, T.F.: Effects of various serotoninergic agents on alcohol intake and alcohol preference in Wistar rats selected at two different levels of alcohol preference. Alcohol & Alcoholism 28: 157 - 170, 1993.

Meert, T.F., Clincke, G., De Korte, I., Gheuens, J.: Ritanserin and alcohol dependence. Alcoholism Clin. Exp. Res., 18: 9A, 1994.

Mellor, C.S. and Sims, A.C.P. (1971). Citrated calcium carbimide-alcohol reaction—its severity and effectiveness as a deterrent. *Br. J. Addictions*, 66: 123 - 128.

Merry, J. and Marks, V. (1972). The effect of alcohol, barbiturate, and diazepam on hypothalamic/pituitary adrenal function in chronic alcoholics. *Lancet*, 2: 990 - 992.

Morrisett, R.A., Rezvani, A.H., Overstreet, D., Janowsky, D.S., Wilson, W.A. and Swartzwelder, H.S. (1990). MK-801 potently inhibits alcohol withdrawal seizures in rats. *Eur. J. Pharmacol., 176: 103 - 105.*

Morrow, A.L., Suzdak, P.D. and Paul, S.M. (1988). Benzodiazepine, barbiturate, ethanol and hypnotic steroid hormone modulation of GABA-mediated chloride ion transport in rat brain synaptosomes. In: Biggio, G. and Costa,E. (eds.). *Chloride Channels and their Modulation by Neurotransmitters and Drugs.* pp.247 - 261. New York: Raven Press

Myers R.D. and Veale, W.L. (1968). Alcohol preference in the rat: Reduction following depletion of brain serotonin. *Science, 160:* 1469 - 1471.

Myers, R.D., Borg, S. and Mossberg, R. (1986). Antagonism by naltrexone of voluntary alcohol selection in the chronically drinking macaque monkey. *Alcohol, 3:* 383 - 388.

Naranjo, C.A. and Bremner, K.E. (1992). Evaluation of the effects of serotonin uptake inhibitors in alcoholics: A review. In: Naranjo, C.A. and Sellers, E.M. (eds.). Novel Pharmacological Interventions for Alcoholism. pp. 68 - 82, New York: Springer Verlag.

Naranjo, C.A. and Sellers, E.M. (1986). Clinical assessment and pharmacotherapy of the alcohol withdrawal syndrome. In: Galanter,

M. (ed.). *Recent Developments in Alcoholism: Combined Alcohol and Drug Abuse, Typologies of Alcoholics, The Withdrawal Syndrome, Renal and Electrolyte Consequences,* vol. 4: pp. 265 - 281, New York: Plenum Press.

Naranjo, C.A., Sellers, E.M. and Lawrin, M.O. (1986). Modulation of ethanol intake by serotonin uptake inhibitors. *J.Clin. Psychiatry,* 47(4 Suppl). 16 - 22.

Naranjo, C.A., Sellers, E.M., Jullivan, J.T., Woodley, D.V., Kadlec, K. and Sykora, K. (1987). The serotonin uptake inhibitor citalopram attenuates alcohol intake. *Clin. Pharmacol. Ther.,* 41: 266 - 274.

Naranjo, C.A., Sellers, E.M., Roach, C.A., Woodley, D.V., Sanchez-Craig, M. and Sykora, K. (1984). Zimelidine induced variations in alcohol intake by non-depressed heavy drinkers. *Clin. Pharmacol. Ther.,* 35: 374 - 381.

Naranjo, C.A., Sullivan, J.T., Kadlec, K.E., Woodley-Remus, D.V., Kennedy, R.N. and Sellers, E.M. (1989). Differential effects of viqualine on alcohol intake and other consummatory behaviors. *Clin. Pharmacol. Ther.,* 46: 301 - 309.

Nutt, D. Adinoff, B., and Linnoila, M. (1989). Benzodiazepines in the treatment of alcoholism. In: Galanter, M. (ed.). *Recent Developments in Alcoholism: Treatment Research,* vol. 7: pp. 283 - 313,New York: Plenum Press.

Nutt, D.J. and Lister, R.G. (1987). The effect of the benzodiazepine Ro 15-4513 on the anti-convulsant effects of diazepam, sodium pentobarbital and ethanol. *Brain Res.,* 413: 193 - 196.

Nutt, D.J., Lister, R.G., Rusche, D., Bonetti,E.P., Reese, R.E. and Rufener, R. (1988). Ro 15-4513 does not protect against the lethal effects of ethanol. *Eur. J. Pharmacol.,* 151: 127 - 129.

Öjehagen, A., Skjaerris, A. and Berglund, M. Long-term use of aversive drugs in outpatient alcoholism treatment. Acta. Psychiatr. Scand. 84(2). 185 - 190(1991).

O'Malley, S.S., Jaffe, A., Chang, G., Witte, G., Schottenfiedl, R.S. and Rounsaville, B.J. (1992). Naltrexone in the treatment of alcohol dependence: Preliminary findings. In: Naranjo, C.A. and Sellers, E.M. (eds.). *Novel Pharmacological Interventions for Alcoholism.* pp. 148 - 157, New York: Springer Verlag.

Peachey, J.E. (1984). Clinical uses of the alcohol-sensitizing drugs. In: Edwards, G. and Littleton, J. (eds.). Pharmacological treatments for alcoholism, pp. 531 - 557, London: Croom Helm.

Pelc, I., Le Bon, O., Verbanck, P., Lehert, Ph. and Opsomer, L. (1992). Calcium-acetylhomotaurinate for maintaining abstinence in weaned alcoholic patients: A placebo-controlled double-blind multicenter study. In: Naranjo, C.A. and Sellers, E.M. (eds.). Novel Pharmacological Interventions for Alcoholism. pp. 348 - 352, New York: Springer Verlag.

Phillips, M. (1992). Depot disulfiram: Pharmacokinetics and clinical effects during 28 days following a single subcutaneous dose. In: Naranjo, C.A. and Sellers, E.M. (eds.). *Novel Pharmacological Interventions for Alcoholism.* pp. 273 - 276, New York: Springer Verlag.

Pohorecky, L.A. (1974). Effects of ethanol on central and peripheral noradrenergic neurons. *J. Pharmacol. Exp. Ther.,* 189: 380 - 391.

Rabe, C.S. and Tabakoff, B. (1990).Glycine site directed agonists reverse ethanol's actions at the NMDA receptor. *Mol. Pharmacol.,* 38:753-757.

Rassnick, S., Pulvirenti, L. and Koob, G.F. (1989). Effects of a novel dopamine agonist, Sandoz 205-152, on ethanol self-administration. *Soc. Neurosci. Abstr.,* 15: 251.

Reid, L.D. and Hubbell, C.L. (1992 . Opioid modulate rats' propensities to take alcoholic beverages. In: Naranjo, C.A. and Sellers, E.M. (eds.). Novel Pharmacological Interventions for Alcoholism. pp. 121 - 134, New York: Springer Verlag.

Ricardo, J.A. and Koh, E.T. (1978). Anatomical Evidence of Direct Projections from the Nucleus of the Solitary Tract to the Hypothalamus, Amygdala and Other Forebrain Structures in the Rat. Brain Research, 153: 1 - 26.

Roy, A., DeJong, J., Ferraro, T., Adinoff, B., Ravitz, B. and Linnoila, M. (1990). CSF gamma-aminobutyric acid in alcoholics and control subjects. *Am. J. Psychiatry,* 147(10). 1294 - 1296.

Rusi, M., Eriksson, K. and Mäki, J. (1977). Genetic differences in the susceptibility to acute ethanol intoxication in selected rat strains. In: Gross, M.M. (ed.) Alcohol Intoxication and Withdrawal, Vol. 3A, pp. 97 - 109, New York: Plenum Press.

Saito, T., Lee, J.M., Hoffman, P.L. and Tabakoff, B. (1987). Effects of chronic ethanol treatment on the -adrenergic receptor-coupled adenylate cyclase system of mouse cerebral cortex. J. *Neurochem.,* 48: 1817 - 1822.

Smith, D., Oie, T.P.S., Ng, K.T. and Armstrong, S.(1980). Rat selfadministration of ethanol: Enhancement by darkness and exogenous melatonin. *Physiol. Behav.,* 25: 449 - 455.

Stibler, H., Borg, S. and Joustra, M. (1986). Micro anion exchange chromatography of carbohydrate-deficient transferrin in relation to alcohol consumption. *Alcohol Clin. Exp. Res.,* 10: 535 - 544.

Strömbom, U. and Svensson, T.H. (1978). Antagonism of morphine-induced central stimulation in mice by small doses of catecholamine-receptor agonists. *J. Neural. Transm.*, 42(3).169-79.

Suzdak P.D., Schwartz, R.D. and Paul, S.M. (1987). Alcohols stimulate GABA receptor-mediated chloride uptake in brain vesicles: correlation with intoxication potency. *Brain Res.*, 444: 340 - 344.

Suzdak, P.D., Glowa, J.R., Crawley, J.N., Schwartz, R.D., Skolnick, P. and Paul, S.M. (1986b). A selective imidazobenzodiazepine antagonist of ethanol in the rat. *Science*, 234: 1243 - 1247.

Suzdak, P.D., Schwartz, R.D., Skolnick, P. and Paul, S.M.(1986a). Ethanol stimulates γ-aminobutyric acid receptor mediated chloride transport in rat brain synaptosomes. *Proc. Natl.Acad. Sci.*, (USA) 83: 4071 - .

Szabó, G., Hoffman, P.L. and Tabakoff, B. (1988b). Forskolin promotes the development of ethanol tolerance in 6-hydroxy-dopamine-treated mice. *Life Sci.*, 42(6). 615 - 621.

Szabó, G., Tabakoff, B. and Hoffman, P.L. (1988a). Receptors with V₁ characteristics mediate the maintenance of ethanol tolerance by vasopressin. *J. Pharmacol. Exp. Ther.*, 247: 536 - 541.

Tabakoff, B., Hoffman, P.L., Lee, J.M., Saito, T., Willard, B. and De Leon-Jones, F. (1988). Differences in platelet enzyme activity between alcoholics and non-alcoholics. *N. Engl. J. Med.*, 318: 134 - 139.

Tabakoff, B., Rabe, C.S., Grant, K.A., Valverius, P., Hudspith, M. and Hoffman, P.L. (1991). Ethanol and the NMDA receptor: Insights into ethanol pharmacology. In: Meyer, R.E., Koob, G.F., Lewis, M.J. and Paul, S.M. (eds.). Neuropharmacology of ethanol. pp. 93 - 106, Boston: Birkhäuser.

Thomson. A.D., Ryle, P.R., World, M.J. and Shaw, G.K. (1984). Treatment and prevention of alcohol related tissue damage: Currently available drug treatments and their future. In: Edwards, G. and Littleton, J. (eds.). Pharmacological treatments for alcoholism, pp. 373 - 404, London: Croom Helm.

Valverius, P., Borg, S., Valverius, M.R., Hoffman, P.L. and Tabakoff, B. (1989). Adrenergic receptor binding in brain of alcoholics. *Exp. Neurol.*,105: 280 - 286.

Valverius, P., Hoffman, P.L. and Tabakoff, B. (1987). Effect of ethanol on mouse cerebral cortical β-adrenergic receptors. *Mol. Pharmacol.*, 32: 217 - 222.

Victor, M. and Adams, R.D. (1971). *The Wernicke-Korsakoff syndrome*, Philadelphia: Davies.

Volpicelli, J.R., Davis, M.A. and Olgin, J.E. (1986). Naltrexone blocks the post-shock increase of ethanol consumption. *Life Sci.*, 38: 841 - 847.

Volpicelli, J.R., O'Brien, C.P., Alterman, A.I. and Hayashida, M. (1990). Naltrexone and the treatment of alcohol dependence: Initial observations. In: Ried, L.D. (ed.) Opioids, Bulimia and Alcohol Abuse and Alcoholism. pp. 195 - 214, New York: Springer-Verlag.

Volpicelli, J.R., Ulm, RR. and Hopson, N. (1991). Alcohol drinking in rats during and following morphine injections. *Alcohol*, 8(4).289-92.

Voltaire, A., Beck, O. and Borg, S. (1992). Urinary 5-hydroxytryptophol: A possible marker of recent alcohol consumption. *Alcoholism Clin. Exp. Res.*, 16(2). 281 - 285.

Weingartner, H., Buchsbaum, M.S. and Linnoila, M. (1983). Zimelidine effects on memory impairments produced by ethanol. *Life Sci.*, 33: 2159 - 2163.

Weiss, F., Mitchiner, M., Bloom, F.E. and Koob, G.F. (1990). Free-choice responding for ethanol versus water in alcohol preferring (P) and unselected Wistar rats is differentially altered by naloxone, bromocriptine and methysergide. *Psychopharmacology*, 101: 178 - 186.

Wilkins, A.J., Jenkins, W.J. and Steiner, J.A. (1983). Efficacy of clonidine in treatment of alcohol withdrawal state. *Psychopharmacology*, 81: 78 - 80.

Wilkins, J.N. and Gorelick, D.A. (1986). Clinical neuroendocrinology and neuropharmacology of alcohol withdrawal. In: Galanter, M. (ed.). Recent Developments in Alcoholism: Combined Alcohol and Drug Abuse, Typologies of Alcoholics, The Withdrawal Syndrome, Renal and Electrolyte Consequences, vol. 4: pp. 241 - 263, New York: Plenum Press .

Woodward, J.J. and Gonzales, R.A. (1990). Ethanol inhibition of N-methyl-D-aspartate stimulated endogenous dopamine release from rat striatal slices: reversal by glycine. *J. Neurochem.*, 54: 712 - 715.

Wright, C. and Moore, R.D. (1988). Disulfiram treatment of alcoholism. *Am. J. Med.*, 88(6). 647 - 655.

Yoshishige, I., Masotoshi, T., Tsuda, A., Tsujimaru, S. and Nagasaki, N. (1985). Attenuating effect of diazepam on stress induced noradrenalin turnover in specific brain regions of rats: Antagonism by RO15-1788. *Life Sci.*, 37: 2391 - 2398.

Zeise, M.L., Kasparow, S., Capogna, M. and Zieglg:ansberger, W. (1990). Calciumdiacetylhomotaurinate (CA-AOTA) decreases the action of excitatory amino acids in the rat neocortex in vitro. *Prog. Clin. Biol. Res.*, 351: 237 - 242.

Zeise, M.L., Kasparow, S., Capogna, M. and Zieglg:ansberger, W. (1992). Calciumdiacetylhomotaurinate (CA-AOTA) decreases postsynaptic potentials in the rat neocortex; possible involvement of excitatory amino acid receptors. *Alcohol and Alcoholism*, 27(Suppl. 1). 58.

Abbreviations

A-I .... Apolipoprotein A-I
A-II .... Apolipoprotein A-II
AA .... Alko-alcohol rats
AANB .... Alpha-amino-n-butyric acid
AC .... Adenyl cyclase
ACTH .... Adrenocorticotropic hormone
ADH .... Alcohol dehydrogenase
ALAT........... Alanine aminotransferase
ALD............ Alcoholic liver disease
ALDH .... Aldehyde dehydrogenase
AMPT .... Alpha-methyl-para-tyrosine
ANA .... Alko-non-alcohol rats
ANT............ Alcohol nontolerant rats
ARC............ Alcohol Research Center
ASAT........... Aspartate aminotransferase
+ASAT.......... Total aspartate
AT .... Alcohol tolerant rats
AVP .... Arginine vasopressin
$[Ca^{2+}]_i$ .... Intracellular Ca^{2+} concentration
cAMP .... Cyclic adenosine monophosphate
cDNA .... Complementary DNA
cGMP .... Cyclic guanosine monophosphate
CDT............ Carbohydrate deficient transferrin
CEPH .... Centre d'Etude du Polymorphisme Humain
cM .... Centimorgan
CNS............ Central nervous system
CR .... Conditioned response
CS.............. Conditioned stimulus
CSF .... Cerebrospinal fluid
CT .... Computerized tomography
DHP............ Dihydropyridine
DNA .... Deoxyribonucleic acid
DRD2........... Dopamine D_2 receptor
DSM-III-R....... Diagnostic and Statistical Manual of Mental Disorders,
                 3rd edition, revised
DT or DTs........ Delirium tremens
DZ .... Dizygotic
EAA............ Excitatory amino acid
EEG .... Electroencephalograph
EPSPs .... Excitatory postsynaptic potentials
FAE .... Fetal alcohol effect
FAS .... Fetal alcohol syndrome
FDG............ Fluoro-deoxyglucose
GABA .... γ-aminobutyric acid
GDH .... Glutamate dehydrogenase
GGT............ Gamma glutamyl transferase
G_i .... Inhibitory guanine nucleotide binding protein

299

G_s .... Stimulatory guanine nucleotide binding protein
HDL-C .... High density lipoprotein-cholesterol
β-Hex .... Beta-hexosaminidase
5-HIAA .... 5-Hydroxyindole-acetic acid
HLA .... Human leukocyte antigen
5-HT .... 5-Hydroxytryptamine (serotonin)
5-HTOL 5-Hydroxytryptophol
IgA .... Immunoglobulin A
IgG .... Immunoglobulin G
Kb .... Kilobase
K_m .... Michaelis constant
KS .... Korsakoff's syndrome
L .... Leucine
LCBF .... Local cerebral blood flow
Lod .... Likelihood of odds
LOD score .... Logarithmic measure of strength of linkage
LS .... Long-sleep mice
LTP .... Long-term potentiation
MAO .... Monoamine oxidase
mASAT .... Mitochondrial aspartate aminotransferase
MCV .... Mean cell volume
MEN .... Multiple endocrine neoplasia
MEOS .... Microsomal ethanol oxidizing system
MK-801 .... (+)-5-methyl-10,11-dihydro-5H-dibenzo [a,d]cyclohepten-
                             5,10-imine maleate (Dizocilpine)
MRI .... Magnetic resonance imaging
MZ .... Monozygotic
NADH/NAD ..... Nicotinamide adenine dinucleotide (reduced form/oxidized form)
NMDA .... N-methyl-D-aspartate
PCP .... Phencyclidine
PCR .... Polymerase chain reaction
PET .... Positron emission tomography
PIIIP .... Procollagen type III-peptide
RFLP .... Restriction fragment length polymorphism
Rh .... Rhesus
SS .... Short-sleep mice
SSCP .... Single strand conformational polymorphism
tASAT .... Total aspartate
THIQs .... Tetrahydroisoquinolones
Type 1 .... Type 1 alcoholics
Type 2 .... Type 2 alcoholics
UCR .... Unconditioned response
UCS .... Unconditioned stimulus
V_{max} .... Maximal velocity
WE .... Wernicke's encephalopathy
WHO .... World Health Organization
WKS .... Wernicke-Korsakoff syndrome
WSP .... Withdrawal seizure prone mice
WSR .... Withdrawal seizure resistant mice

Index

List of Authors

John B. Saunders, MD
Centre for Drug and Alcohol Studies
Royal Prince Alfred Hospital
Departments of Medicine and Psychiatry
University of Sydney
New South Wales, Sydney
Australia

Torsten Ehrig*, PhD
Ting-Kai Li, MD
Department of Biochemistry and Molecular Biology
Department of Medicine
Indiana University School of Medicine
545 Barnhill Drive
Emerson 421
Indianapolis, Indiana 46202-5124
USA

*Present address:
Guggenheim 1417
Mayo Foundation
Rochester, Minnesota 55905

Itaru Yamashita, MD
Tsukasa Koyama, MD
Tetsuro Ohmori, MD
Department of Psychiatry
Hokkaido University School of Medicine
West 7, North 15
Sapporo 060, Japan

Abbas Parsian, PhD
C. Robert Cloninger, MD
Department of Psychiatry
Washington University School of Medicine
Box 8134
4940 Children's Place
St. Louis, Missouri 63110-1093
USA

David I. N. Sherman, MB BS MRCP(UK)[1]
Roberta J. Ward PhD
Roger Williams, MD FRCP FRCP(E) FRACP FRCS[1]
Timothy J. Peters, PhD DSc FRCP FRCP(E) FRCPath
Department of Clinical Biochemistry
[1]Institute of Liver Studies
King's College School of Medicine and Dentistry
Bessemer Rd
London SE5 9PJ
United Kingdom

Mikko Salaspuro, MD
Research Unit of Alcohol Diseases
University of Helsinki
Tukholmankatu 8 F
00290 Helsinki
Finland

Ilana B Glass-Crome, PhD
The Medical College of Saint Bartholomew's Hospital
University of London
Department of Psychological Medicine
West Smithfield, London
ECIA 7BE
United Kingdom

J. E. Dildy-Mayfield, PhD
R. A. Harris, PhD
Department of Pharmacology
University of Colorado Health Sciences Center
4200 East Ninth Avenue, C-236
Denver, Colorado 80262
USA

M. Vogel-Sprott, PhD
Department of Psychology
University of Waterloo
Waterloo, Ontario N2L 3G1
Canada

P. L. Carlen, MD FRCP(C)
Enrique Menzano, MD
Playfair Neuroscience Unit
Room 12-413
The Toronto Hospital, Western Division
399 Bathurst Street
Toronto, Ontario M5T 2S8
Canada

Peter Valverius, MD PhD
Stefan Borg, MD PhD
Department of Psychiatry at St. Göran's Hospital
Department of Clinical Neurosciences
Karolinska Institute
PO Box 12557
10229 Stockholm
Sweden